ALICE LYNCH

Endo Smart

A Guide to Understanding and Managing Your Health

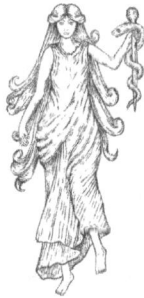

Reviewed by Dr Tatjana Gibbons

First edition

ISBN (paperback): 978-1-0683223-5-8
ISBN (hardcover): 978-1-0683223-2-7

This book was professionally typeset on Reedsy.
Find out more at reedsy.com

Contents

Foreword   vi

Acknowledgments   ix

The Beginning   x

I   Part One

1   Introduction   3
2   History of Endometriosis   7
3   My Story   11
4   What Is Endometriosis?   24
5   What Is Inflammation?   28
6   What Are Adhesions?   30
7   What Are the Types of Endometriosis?   32
8   What Causes Endometriosis?   35
9   What Are the Stages of Endometriosis?   47
10 What Are the Symptoms of Endometriosis   50
11 What Is a Flare-Up?   62
12 Bowel Endometriosis   64
13 Rectovaginal Endometriosis   66
14 Extragenital Endometriosis   70
15 Tilted Uterus   74
16 Frozen Pelvis   76
17 Adenomyosis   80
18 Biochemistry of Endometriosis   83
19 Microbiology   89
20 The Nervous System   93

21 Endometriosis Brain   95
22 Comorbidities   97
23 Fertility   131
24 Is Endometriosis Preventable and What Are the Risk Factors?   142
25 Menopause   146
26 Endometriosis in Infants, Children, and Adolescents   149
27 Endometriosis in Biological Males and Transgender Men   151

II   Part Two

28 How to Get Diagnosed   155
29 Endometriosis Diagnosis   159
30 Meeting the Gynaecologist   164
31 Non-Invasive Diagnostic Procedures   166
32 Diagnostic Surgery   174
33 Specialist Endometriosis Centres   178
34 Why is Early Diagnosis Important?   180

III   Part Three

35 Introduction   185
36 Cures & Myths   189
37 Pain Medications   192
38 Hormone Treatment   195
39 Endometriosis Surgery   209
40 Hysterectomy   223
41 Surgery Care   227
42 Do You Need Surgery?   239
43 Fertility and Surgery   242
44 Management Outside of Surgery & Hormone Treatments   248
45 The Four Pillars of Health   250
46 The Four Pillars of Health – Nutrition   251
47 FODMAP Diet   294

48 Histamine & Allergies   299

49 Diet Summary: Key Takeaways for Endometriosis Management 309

50 Alcohol   312

51 Supplements   316

52 The Four Pillars of Health - Movement   353

53 The Four Pillars of Health – Sleep   369

54 The Four Pillars of Health – Wellbeing   375

55 Alternative Medicine   385

56 Herbal Medicine   387

57 Traditional Chinese Medicine (TCM)   399

58 Acupuncture   405

59 Homeopathy   409

60 Meditation   412

61 Other Treatments   415

62 How to Deal with the Day-to-Day   426

63 Toxins to Avoid   432

64 Medical Research   441

65 (Not) The End   447

References   451

Foreword

As a doctor in the UK, I've witnessed the spectrum of care and information people with endometriosis are given, and the critical need for clearer answers to people's questions. Even seemingly the most basic question someone might ask, "Why does endometriosis occur?" is still heavily debated as there are various theories out there, which you will hear about later. I've read papers from as far back as the 1960s on the 'endometriosis enigma', and although we have many more studies available, we still today have papers published 'on the enigma that continues to be.' This is what drives so many of us working on endometriosis research; there's still so much to uncover, and each scientific discovery brings us closer to providing solutions and the best possible care for those living with the condition.

I came to understand the complexities of endometriosis through a story that many of you will have heard before. As a teenager, one of my closest friends, the life and soul of every event, who radiated such beautiful energy, started struggling more and more with pain. Sometimes when I saw her, she would be drained of everything, and I felt so helpless, as we didn't know what was wrong with her. I then started medical school and thought it would teach me what I needed to figure it out myself. But even the doctors she saw didn't have answers, and her test results were normal. That was until she had a diagnostic laparoscopy that found endometriosis. As I read more into endometriosis, everything started to make sense, but of course, her symptoms weren't as black and white as the textbooks made it sound. The more I read, the more I realised how little we actually know about this condition — even though it affects millions of people. The more I learnt, the more questions I had. If I was finding it all so complicated trying to understand the information I was getting about endometriosis, I didn't know how people living with it were coping. I realised there is a profound need for endometriosis to be demystified.

I'm Tatjana, a British-Danish doctor; I received my medical degree and a Bachelor of Science in Reproductive Medicine from Imperial College London. I was raised by the most incredible woman, who, despite having me at 15 years old, taught me right from the start the strength that women possess and how important it is to support each other in this world, which can sometimes make it hard to shine as brightly as we deserve. I realised that becoming a doctor and focusing on Women's Health could be my way to help other women when they need it most. Plus, as you will see in this book, our bodies are pretty incredible, it's worth learning about them!

I have been privileged to spend the last four years leading various research studies at the University of Oxford endometriosis research group (Endometriosis CaRe) as part of my PhD. You will hear about one of the studies later in the research section. I've learnt so much during this time, but it is a true skill to be able to critically analyse, summarise and explain research in a way that is less dry than a journal article. This is a skill that your author, Alice Lynch, has mastered.

I had the pleasure of meeting Alice through Instagram. I was so impressed with the evidence-based content she created and was so relieved to see there was a place for people to find the information they needed. But it is a shame that despite endometriosis affecting and impacting so many people's lives, often, the best sources of information come from social media, not the healthcare providers you meet. That being said, endometriosis is a complex enigma and a disease that can't be fully explained in a 10-to-15-minute consultation.

For those who want to know the ins and outs of the condition and the potential impact it may have on them personally, a book such as this is invaluable. There is now a lot of information out there, but it is still very difficult to know how to interpret it. Alice has spent an impressive amount of time figuring that out for you and providing you with the most up-to-date information in the field, always backed up by sound research, and has been careful to interpret it as it should, avoiding the pitfalls that easily arise. It's been an honour to work with Alice and review the content of this fantastic book.

I'm excited for you, getting to read the book for the first time. So, get cosy (or hygge, as we Danes say) with matcha or your drink of choice and dig in!

Acknowledgments

I want to express my sincere gratitude to Dr Tatjana Gibbons for her invaluable expertise, guidance, and support throughout the editing process of this book. Her kindness matches her impressive career, and I am truly thankful for her taking the time out of her busy schedule to work on this project with me. Her role as subject matter expert greatly enhanced the quality of the content, ensuring its accuracy and relevance. I am deeply appreciative of her insights and willingness to contribute to this work.

The Beginning

"Knowing yourself is the beginning of all wisdom."
— Aristotle

If you've opened this book, chances are curiosity or hunger has led you here, maybe both. One thing is certain: you desire to learn more about endometriosis. Whether you're grappling with a new diagnosis or have been dealing with this disease for years, or even if you simply suspect you have it and want to learn more, this book will have something for you. If you are reading this to gain a deeper understanding of a loved one's experience, that is beautiful and appreciated. I hope the following pages provide the answers and information you need to truly comprehend the complexities and nuances of endometriosis... Well, at least as far as current research allows us to do anyway. You will notice from the evidence presented in this book that although there are many studies to discuss, there remains a lack of high-quality research into endometriosis, resulting in significant knowledge gaps. Where research is lacking, so too is proper education on the subject. Although numerous factors have contributed to the underfunding of research, a significant issue is the gender health gap. Shockingly, less than 2.4% of publicly funded research in the UK is spent on women's reproductive health and childbirth,[1] despite 1 in 3 women facing a gynaecological or reproductive health concern.[2] To make matters worse, women have historically lacked representation in studies, meaning research was carried out primarily on men. Notably, women were less likely to be included in studies if they were pregnant, from ethnic minorities, lesbian, or bisexual.[3] Despite efforts to improve the gender gap in research, progress is slow, and women are still underrepresented in clinical trials. Only once the data gap is closed can we truly understand how diseases affect genders differently, as well as improve our knowledge of female-specific conditions.

My journey with endometriosis, or "endo" as it's often called due to its lengthy, six-syllable name, has been one of trying to find answers and solutions. I wanted to understand what doctors were telling me with their medical jargon and investigate what they couldn't explain or didn't have time to answer. Since my diagnosis, I have been repeatedly asked by friends and family to speak to people who had or thought they had endo to give guidance and share insights I had acquired on my own journey. I enjoyed helping these women, but it also made me aware there was a lack of comprehensive information available in one place that educated, provided answers, and empowered women with the knowledge to understand their disease from start to finish, diagnosis to management — from someone familiar with the intricacies of living with endometriosis. Having a chronic condition like endo can be a trying experience, particularly when you don't understand what is happening with your body. Not having the knowledge to explain why and how you feel the way you do can exacerbate the situation. I know it sounds dramatic, but before my diagnosis, the rapid escalation of my symptoms and the absence of a clear explanation led me to think that I must be dying. It can be an all-encompassing experience affecting your entire being, and I didn't know of any conditions that could explain everything I was feeling. After receiving a diagnosis and having a title for what you have been going through can bring about a great deal of relief, but it doesn't provide healing. The scarce education and societal awareness regarding the effects of endometriosis on the body often leads to disheartening experiences, with many of us not having a good insight into what the path to recovery looks like. Someone may assume a single surgery will change their life and make things better, only to discover they need a handful of surgeries, hormone therapy, and lifestyle changes before improving their condition. Notably, a lack of education is available on how to live with and manage this chronic disease, especially as surgery isn't always accessible or successful in relieving symptoms.

The type of medical treatment someone receives varies depending on their symptoms, where they are in their journey, where they live, and the hospital they attend. The common avenues of treatment include hormonal medications and surgery. Simply, very little information is provided when diagnosed about what the disease is and how to manage it outside of these options. When newly diagnosed with type 1 diabetes, patients are offered classes to help them understand and manage their disease. Individuals with endometriosis also deserve this basic insight. I had the desire to create a book to hold the information I wish I had when I was first diagnosed and the knowledge I found myself seeking six years later. I was fed up with reading online or having to explain my disease as "they think endometriosis is like endometrial tissue...but it's not" or "there are some theories as to what causes it...but they're not sure". I wanted to know what these statements meant. I wanted answers. Given the lack of research and the enigmatic state of the disease, this is a difficult challenge. Furthermore, considering the vast ways this disease manifests in each person, every aspect cannot be covered within just one book, so I apologise if there are specific questions not covered. Despite this, I hope the contents of this book enable each of you to better understand your disease, make choices, and discover the self-management tools that will work best for you. Better yet, I hope it provides more answers than you even knew to ask.

As endometriosis is experienced differently by each of us, the effectiveness of treatments will vary too. Unfortunately, even if surgical treatment makes you feel like you are back to normality, this is not a cure for this disease. There is no cure to date. No one knows if their endometriosis will come back or impact their health in other ways. You see, this disease is not confined to the pelvis; it can have a rippling effect, causing changes throughout the body. With that in mind, this book aims to equip readers with a holistic understanding of their condition so that they better know how to address the impact of endo on their past, present, and future. With no known cure, managing endometriosis involves navigating a complex journey that extends beyond medical interventions. Knowledge is power so they say, I hope this book achieves at least that. Giving you the knowledge to regain power in your life.

I collated a wealth of information from thousands of sources to bring this book to life. This is a complicated disease, and I understand why health websites don't provide information unless it's sufficiently proven through medical research. I mean, nor are they able to due to the bureaucratic governance between research and medical advice or practice. This is an important custom which regulates the treatment of care and prevents maltreatment of patients. However, it's hard to expect people to wait for research to catch up and provide the solid, conclusive answers we've been waiting for. We have this disease now, and it's impacting our lives no matter what. This book seeks to bridge that gap, offering insights for individuals who want to understand this disease and get informed on the scientific literature out there, whether that's why they have certain symptoms or safe ways to manage the condition. It can be a full-time job keeping up with the ever-evolving information, so this is for those who may not have the time to sift through countless websites to gather answers on a particular question, ...still struggling to find what they are after. Most people don't read medical papers, but helpful or fascinating data can be found within them.

In the UK, the average duration before someone receives a diagnosis is around eight years.[4] This statistic has not changed much since my diagnosis six years ago. Yet the social movement that has transpired across the world makes me believe that 'Endo Warriors' are championing the revolution of making us heard, acknowledged, and trusted. Many of us have struggled to find support and compassion from friends, family, colleagues, bosses, or teachers. Our symptoms have not been taken seriously or possibly ignored. The endometriosis community has been raising awareness for this disease so that we trust someone who says their periods make it impossible for them to work or function; we are no longer labelling them as lazy, weak, or dramatic. We are empowering ourselves to face the world without receiving prejudice and stigma and instead meeting empathy. We are getting recognised for the challenges we face. I want to thank the healthcare professionals who are listening to us, taking action, and helping people get diagnosed. I want to thank clinicians, researchers, and other practitioners who specialise in this field and have made it their life career to help all those with this disease. Even if the disease is not generally considered deadly, you are saving lives!

In this book, I sometimes use the term woman/women when describing those impacted by endometriosis. I want to acknowledge this disease affects women, men, and children, as well as those who are trans or non-binary. You do not have to have a womb to experience this disease, and there are also many people in society suffering who do not identify as or were born female. Please know that it goes without saying everyone is welcome here and everyone is acknowledged. The research in this book focuses predominantly on cisgender women so in instances where I reference or discuss a study, I will use the gendered term as provided so as not to change the meaning of the paper. There is already a scarcity of studies centred on females in the realm of science with a prevalent male bias; even mice used in lab experiments are primarily male. You will see the effects of this particularly the comorbidities chapter, as many diseases mainly affecting women are under-researched. Unfortunately, there is an even wider gap in research when it comes to including gender-diverse individuals and those from ethnic minorities. With improved efforts from agencies to push for inclusiveness it is my sincere hope that over time, this disparity will diminish, allowing for a more inclusive approach where research is not concentrated on heterosexual white cisgender men.

Beyond gender-related concerns, it's essential to acknowledge that research often delineates patterns within a specific sample of individuals. Consequently, the findings discussed may not only always resonate with your own experiences. I hope, however, you do find yourself represented within this book, and where you are not, you at least find the material as interesting as I did in researching and writing it.

The reader is advised that this book is not intended to be a substitute for an assessment by, and advice from, an appropriate medical professional. All new, persistent, or concerning symptoms should be evaluated by a doctor. Treatments also vary in their effectiveness for each person.

I

Part One

1

Introduction

"No woman has ever benefited by learning less about her body."
— Dr. Jen Gunter

An estimated 10% of females of reproductive age have endometriosis,[1] that's 190 million people worldwide. This is not a small issue. To put this figure into perspective against other widely known and better-understood diseases, there were 19.3 million new cancer cases around the world in 2020,[2] 8.4 million people were living with type 1 diabetes in 2021,[3] and a relatively minute 162,428 people on the planet have cystic fibrosis.[4] This is a pretty impressive secret, considering many have still never heard of it. So, let's start by providing an overview for those first encountering the disease. Endometriosis, pronounced **en-do-meet-ree-oh-sis,** is an oestrogen-dependent, proinflammatory, chronic, 'gynaecological' disease, mainly affecting females, typically of reproductive age. I know that's a lot of words, but we will break them all down. It's not a cancer, nor an infection. It's a disease most associated with pain and bleeding but it can cause a great number of debilitating symptoms that reduce a person's quality of life. It can impact fertility, so some people may be diagnosed when seeking fertility treatment, others may be diagnosed based on symptoms. It's often listed as one of the top 20 most painful conditions. There is no cure, and the current treatments can be invasive, ineffective in relieving the symptoms, or come with unpleasant side effects. Although often related to pain in the pelvic organs, it's also a system-wide hormonal disease affecting various body systems with links to allergies and anxiety. It's also found in infants and cis men, but this is very rare.[5]

Endometriosis costs the UK economy an estimated €9.9 billion a year, whilst the USA faces a €49.6 billion annual burden.[6] Majority of this expense comes from productivity loss due to decreased quality of life rather than direct treatment. This huge cost represents individuals who want to be healthy, thrive, and work. Many find they must change jobs, work part-time, or stop working in order to find a suitable job that can fit together with the unpredictable symptoms of endo, or to relieve the stress and demands of a job that has now become unachievable to meet. This is important to recognise, as many women with the disease experience limitations in their career development due to loss of time at work and productivity loss.[7] This can be devastating. It can also strain relationships with co-workers and create issues with bosses, particularly if someone is struggling to communicate effectively. Poor communication in the workplace can stem from individuals not feeling safe or comfortable talking about the intimate details of their health. A gynaecological disorder might be considered embarrassing for some to address, particularly as it's still not widely known or understood, so it may involve having to explain what it is. There is also judgement, or fear of judgement from those at work, that hinders a person's career. Feeling that those around you view you as not pulling your weight or taking too much time off can add stress to an already difficult time. Between dealing with crippling and debilitating symptoms, attending doctors' appointments, and requiring time off for surgery, there is often a valid reason for someone not being able to put their best foot forward and instead for them to retreat to deal with what's happening with their body. Of course, there are also many bosses and colleagues who are supportive of their peers with endo. Most of us do not have the luxury to stop working altogether when our health deteriorates, so for those who show grace and compassion to an endo sufferer as they try to continue with their career, we salute you. It does not go unnoticed or undervalued. Even if there is support from the workplace, it might not be enough as studies show endometriosis still impairs the professional life of many, as ultimately, they are less able to work in their desired profession.[7] Investment in research on effectively treating endometriosis (and maybe even one day cure it) is critical in reducing this economic cost and allowing people to prosper in the life they choose.

Endometriosis affects all ages; there is a misconception the condition primarily affects 30 and 40-year-olds. However, improvements in awareness and diagnosis show this is not the case; no one is too young to have endometriosis. A cohort study found 67% of people are diagnosed before 40 years of age.[8] This figure will likely increase due to rising awareness as many start experiencing symptoms in adolescence. Endometriosis also affects all ethnicities. It used to be thought endo affected certain ethnicities more than others. Statistics show Asian women are approximately 60% more likely to be diagnosed than White women, whilst White women are around 50% more likely to be diagnosed compared to Black or Hispanic women.[9] Whilst other diseases are more prevalent in certain ethnicity groups, with endometriosis, other factors have likely contributed to this disparity in diagnosed cases. Firstly, some individuals may find talking about their periods or sex life awkward, taboo, or in some religions or cultures, it is unacceptable. Therefore, many may find it hard to communicate their feelings or learn if their experience is not normal. For instance, someone may only become aware something is wrong, such as the heaviness of their periods or the painful sex they experience, through having discussions with family and friends. However, if these conversations are off-limits or non-existent due to cultural reasons, it impedes the awareness and understanding needed to seek medical assistance. Periods are often taught to us as being painful, making it harder to determine if our pain goes beyond the norm. Even if someone feels something is wrong, there may be pressure not to discuss their problems or further cultural barriers that deter them from seeking help. For others, it's a very different issue, with healthcare disparities perpetuating a lack of diagnosis instead. Firstly, gender bias exists towards women's pain compared to men's pain. A study showed that when male patients expressed the same amount of pain as female patients, the observers viewed the females' pain as less intense.[10] If you pair gender bias with the racism, hidden biases, or damaging stereotypes that BAME communities face in healthcare settings involving pain tolerance, pain perception, and pain treatment,[11] it becomes easier to piece together how disparities in diagnoses may be inaccurately represented, particularly in Western countries. The variance in ethnicity and diagnosis rates could also be influenced by varying healthcare standards or access to care in parts of the world. Endometriosis is largely unheard of and renowned for taking nearly a decade on average to diagnose. Moreover, it often requires highly trained surgeons to perform an expensive, invasive surgical procedure to diagnose, and that's if they even know what they are looking for. For many, the option of surgical diagnosis might not be available. There is insufficient research into why endometriosis has a high prevalence in South Asian women; it's suggested a high soy intake in their diet,[12] high levels of pollution,[13] or having a lower Body Mass Index (BMI) are possible causes.[14] Yet none of the studies exploring this were conclusive. Other general risk factors include starting your period at an early age, having a short menstrual cycle, never giving birth, having a family history of the disease, or going through menopause late. Women all over the world are delaying having children until later in their lives. In the UK, 50% of women aged 30 are childless.[15] Could this explain one reason for the high rates of endometriosis? It's food for thought, but we will get more into the reasons later.

2

History of Endometriosis

Endometriosis only gained traction in public discourse in the 21st Century. Even just ten years ago, it seems only a minority of people had heard of it, mainly scientists, gynaecologists, and the people fortunate enough to have received a diagnosis. Despite a considerable rise in awareness thanks to individuals advocating in mainstream or social media, there is still a substantial lack of knowledge on the disease. This validates the condition has been largely ignored or forgotten about, or could it perhaps indicate this is a modern disease? Endometriosis is considered ahistorical, with many medical books, even up to 1985 failing to include it.[1] For a disease affecting 1 in 10 females that causes a plethora of symptoms, it seems bizarre it's not more documented or widely known. It's natural to assume historic sexism meant women were not taken seriously, so social issues were capable of bottlenecking the discovery of the disease. Instead of doctors recognising something was wrong, women were instead labelled as having a low pain tolerance, exaggerating, or simply reacting inappropriately to menstruation. Despite a gap in recent modern medicine attention and recognition, it's believed to have been written about in modern European history approximately 300 years ago.[1]

A German physician named Daniel Shroen first described the disease in 1690 as a common female disorder, whereby sores or "inflammations" were found in the pelvis with the tendency to form adhesions.[2] Although this issue wasn't yet given a name, over the following centuries, papers were published across Europe, developing details and advancing our understanding of the disease. This slow but important journey, piece by piece, built up the story of what we know today. Some findings include: William Broughton, a physician from Scotland, wrote in 1755 that lesions could penetrate the rectum,[3] whilst in 1779, English physician Philibertus Hoctin noted the main symptom of the disease was intense pain resembling labour,[4] and in 1899 endometriosis cysts were first described which would later be named endometriomas.[5] In 1860, a pathologist named Karl von Rokitansky was the first to explain how the disease might develop in the body, describing it as "active endometrium outside the uterine cavity".[6] He was also the first to describe adenomyosis, a similar disease found in the uterus.[7] It was in 1927 that an American gynaecologist called John Sampson introduced the term "endometriosis" and described his theory on the cause of the disease.[8,9] Throughout the rest of the 20th Century, vital improvements were seen in diagnosis and laparoscopic surgery techniques. Scientists identified characteristics such as genetic and immunological factors and gained an understanding that hormonal treatments such as birth control pills could alleviate symptoms.

Although the name 'endometriosis' was coined in Europe around 100 years ago, it may have been described as far back as the Ancient Egyptians. Doctors in Ancient Greece also described symptoms of the disease 2,500 years ago. The Hippocratic Corpus, a collection of medical books written in Ancient Greece, includes a book called *Diseases of Women*. Many symptoms of endometriosis are detailed within it; however, the explanations for them are peculiar and reflect the understanding of the human body at the time. The symptoms are attributed to conditions such as 'a wandering uterus' or 'The Disease of Virgins'. We now know these concepts are not correct; we do not have the Disease of Virgins still today, so we can question if these women did in fact have endometriosis instead. Hippocratic doctors wrote the following descriptions of the sick women, does this sound like endometriosis to you?[10]:

8

Inflamed

...suffers pain in their whole body

Sometimes the menses break out in a mass through the vagina, and what comes out has a fleshy appearance, as if it were from an abortion, and is dark in colour.

When she has intercourse with her husband, she will suffer a pain that seems to indicate that some object is lying there

A weight is present in her body, and it protrudes, rising up just as in a woman who is pregnant

She suffers heartburn... and pain from time to time occupies her belly down from the naval, her groyne, and lower back

She suffers the most when her menses are approaching

Unless treatment is applied, her pain will increase in time [to] between the menses, she will run the risk of becoming barren due to the disease and its chronicity.

The menses are very black... both seeds of the male and female are weakened and the woman does not become pregnant.

In women whose cervix has turned to the side and is leaning against the hip

These descriptions, albeit very old-fashioned, sound like endometriosis... painful periods, bloating, painful sex, dark menstrual blood, inflammation, infertility, pain, and distortions to the pelvis due to adhesions. If these women were suffering from endometriosis, it would confirm this is not a modern disease. So, you may be wondering (like I was) if doctors described it 2,500 years ago, what happened to this knowledge and to these women. Well, evidence suggests it comes down to women being misdiagnosed with a disorder you may have heard of called hysteria. If this is true, in the appropriate and immaculate words of Dr Cameron Nezhat, "this would constitute one of the most colossal mass misdiagnoses in human history, one that over the centuries has subjected women to murder, madhouses and lives of unremitting physical, social and psychological pain".[11] We have been born into this world at a fortunate time where this is no longer the case or outcome for women struggling with the disease. We are fortunate the women who lived before us fought for our rights and protested for the social change that disempowered men from putting women in insane asylums for having a disease that doctors couldn't explain or because it made them impractical women, a.k.a unable to have sex without pain or bear children for their husbands. The understanding, awareness, and treatment of endometriosis has come a long way, but at the same time, we are only halfway. Many critical questions are still left unanswered about this mysterious disease. Fortunately, advances in research and funding are on an upward trend. Despite the progress, endometriosis remains a complex and challenging condition to diagnose and treat. Many individuals experience years of pain or infertility before receiving an accurate diagnosis, and there is still much to learn about the best ways to manage the condition. Nevertheless, ongoing research and advocacy efforts are helping raise awareness of endometriosis and improve the lives of those who suffer from it. This will no longer be a hidden global pandemic.

3

My Story

"You don't write because you want to say something.
You write because you have something to say."
– F. Scott Fitzgerald

I once received a little card with the quote above written on it when I placed an order from Papier. When I first read it, the words resonated with me. Looking back, it's hard to tell why, but I kept the card, keeping it in view by placing it on top of my mirror. I guess in the back of my mind, I had always wanted to write this book, but I was in the energy of *"I want to say something"*, so I waited, burying the notion along with all my other ideas about wanting to start a career in women's health. At some point a seed was planted, one that grew over years, snowballing with this desire and drive to change career paths, choosing one that could serve those with endometriosis. Even so, I kept putting it off, telling myself "I'll do it…, but not now". However, during the COVID lockdown, dismissing this calling no longer felt right; I didn't want to wait any longer, so I signed up for five years of full-time study to become a dietician.

I was motivated by a deep desire to help people, but after nearly three years of study, I made the difficult decision to leave my course. I was riddled with anxiety, my nervous system was shot, and I felt unable to continue down that path. As you may recall, many women change careers because of endometriosis; this was an example of this. I was caught in a tide where my deregulated nervous system was fuelling my anxiety, and high anxiety levels had triggered histamine intolerance. I struggled with gastrointestinal issues, often throwing up after meals, and suffered from red hot flushing on my face, neck, and chest in response to certain foods or even mild stress. If you have ever experienced these sorts of issues, you will know how debilitating they can be. During this period, I was also diagnosed with nut allergies, so combined with the other problems I was facing, it led to a fear of eating at university or in public, feeling paranoid about triggering an allergic reaction. When you are dealing with elevated amounts of histamine in your body, it can further contribute to anxiety, so you see, I was in a miserable cycle where histamine triggered anxiety, which, in turn, worsened my histamine symptoms. It was a challenging period in my life — not the worst, but I needed to take a break from an environment that felt like I was living in perpetual survival mode.

Still wanting to help women, I began searching for other ways to do so. I'd learned a lot in my studies, and I didn't want to abandon that knowledge but rather use it to make a meaningful impact. Around the same time, several friends were either being told by doctors that they might have endometriosis or were undergoing surgeries, so I found myself increasingly speaking to women, offering advice, and sharing what I knew. I realised that since the time I was diagnosed, despite a massive increase in awareness, there were little to no improvements in the guidance available to patients. People still faced a dire lack of understanding of the disease at all stages of their endo journey. I knew then my purpose was to write this book, not because I wanted to say something, but because I had something to say.

This book is not about my story, so you may be wondering why there's a chapter focused entirely on my experience. When I was first diagnosed, like many people, I had so many questions, yet finding the answers was nearly impossible as endometriosis was not as well-known as it is now. My journey since then has confirmed that getting the answers you need is often difficult. This disease impacts the body in so many ways, so expecting doctors to have the best advice on how to cope with every specific symptom you have is a lot to ask, considering all the other conditions they must know in depth. I realised doctors didn't always have the knowledge or time to provide me with the information I sought. Not because they weren't great doctors or didn't have a wealth of information that helped hundreds of people each day. They were already helping me so much, but there was simply a gap of additional support I needed. Desperate for answers, I found the best way to get advice was by connecting with other women on forums like 'HealthUnlocked'. No one I knew had this disease to share my experience with, yet I could go to these forums to find answers, guidance, and reassurance from others suffering from the same challenges. It can be isolating going through something that you, nor the people around you understand, but communities like these allow people to find solidarity and even comfort. I also learned a lot about other people's experiences and how they differed from mine, which is important as this disease is very individualised. No two stories are the same; the way the disease manifests, the symptoms that occur, and how it affects people on a day-to-day basis can vary significantly. The understanding of endometriosis is still largely driven by storytelling to gain insight into the common ways it affects us and our lives. Whether this information is shared through conversations, social media, medical research, or found in forums or books, each story adds to the discussion. So, that was a roundabout way of saying I have included my story, not as a focal point, but in the hope it may resonate to those with a similar story.

I would like to emphasise that while online communities can be invaluable, there is still misinformation available online, and the voice of others should not overrule your trust in a gynaecologist or doctor who is a highly trained professional with years of medical experience. There has been a lot of progress in awareness of endometriosis, so doctors may now be better equipped to answer these questions.

* * *

I was diagnosed with endometriosis in 2018, before the world had the wave of women championing, speaking out, and raising awareness. On the day I found out, I didn't know how to pronounce the word, let alone have any understanding of what it meant for me and my body. I was at my local hospital's gynaecology ward in London, lying on the bed in a dark consultation room, with a phallic-shaped camera between my legs, protected with a condom and doused in lube-like jelly much to my bemusement, perhaps immature. Still, it humoured me enough to distract me for a few minutes. Another specialist was called into the room to confirm the ultrasound findings. I had no idea what they were looking at or discussing; I just knew I felt an uncomfortable pain from the camera and was lying there waiting for the scan to be over. The doctor proceeded to inform me I had endometriosis, kissing ovaries that were located behind my uterus, and a chocolate cyst around the size of a tennis ball on my left ovary. These words sounded very romantic, but I was pretty confident they weren't anything to celebrate. She then informed me that surgery was an option, however, there was a risk of losing my ovary so she would not advise me either way... "it had to be my choice". Then she left the room. I was 23 years old, I was by myself and had no understanding of what I had or the right thing to do. Despite this, I had to decide right then and there if I wanted to have surgery that could risk losing my ovary. I knew of course I didn't want that, but I also recognised it might be my only way out of the symptoms I had been experiencing. Fortunately, the other clinician said, as she pressed away on the computer keyboard in the corner of the room, that she thought I should go ahead with the surgery. Hearing her advice immediately affirmed I was happy to proceed and I am still grateful she gave me the reassurance I needed. I had been on a long journey of health issues, numerous appointments, and frankly...despair. If surgery offered any solution to fix all of that, then I would take it. I left the hospital room with an operation booked and a heavily re-photocopied leaflet on endometriosis the gynaecologist handed to me. This was obviously to replace the role of anyone explaining to me what they just diagnosed me with. When I got home, I scoured the internet, reading every link on countless Google search pages to gather all the information I could. I quickly recognised that endometriosis seemed like a forgotten disease, with health websites listing that they didn't know what it was, what caused it, or how to cure it. Even the treatment options were unhelpful, suggesting surgery, the pill, or paracetamol. Having non-curative surgery so young was scary, whilst the pill and painkillers seemed to be ways to mask the issue rather than treat it. I also knew from experience that paracetamol didn't sufficiently curb the pain. I needed more answers and realising that no one else would hand-feed me the information, I decided to educate myself. I was seeking greater insight into the condition than the standard vague buzzwords commonly listed on websites such as 'painful and heavy periods', 'pelvic pain', and 'infertility'. I read books such as *The Doctor Will See You Now* by Dr Seckin, health pages, blogs, and researched medical papers to get the understanding I needed. This helped when having to inform and educate everyone around me about endometriosis, which was at the time a very unknown disease. Not one person had heard of it.

Statistics say it takes on average eight years to be diagnosed with endometriosis. I was fortunately not one of them. When a scan shows your ovaries glued together, a doctor is going to offer help. With hindsight, I first noticed the changes to my body when I was 20, just three years before my diagnosis. I had come off the pill, which I had been on since I was 16 due to developing severe acne in my later teenage years. I wanted to give my body a break, but I found my periods steadily became more painful and exhausting. I was at university, so I was often able to get away with spending the first day of my period in bed. I started getting severe yo-yo bloating which could be painful at times. The doctor diagnosed me with Irritable Bowel Syndrome (IBS) and prescribed Buscopan® which did nothing to help...unsurprisingly. I also started experiencing excruciating knee pain for no explicable reason. I even begged my doctor for a knee x-ray after two years because I couldn't fathom how so much pain had no cause. My knees were clinically perfect, and I would only discover years later that this, as well as severe bloating, was a symptom shared by other people with the disease I would soon be diagnosed with.

It was in 2017 that I started to recognise something really wasn't right with my body. I hadn't been sexually active in a while, but I met someone and as the relationship evolved into an intimate nature, symptoms started unravelling in a new way. I started spotting every week, which was new for me, but it didn't seem like anything crazy to worry about, plus my friend reassured me she had it from time to time. Within a month it became a daily occurrence, so I started wearing sanitary towels every day. You would think this would be enough to make me call a doctor, but in isolation it didn't seem like a big enough problem. Then there were two particular experiences where sex proceeded with an intense, overwhelming haze of abdominal pain. So intense that it crippled me into laying in the foetal position on the bathroom floor waiting for it to end. The first time it happened, the sensation was so dreadfully unfamiliar that I almost called an ambulance. Thankfully, the pain subsided so I was able to sleep it off, but it did leave me bewildered and unsure of what to make of it. Taking painkillers to have sex became my new normal, as did bleeding from or during sex. It's an incredibly sad moment in life when you realise that for some unknown reason, sex now equals agony. It took longer than it should for me to visit the doctor because I thought for women, bleeding is natural, as is pain. Over time, the symptoms progressed with nausea, frequent UTIs, and painful urination. I had never experienced nausea before and I kept running to the bathroom at work to throw up, but nothing would ever relieve it. After ruling out pregnancy, I went to the doctor who carried out a smear, blood tests, and a pelvic examination. When I returned to discuss my results, he was concerned and referred me to a gynaecologist. I had cervical ectropion, which is a benign graze-type appearance of the skin on the cervix. This can closely resemble the early stages of cervical cancer; plus, other test results meant it needed to be ruled out. Cervical ectropion can be caused by high levels of oestrogen and is sometimes found in individuals with endometriosis — so some of you may have shared this type of experience. I told my parents, and as I was living in Australia at the time, they insisted I come home to sort out my health. I made a GP appointment on my first day back in England and listed out everything I had been experiencing. I found this note on my phone that I wrote before being diagnosed. It shows how this disease can affect so many aspects of our health. It's not limited to the pelvis, and there are *many* types of pain associated.

Bloating: Permanent bloating in the lower stomach.

Lower Abdomen Pain: There's a heavy feeling like I have to hold myself up. Sometimes, it can be crampy, like period pain. Other times, I experience bad, sharp, stabbing pains.

Lower Back Pain

Pain in Hips: Particularly deep in the right side.

Tiredness

Knee Pain: I'm unsure if it's related, but it's really painful.

Full Leg Pain: I'm so sore and achy — it feels like a constant flu.

Recurring Water Infections

Painful Bowel Movements

Indigestion

Pain During Sex

Nausea: it's all the time but comes in waves.

Periods: Irregular, heavy, pain varies — can be excruciating where I am unable to walk straight.

Acne: Do I have a hormone problem that could be causing the issues with my periods?

Allergies: I developed hay fever and oral mouth allergy syndrome at 18 — this is not directly relevant, but it seems that at 18, my immune system started changing.

I felt like a hypochondriac. My body was going through all these changes that didn't seem related, nor were they individually a cause for major concern. Still, I summarised everything to my doctor, although I worried I was overwhelming them with a long list of random symptoms. Yet, deep down, I also knew each symptom was an important piece of the puzzle. Due to the cervical ectropion and abnormal smear results I received in Australia, I was referred for a colposcopy, where they cauterised my cervix. After my treatment, I returned for my follow-up smear, which came back with normal results. It will always be happy news knowing you don't have cancer, but as weeks passed without any improvements in my health, it became clear something was still wrong. The fatigue reached new extremes; merely walking down the road would exhaust me to a point where the concrete pavement looked like a comfortable place to lie-down. I had a chronic aching in my hips and deep in my groin that never left. The nausea was fierce and overwhelming, and I often looked pregnant with a rock-hard stomach, which meant I had to wear loose, less restrictive clothing. My mental health also started to deteriorate. I had my first panic attack on a tube on my way home from work. I didn't know what was happening; I had always been self-assured and confident. I had experienced nervousness of course, but had never truly understood what anxiety meant. I believe my first panic attack stemmed from my body and not my mind, a mix of utter exhaustion and stress hormones perhaps, but thereafter that combined with the fear of ever having a similar experience again, manifested into chronic anxiety. I lost trust in my own body. I began doubting my ability to breathe by myself and became claustrophobic, unable to get on busy trains or tubes. I didn't even have faith in my body to walk down a flight of stairs without holding on to the rail and staring at every step to make sure I didn't miss it. I couldn't make sense of what was happening to me; I feared I was possibly losing my mind or...there was another logical explanation that I just needed to figure out. So, I went back to the GP, this time focusing on abnormal bleeding. I didn't mention any other symptoms because I didn't know if they were related, but I did know the bleeding was not normal. I didn't want them to think I was being dramatic in wanting to see a gynaecologist when some of my symptoms were knee pain and indigestion. I had recorded my periods and bought a letter from my Australian doctor requesting my referral to a gynaecologist. Thankfully, the GP agreed without question. The day of my appointment came, and within an hour of arriving at the hospital, I had my answer and a name for what I had been experiencing.

* * *

Leading up to my operation, I had a consultation at the hospital. My auntie came along with me, concerned about the anxiety I was experiencing. It was completely unlike me, so she wanted me to address it and get advice. Unfortunately, when I raised the issue with the doctor, they completely and thoroughly dismissed any association between anxiety and endometriosis. I ended the conversation because I didn't want to make a fuss, but I knew in my heart there was a link. I knew my body well enough to know it was all related somehow, even if the doctor we met that day didn't know. I think it's important to see how far we have come in our understanding in such a short space of time, as progress has been made in this area since then. Afterwards, we met with my surgeon, who stated one of the most effective ways to treat endometriosis was to have a baby, so asked whether I would choose that option. I was 23 years old; I had basically just finished university and was also single. Having a baby was nowhere on my agenda. I straightforwardly responded with a no, so he swiftly moved on to the next best option for me, which was surgery.

On the morning of my first-ever operation, my mum dropped me off at the hospital as patients had to go in alone. The staff were lovely and made me feel very comfortable, particularly a nurse named Orla, whom I wish I could thank again for making my experience. The surgeon came and explained they would treat my cyst and remove any other visible endometriosis. During surgery, they found a 6cm endometrioma on my left ovary, lesions on my abdominal wall and uterus, scar tissue, as well as uterosacral and rectovaginal endometriosis, which had caused my rectum to be displaced to the right. When I awoke, they confirmed I was able to keep my ovary, which gave me a massive wave of relief before announcing I would need another operation. The recovery took around three to four weeks to feel normal again. I will share what to expect during surgery as well as tips and advice later in the book.

At the time, I was working for my dad's company, gratefully, because I don't know how I would have sustained working anywhere else due to the amount of time I needed off for medical appointments and from my symptoms. One day, my dad called me into his office, and all it took was a simple "What's up?" from him in a concerned voice for me to break down in tears. I thought my surgery would solve everything I had been feeling or at least provide freedom from the hell I was living in. Yet I felt pretty much the same, *always* in pain and *always* tired. Fortunately, my follow-up appointment was shortly after, and they explained I would be able to have a second surgery in four months to treat my rectovaginal endometriosis (which explained why going to the toilet felt like a sharp kitchen knife slicing through me). We discussed the risks of surgery, which included cutting my ureters, bowel injury, and requiring a stoma. A stoma, for anyone who doesn't know, is when your bowel is diverted so that faeces are removed from the body via the stomach into a bag. The risks were daunting, but my surgeon reassured me it was very unlikely, so I agreed, now determined to have a surgery that provided the healing I was desperate for. He informed me I was to start hormone therapy using a drug called Prostap®, which is commonly used for breast and prostate cancer, putting you into temporary menopause. I had read online forums about this drug and there were many horror stories. I asked if I could decline the hormone therapy, but he said he wouldn't operate on me if I didn't take it and to not listen to the stories. I knew I wanted the operation, and I trusted my surgeon, so I started monthly injections of hormones alongside add-back therapy, which consisted of daily Hormone Replacement Therapy (HRT) tablets called tibolone. Add-back therapy is commonly taken alongside hormone therapy injections, aimed at lessening the severe side effects it can cause. These medications use steroids, so naturally, I gained some weight, but I didn't care, it was the absolute least of my worries. The hot flushes, on the other hand, were intense, and I would constantly break out in an uncomfortable and uncontrollable heat. In the middle of winter, I would walk around outside in a t-shirt because if I put on any layers, I would soon feel like I was on fire. The intolerance to rapid heat changes has never entirely gone despite only being on hormone therapy for three months. At that time, I felt like my whole life was spent at hospital or doctor's appointments, seemingly there every week for a check-up, scan, blood test, injection, or some other kind of appointment..., but it would soon be over.

For my second surgery, I stayed in the hospital the night before and had to do a bowel cleanse. This is where you take a strong laxative to ensure you have empty bowels for the surgery. I was slightly concerned and had imagined horrible scenes, but it was fine — thankfully. The following morning, I was told I would be the first person in surgery, so I got prepped in my gown and stockings and was wheeled to the theatre. My surgery lasted four hours. Later in the afternoon when I was back on the ward, my surgeon came to visit me, and even in my morphine anaesthesia haze, I could tell he was pleased. He said there was a significant amount of endometriosis, more than expected, but my surgery had gone perfectly; the endometriosis was gone, and no colostomy or stents were required. Hurrah!

After the surgery, I was allowed codeine but unfortunately, the night nurse on the ward didn't read this on my chart. As the morphine wore off, the pain kicked in with a vengeance, so I asked if I could have something for it. I cannot remember if I was given paracetamol or not, but either way, it wasn't enough and I cried all night in pain. I couldn't move any part of my torso from my shoulder to my hips without it setting off a new rampage of torture. At that point, I didn't know I was allowed codeine so I didn't ask for it. Thankfully, a re-visit from one of my surgeons the next day rectified that. If you ever have surgery, always check which medications you are allowed to prevent this from occurring to you too. After that, I went home and took around four weeks to recover.

My second surgery changed my life forever. I will always remember the day I started skipping home, *yes*, skipping, from the train station to my house after a day of work because I felt so good. I felt normal, I had energy, and I was back. I was so elated from a lack of any feeling in my body — no pain, no nausea, and no tiredness. I have been very lucky because I had an excellent surgeon, but with endometriosis, surgery is not a cure. I still wanted to learn everything I could about the condition and how to manage it to ensure I never went back into the hole I was in before. This book is an ode to that mission, and I want to help every other person I possibly can along the way.

When I went for my post-surgery check-up, I met with a specialist nurse. Again, I was faced with the same conversation about my plans for babies. The nurse asked when I planned to have children, I wasn't sure, so she probed whether I wanted children. After confirming that I did, she started again, querying about when I planned on having them. I explained that I was single and only 24, so I didn't know. She responded, "If you were in a relationship tomorrow, when would you plan to have children?" At this point, slightly bewildered by the questions, I declared "I really don't know!". She looked at me and responded "ok, that's fine, but if you want them don't wait until you are 30". These words have haunted me throughout my twenties, and now that I've reached my thirties, I have moments of fear that I am taking too long and will live to regret it. Although I do believe that working on a gynaecological ward, seeing women day in and day out struggling to get pregnant, the nurse was probably just trying to help warn me, however, it's a horrible stress to put on young women.

Regardless of a few strange encounters along the way, I am so grateful for the care that I received because my surgeries transformed my life. I mostly feel like a normal healthy person who is energised and pain-free. I have researched ways to try and prevent endo growing back and have tried multiple alternative medicine options to alleviate side effects of the disease, including yoga, nutrition, meditation, acupuncture, reflexology, hypnotherapy, Chinese herbs, and Western herbs. I am on the pill at the gynaecologist's recommendation, but I don't take it back-to-back as I found the bloating too severe. I still get endo belly and wear clothes to suit my body that day or undo the top button of my jeans if it flares up. I still get bad periods, pain, or days when I feel incredibly inflamed. I have also struggled with allergies and anxiety and have a fibroid in my uterus — all comorbidities of endo. Although these are all ways that I am still reminded some days that I have a disease, my recovery has been nothing short of amazing. I will take all those feelings and side effects in comparison to how I felt before my surgeries. With this disease, you need to accept your new version of health because getting down about things outside of your control tends not to be very helpful. I believe a positive mindset is essential in regaining your life. Seeking good health and knowledge has been my tactic for coping, making sure I take it day-by-day or month-by-month and having a routine to support my body the best I can. If you are reading this book, I presume you are the same, someone who wants to know as much as they can about endo so they can support their body as much as possible. I hope this book provides the information you are after and is a helpful step in your endo story.

Love, Alice

4

What Is Endometriosis?

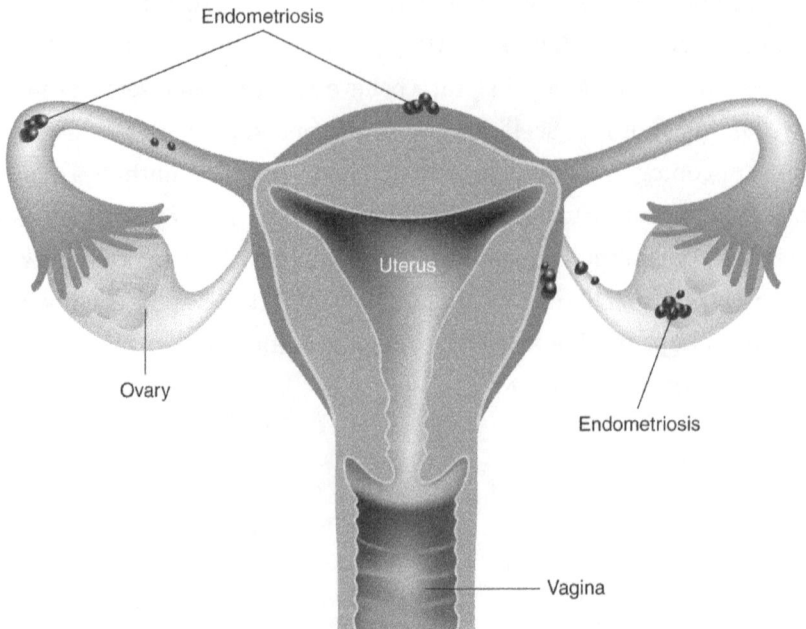

Endometriosis is a condition whereby tissue similar to endometrial tissue (the innermost lining of the uterus that is shed during a period) grows outside the uterus, called nodules, lesions or implants. It's typically found within the pelvic cavity but can be found in other areas.

Most common locations:
Peritoneum (a sheet of tissue lining your abdomen and abdominal organs)
Outer surface of the uterus
Ovaries
Fallopian tubes
Uterosacral ligaments

Less common areas include:
Rectovaginal septum
Bladder or urinary tract
Intestines
Appendix
Kidney
Vagina
Liver
Gluteal muscles
Diaphragm
Lungs
Abdominal scars (e.g. caesarean scars)

Endometrial tissue (not endometriosis) is a normal formation in the female cycle. Every month it grows in preparation for pregnancy, but if you do not become pregnant within that cycle, the endometrium is shed during menstruation. This is what your period is, it's a mix of blood and tissue that would have supported the implantation and growth of a fertilised egg by providing oxygen and nutrients. After your period, the endometrium grows back ready for the next cycle, a process controlled by our hormones.

Oestradiol (a type of oestrogen) is a hormone primarily made by the ovaries which stimulates a new lining to grow and thicken each month to prepare once again for a possible pregnancy.

Endometrial glands and stroma are vital structures within endometrial tissue that allow it to carry out its functions. Those with endometriosis have tissue similar to endometrial tissue, *but which is not endometrial tissue*, growing outside the uterus. These lesions also contain endometrial glands and stroma, which is why it's described as an endometrial-*like* tissue. Diseased endometriosis tissue can range from tiny dots to a few centimetres in size. The lesions develop their own blood supply to help it grow and nerve supply to communicate to the brain.[1] Due to the similarity to endometrial tissue, the misplaced lesions also respond to the menstrual cycle, growing and bleeding each month in response to oestrogen. Yet when it's time to shed, unlike your period, it has nowhere to go. This can stimulate inflammation and hormone dysregulation. In a normal period, pain is caused by the contraction of the uterus, whereas in endometriosis, this can be combined with pain produced from an array of complex mechanisms that have developed due to the presence of this tissue. We will break these down throughout Part 1. There are different types of endometriosis and different stages of the disease. In mild cases, small amounts grow on the surface of the peritoneum, whilst in severe cases, endometriosis may grow similar to a tumour, growing through tissue layers and in some instances, causing abnormal functioning of organs. It can also prompt scarring, sometimes resulting in organs sticking together.

Endo is a disease, not an infection. It cannot be passed on and you cannot infect someone else with it.

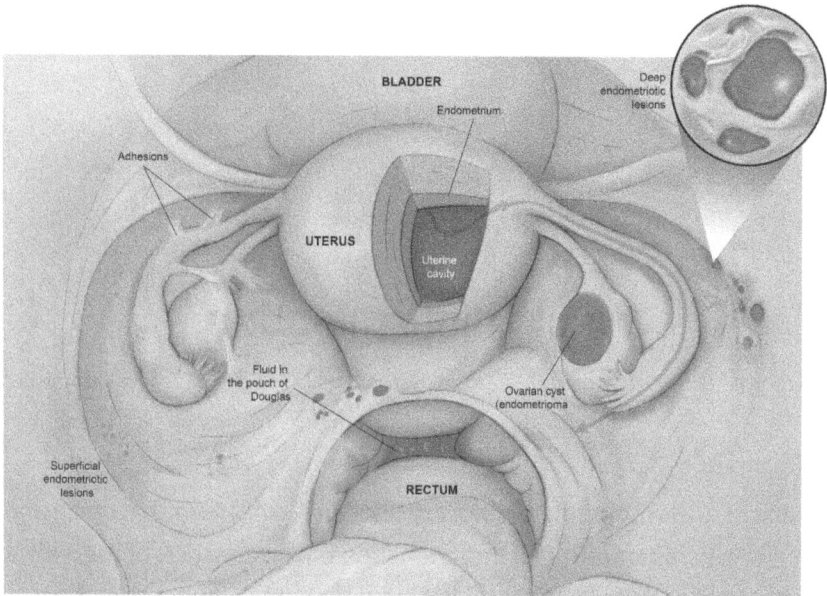

Inspired by Natalie Koscal's illustration for Zondervan et al.[2]

5

What Is Inflammation?

Endometriosis is an inflammatory disease, but what does that mean and what is inflammation? Well, inflammation is a normal part of the body's immune and defence system. It's how the body fights off pathogen-causing viruses or allows our bodies to heal from a cut and repair itself. Inflammation has a bad rep, but it's a good thing! We wouldn't survive very long without it. Acute inflammation is a short-term response when the body reacts to injury or a pathogen, working to destroy and remove it from the body. However, chronic inflammation is long-term, experienced over months or years, which has the potential to cause other issues in the body. On a basic level, inflammation causes redness, warmth, swelling, and pain, all side effects of the healing process. When it occurs chronically, these symptoms can significantly impact a person's health. Beyond the physical discomfort, individuals may experience knock-on effects such as fatigue, stemming from the body needing more energy to repair itself, and mental fatigue due to persistent pain. Unfortunately though, it goes deeper than that, chronic inflammation can cause the body to accidentally attack healthy tissues, leading to greater pain or even the development of disease.

During the menstrual cycle, inflammation naturally occurs as the immune system works to shed and release endometrial tissue from the body, and then facilitate the repair and regeneration of the womb for the next cycle. In the case of endometriosis, the diseased tissue also thickens and becomes inflamed, but with nowhere to go it cannot exit the body. Over time, the localised inflammation can cause irritation to neighbouring areas as immune cells aggravate healthy tissue. This can promote greater issues as the inflammation can lead to scar tissue and adhesions in the pelvis.

Endometriosis also causes an inflammatory immune reaction, meaning the inflammatory nature of the disease causes an imbalance in the immune system. Although, it's not entirely clear on whether it's actually a dysfunctional immune response that allows endometriosis to begin in the first place.[1] A chicken and egg scenario. It's thought the dysfunctional immune system leads to dysfunctional immune cells that are unable to clear endometriosis tissue, whilst simultaneously facilitating the growth and survival of endometriosis lesions.[1] This is far from ideal. The dysfunctional immune cells contribute to chronic local inflammation as well as systemic inflammation[2] — this is when the immune system is constantly defending the body. Endometriosis, therefore, is not just a disease affecting the pelvis, it's considered a systemic disease which can affect several tissues and organs, causing a multitude of side effects.

6

What Are Adhesions?

Have you ever heard of adhesions? They are not a household term, but they affect many people for different reasons, sometimes having a significant impact on their lives. Adhesions are a type of sticky scar tissue that allows it to act as superglue, causing thin or thick fibrous bands to connect two parts of the body that would otherwise not be joined together. Inflammation can be a direct source of adhesion growth. Active endometriosis also promotes peritoneal inflammation, creating an environment that fosters the formation of adhesions.[1] This relationship is evident as around 70% of patients have adhesions in their abdominopelvic cavity on their first operation.[2] Surgery is another cause for adhesion growth, so it's best to avoid more operations than what is necessary. In some instances, this connection between endometriosis and inflammation contributes to advanced adhesion growth and extreme cases like frozen pelvis, although don't worry, such cases are rare. Adhesions will form anywhere in the pelvic cavity and can affect all organs, including the ovaries, fallopian tubes, rectum, uterus, and bladder. Sometimes, they lead to complications by changing the anatomy of the pelvis. For example, they may cause kissing ovaries (when the ovaries move closer so that they are in close proximity or touching one another), or they might attach your uterus to other organs or the abdominal lining. When this happens, it can change the location of the uterus by pulling it out of place or altering its shape. This is true of any organ they impact. Furthermore, adhesions may exert tension on nerves, resulting in pain.

Adhesions can cause their own symptoms such as[3]:

Cramping

Painful Intercourse

Nausea

Bowel Obstruction, Constipation, or Loose Stools

Stabbing Pains

Decreased Libido

Infertility

Chronic Bloating

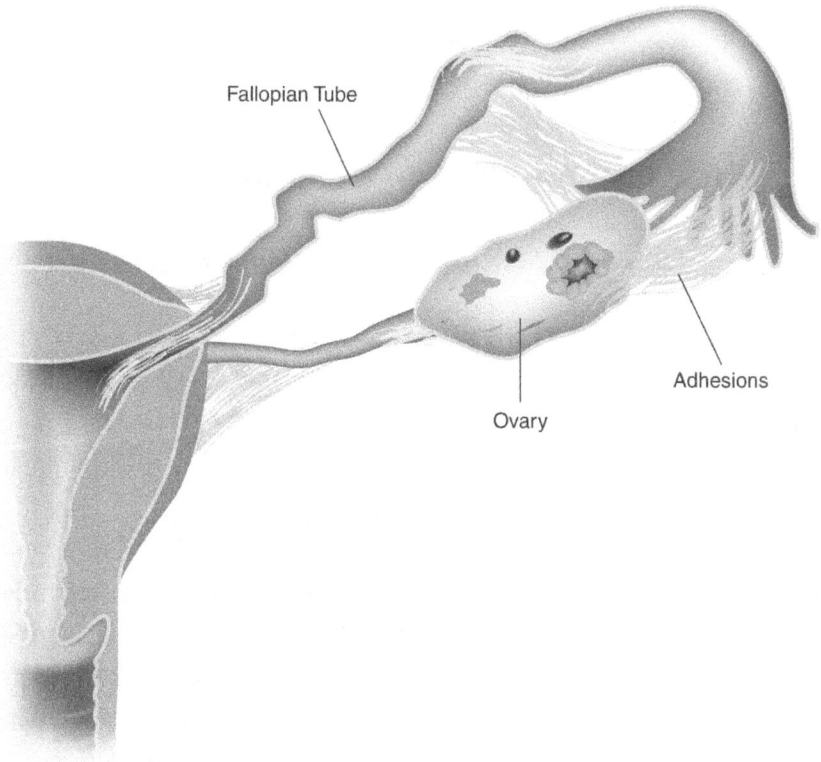

Fallopian Tube

Adhesions

Ovary

7

What Are the Types of Endometriosis?

Endometriosis is classified into three phenotypes, depending on the location and depth to which the lesions grow. A phenotype is just a fancy term for subcategories.

The Three Phenotypes of Endometriosis

Superficial Peritoneal Disease (SUP) or Superficial Disease

Superficial endometriosis is the most common form, affecting around 80% of cases.[1] These lesions are typically small and flat and sit on the surface of organs or tissues.

Ovarian Endometrioma (OMA) or Endometrioma

Endometriomas, also known as chocolate cysts, are found in the ovaries and affect between 17 to 44% of people.[2] They occur when a lesion invades the ovary and develops a blood-filled cyst. This blood darkens with time, inspiring the name 'chocolate' cysts. This dark brown fluid contains fragments of endometriosis tissue. When found, they typically suggest a more severe state of the disease. Endometriomas can be as small as a pea or grow bigger than a grapefruit. Fortunately, they can usually be detected with an ultrasound or MRI; however, they will still often require surgery for treatment, particularly if causing symptoms like pain or there is a risk of rupture. This shouldn't cause you to worry though, less than 3% of endometriomas will rupture and typically occur in cysts larger than 6cm.[3]

Deep Infiltrating Endometriosis (DIE) or Deep Endometriosis

DIE is the most aggressive phenotype — a horrible abbreviation I'm sure we can agree. It affects 20% of women who suffer from endometriosis.[4] DIE lesions invade tissue or organs, growing deeper than superficial lesions. These lesions are classified as penetrating over 5mm into a tissue surface.[2] They grow in many areas, including the rectal wall, ureters, and bladder. Due to their invasive nature, this type of endometriosis can cause severe symptoms like pain, but also gastrointestinal and urological tract abnormalities. Medical treatment or surgery can be used to treat them.

* * *

Although ovarian endometriomas and deep endometriosis are associated with more severe forms of the disease, this does not always correlate with the symptoms experienced. It's thought that the location of the lesions and the body's inflammatory immune response are mostly responsible for the symptoms of endometriosis. However, pain is complex, with pain perception and pain mechanisms also playing an important role. Due to the diverse natures of these phenotypes, it's been proposed they represent three different diseases that are similar yet are grouped under the term endometriosis.[5] This is due to the varying molecular changes and genetic or epigenetic factors required to occur. Endo tissue can also come in different colours; lesions can be clear, blue, yellow, black, white, red, brown, or mixed. You will never need to know the colour of your lesions, but this knowledge helps researchers determine patterns and characteristics within the different colours to further understand the condition. It's

33

thought white lesions are older, whilst clear and red lesions are newer.[6] In teenagers, clear lesions are commonly found, making them harder for surgeons to see.[7] There are diverse manifestations of the disease. Whilst superficial disease and endometriomas are easier to summarise, lesions that are associated with the DIE phenotype introduce a level of complexity, varying in their location and impact. Furthermore, endometriosis affecting non-reproductive organs, such as the bowel, is not always considered deep, yet can cause debilitating symptoms for individuals outside of the typical period-associated manifestations.

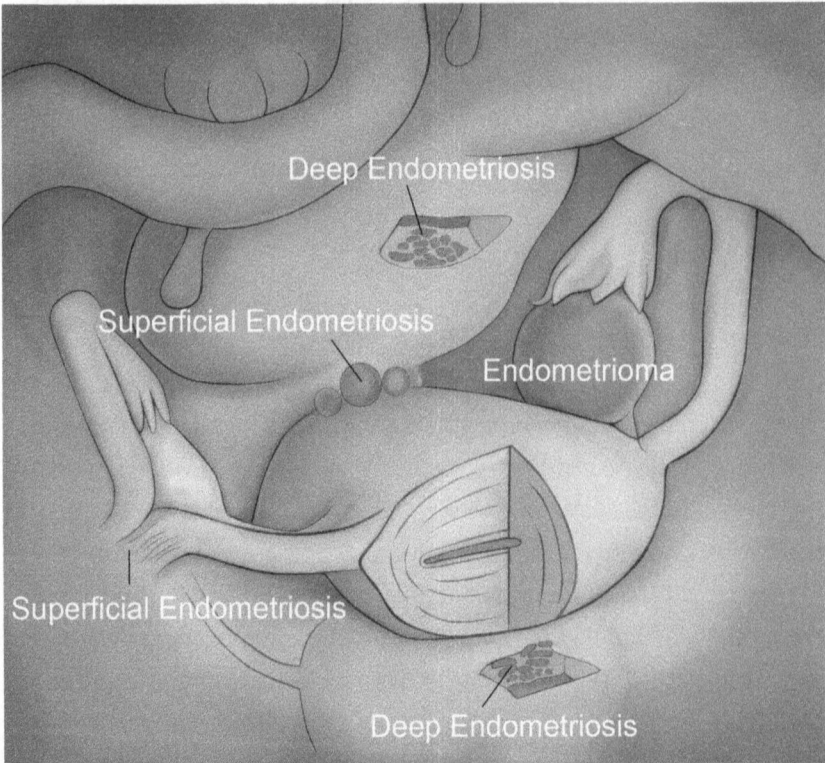

Inspired by Lydia Gregg's illustration for Johns Hopkins University School of Medicine[8]

8

What Causes Endometriosis?

The cause of endometriosis is unknown.

Aetiology is the word used to explain a cause or set of conditions that create disease. The scientific community has proposed several theories to explain how endometriosis manifests in the body. These have been challenged and developed over the past hundred years. Newer evidence can support an existing theory, raise issues, or provide new components to a theory that complements it. Endometriosis is a complex disease, and the answer is still not clear on what causes it. The possibility that different types of endometriosis develop via different mechanisms and may be separate diseases, means some theories work for certain types but not others. Therefore, still no single theory explains all cases and types of endometriosis. Some individuals may want to wait for the perfect answer, whilst others (like myself), do not want to have to possibly wait another hundred years. The following information will help you make sense of your disease with what scientists know now.

The Main Theories of Aetiology

Sampson's Theory - Retrograde Menstruation

Sampson's theory is that retrograde menstrual flow allows the transplantation and implantation of endometriosis lesions. This means period blood flows up the fallopian tubes and into the pelvis rather than down and out through the vagina as it would during menstruation. This theory is rooted in Sampson's observations from the 1920s when he found endometrial tissue coming out through the fallopian tubes and into the pelvic cavity.[1] It makes sense that menstrual blood going into the pelvis rather than exiting the body could potentially cause health problems. However, the issue with this theory is retrograde menstruation is reported in 76-90% of healthy menstruating women.[2,3] These figures are based on menstrual blood found in the peritoneal fluid during laparoscopy procedures. This makes it remarkably common to have blood in the pelvis — but is it *definitely* coming from the uterus? To understand this, doctors carried out a test where they occluded (closed) the fallopian tubes.[2] This resulted in a drop to just 15% of people having blood in their pelvis, supporting Sampson's theory that blood travels from the uterus, through the fallopian tubes, then enters the pelvis...thus retrograde menstruation is possible and common. Yet 76-90% of females don't have endometriosis, only 10% do. This leaves us with more questions. Why does the disease develop in some and not others? The cause of the disease cannot be as simple as retrograde menstruation, otherwise, more people would have it. Maybe there is an association between the *amount* of retrograde menstruation and the subsequent risk of disease. So, those with a larger amount of blood in the pelvis may be more likely to have endometriosis due to a greater chance of lesion implantation.[4] Although this isn't clear, Sampson's theory is the most widely accepted and supported by the science community as it has the most evidence to validate it having a role. Nonetheless, it's over-simplistic, and many additional factors to this theory are continually discussed in research to determine what happens next.

Meyer's Theory - Coelomic Metaplasia

Meyer's theory, proposed in 1919, suggests the pathogenesis of endometriosis originates from coelomic metaplasia.[5] Don't worry, no one expects you to know what that is — I will explain. Coelomic epithelium is the layer of tissue in embryos that transforms, developing into various structures like the peritoneum or pleura (the tissue surrounding the lungs). According to this theory, the disease is initiated by specialised cells on this lining transforming into endometrium-*like* tissue, possibly through hormonal or immunological factors.[6] This basically means normal cells could *change* into endometriosis tissue. This theory is particularly valuable in explaining the occurrence of endometriosis in prepubertal girls and men. However, adolescent endometriosis may be a distinct condition from endometriosis found in teenagers and adults, as it may not be advanced or encouraged to grow by oestrogen.[7] Meyer's theory also provides insight into the presence of endometriosis in unusual places such as the pleura. Yet if this were the primary mechanism behind endometriosis development, you would expect higher prevalence in strange places to be found.[8]

Halban's Theory - Lymphatic and Haematogenous Spread

In 1924, Halban's theory proposed benign metastasis occurred through lymphatic and blood vessel dissemination of endometrial cells to distant sites in the body, causing the spread of endometriosis.[9] In layman's terms, this theory suggests endometriosis is caused by endometrial cells spreading from the uterus to other parts of the body where it's not meant to be, via our blood supply and lymph nodes. This theory addresses the perplexing occurrence of endometriosis in remote and nonpelvic sites such as the lungs and brain.[8] Its validity is supported by the discovery of endometriosis in lymph nodes and blood vessels, indicating a potential pathway for its spread.[10] Furthermore, Halban's theory helps elucidate the recurrence of endometriosis after surgical removal of the lesions, as lymph nodes play a crucial role in the spread of other diseases like cancer. The pathology of deep endometriosis is similar to that of cancer, however, there is no evidence that endometriosis can accomplish the sophisticated mechanisms seen in cancer required to metastasise through the lymph nodes.[11]

Stem Cell Recruitment Theory

Stem cells are special because they have the unique ability to transform into many different types of cells, whether a hair cell on your head or muscle cell in your heart. Stem Cell Recruitment was theorised in the early 2000's, suggesting stem cells originating from the endometrium or bone marrow may differentiate into endometriosis at different sites in the body.[11] For instance, through retrograde menstruation (we are combining the theories here), stem cells leave the uterus where they change into endometriosis cells.[12] This process would likely be facilitated by other factors such as genetics, inflammation, and the immune system.[11] The stem cell theory could support the cause of endometriosis in men, as well as deep lesions of endo. However, this area needs more research as its not fully understood.

Other Factors for Endometriosis Development

The most widely accepted theory is Sampson's theory of retrograde menstruation, even though it is overly simplistic. It only explains the physical relocation of endometrial tissue into the pelvic cavity yet does not explain the manifestation of endometriosis lesions. Sticking to this theory, the question remains: how does the misplaced menstrual blood turn into endometriosis? Numerous medical papers discuss the possible pathophysiology of endometriosis after retrograde menstruation. As you will see, many theories exist for this poorly understood disease, and one theory isn't able to cover everything. Even so, they help tell a story of how endometriosis cells escape surveillance by the immune system whilst simultaneously promoting its growth. Immune surveillance is the process carried out by the immune system to detect and destroy things that shouldn't be there, namely viruses or cancer cells. In the case of endometriosis, immune surveillance should detect these cells and get rid of them, but it doesn't. This dip in immune surveillance allows the disease to continue growing. There are four hallmarks of the disease that may cause lesions to develop in some but not others.[6] These are the most supported by scientific research:

Genetic Predisposition

If you have a family member with endometriosis, your risk increases, particularly for a first-degree family member such as a mum or sister. However, only 7% of women have endometriosis associated with a genetic predisposition.[13] A genetic predisposition for a disease means certain genes are passed on, making a person more susceptible to developing a disease. It doesn't mean an individual will *definitively* develop the condition. Other factors must come into play for the disease to manifest. Researchers do not fully understand the genetics of endometriosis due to its complexity. It's believed a polygenic/ multifactorial mode is inherited, meaning a combination of multiple genes, and the influence of the environment on those genes determines whether the disease forms in a person.[14] Interestingly, when endometriosis is found in multiple family members, it tends to be with more severe forms of the disease.[14] This suggests that severe states of the disease increase genetic propensity.

It's important to consider the shared environmental exposures and lifestyle factors within families, such as diet[15] and stress, that may also contribute to this association. This means a pattern may appear in families as the individuals have comparable lifestyles, and the combined effect of their shared lifestyle factors potentially increases their endometriosis risk.

Oestrogen-Dependence

Endometriosis is known to be oestrogen-dependent, meaning oestrogen stimulates the pathological process of growth. This hormone enables endo to attach to the peritoneum, create a blood supply, and survive.[6] Oestrogen also promotes inflammation and symptoms like pain.[16] Endometriosis tissue has over 100 times more oestrogen *receptors* than normal endometrial tissue.[16] The abundance of receptors provides numerous binding sites for oestrogen to interact with the cells. This abnormality potentially explains why the remaining 90% of women who experience retrograde menstruation do not develop endometriosis. It's believed these molecular defects found in misplaced endometrial tissue allow the establishment and survival of endometriosis.[16] What's more, *aromatase,* the enzyme responsible for converting hormones into oestrogen, is found in significant quantities in endometriosis lesions.[17] Aromatase, therefore, empowers lesions to produce their own local oestrogen, reducing their reliance on the oestrogen produced by the ovaries — meaning the lesions are effectively feeding themselves.

> **Receptors** are like special locks on the surface of cells, and hormones like oestrogen are keys. When these keys and locks bind, they trigger a reaction to take place. This process is vital for maintaining balance throughout the body.

Progesterone Resistance

Due to the significantly elevated ratio of oestrogen receptors in endometriosis lesions, progesterone receptors are often deficient. This imbalance leads to progesterone resistance, a condition where the cells become less responsive to progesterone's regulatory effects.[18] Consequently, symptoms such as inflammation and pain may manifest as progesterone plays a crucial role in dampening inflammation by suppressing several inflammatory pathways.[19] Therefore, chronic inflammation can induce a progesterone-resistant state and vice versa — perpetuating the disease process.[20] Due to the impaired responsiveness of progesterone, treatments targeting this hormone can sometimes be ineffective in managing the condition.[18] It remains unclear whether the issues with progesterone receptor expression are a cause or consequence of the disease.

Inflammation

Endometriosis can cause a chronic inflammatory state, which unfortunately fuels the progression of the disease, exacerbating its associated symptoms, notably pain. Nerves within lesions may exhibit hypersensitivity to inflammatory stimuli, resulting in an exaggerated inflammatory response that may perpetuate endometriosis pain symptoms.[21] A positive feedback loop between oestrogen and inflammation further compounds the heightened inflammatory state.[6] Increased inflammation triggers elevated oestrogen production by the body, and in turn, oestrogens stimulate more inflammation. It achieves this by stimulating immune cells to secrete inflammatory proteins, such as cytokines.[22] Consequently, the continuous cycle of oestrogen-induced inflammation and inflammation-driven oestrogen production is thought to lead to scar tissue formation and adhesions, further complicating the disease pathology. Moreover, it's suggested inflammatory cytokines play a role in reducing the number of progesterone receptors, as discussed previously.[23] This reduction in progesterone receptor expression contributes to resistance, exacerbating the inflammatory response and perpetuating the disease process.

Additional Hypotheses

Immune System Problem

As previously discussed, a healthy immune system is adept at differentiating between healthy tissues from those that are damaged, dead, or foreign, then effectively eliminating these unwanted cells. However, there is evidence of defective immune surveillance in endometriosis,[24] indicating the immune system fails to identify and eradicate endometriosis tissue. Instead, it inadvertently promotes inflammation and the growth of lesions, facilitating disease survival. The dysregulated immune function suggests endometriosis should be classified as an immune disease, albeit distinct from an autoimmune disease (where the body attacks its own tissues). Endometriosis is not classified as an autoimmune disease, but there is an increased risk of developing autoimmune conditions, as detailed in Chapter 22.

Bacterial Contamination

It was previously believed the uterus was sterile, devoid of bacteria or other living microorganisms. However, more recent studies debunked this notion. The type of bacteria found in locations like the vagina, cervix, endometrium, peritoneum, and faeces differ in people with and without the condition. A range of different bacteria have been observed at either lower or higher levels at these sites in those with endometriosis. Although the findings are inconsistent — likely due to the small number of patients involved in each study.[25] The bacterial contamination theory was born after finding high amounts of E. coli bacteria in the menstrual blood of endometriosis patients.[26] Other gynaecological diseases are associated with bacterial infections, like gonorrhoea and chlamydia. If a person sexually contracts a bacteria called Neisseria gonorrhoeae, it changes the microbiome in the reproductive tract and endometrium, leading to the development of gonorrhoea. This bacterium tricks the immune system, allowing it to enter human cells, where it's cloaked and protected from detection by our immune system. This bacterium can then interact with various immune cells and induce inflammatory reactions in the body. So, from this, we already know that changes in bacteria within the endometrium microflora can inhibit the immune system and cause inflammation. This poses the question, could an imbalance in the growth of different types of bacteria be instrumental in creating inflammation, thereby facilitating the growth of endometriosis, or at least contributing to its development?[27] This research adds another branch to the multifactorial disease and its potential aetiology. More investigation is warranted to determine the validity of this theory and its implications for understanding and managing the disease.

Pelvic Inflammatory Disease (PID)

PID is an infection in the female reproductive system affecting the womb, fallopian tubes, and ovaries. Typically, PID is caused by Sexually Transmitted Infections (STI) wherein bacteria enter the vagina and ascend to the uterus. PID is primarily caused by gonorrhoea and chlamydia, which is transmitted through unprotected sex. These conditions are treated with antibiotics and prevented using condoms. However, PID is not always caused by an STI. Normal vaginal bacteria can also lead to PID by spreading up to the pelvis. PID alters the microbiota of the vagina, leading to an overgrowth of harmful microorganisms ascending to the uterus. The immune system often responds by inducing inflammation, which may inadvertently support the implantation of endometriosis lesions. Studies support this possibility as there's an increased risk of endometriosis in patients with a history of PID.[28] Sometimes, inflammation from PID causes significant lower abdominal pain, whilst others can be asymptomatic. Regular testing and treatment for infections are crucial to prevent inflammation from causing damage to reproductive organs and to preserve fertility. STI testing can be performed by your doctor, at a family planning clinic, or with home testing kits.

Maybe She's Born with It

Although rare, endometriosis tissue has been found in female foetuses, giving rise to the embryo genetic theory.[12] This theory suggests that misplaced endometrial glands or cells occur during foetal development. These cells respond to oestrogen; however, they lay dormant until puberty starts, when oestrogen is released by the ovaries, causing the proliferation of the endometriosis tissue.[12] This would mean a person is born with endometriosis. The research supports this theory for some subtypes of endometriosis, but not all of them.[29]

* * *

When used collectively, these theories provide insights into how en-dometriosis tissue possibly avoids clearance by the immune system and apoptosis. Apoptosis is the term for programmed cell death, which occurs naturally in healthy cells at the end of their life cycle. When apoptosis doesn't happen, *like in cancer cells*, it can lead to tumour growth as cells start growing out of control rather than dying. Endometriosis evades normal immune system surveillance, allowing it to infiltrate the peritoneum. Subsequently, lesions acquire a blood supply, enabling their survival and continued growth. An apparent change in the endocrine (hormone) and immune systems is also observed in individuals with endometriosis, which the theories shed light on. Overall, the cause of endometriosis is considered multifactorial, with numerous factors contributing to the development of the disease. The integration of these theories highlights the complex interplay between various physiological systems and pathological processes underlying endometriosis. It may seem weird that a disease has such a long list of possible causes. A way to understand all the information and make sense of why there are so many different theories is to reflect on your understanding of cancer, which is frequently mentioned in endometriosis studies due to similarities. It's accepted by society that there is rarely a single cause of cancer development in an individual. Carcinogens such as smoking, air pollution, poor diet, or UV damage may increase the risk of developing cancer, but it does not guarantee it will happen. Plus, cancer wouldn't appear a moment after you have a cigarette or in the evening after getting sunburnt. Cancer can be a lengthy process due to multifactorial damage from many contributing factors, an *unfortunate* but perfect storm as such. Cancer can also be genetic; if a female carries the BRCA1 or BRCA2 gene, it increases their risk of breast and ovarian cancer, yet we understand not all cancers are genetic, nor does everyone with these genes get cancer. We also recognise that cancer is an umbrella term for over 200 separate diseases depending on their location and features. You see, this all seems logical when it comes to another disease we know about. With endometriosis, it's helpful to understand that the different types might develop in several ways and from various causes. Like cancer, all theories may be accurate to a degree because there may be several pathways that lead to endometriosis developing. The disease manifests differently in each person due to unique environmental, genetic, and epigenetic triggers.[30] Epigenetics is the study of how environmental factors such as malnutrition and toxins (including pollution), as well as behavioural factors such as stress or alcohol consumption, can cause changes in how our genes work. Unlike genetic changes, epigenetic changes can be temporary and reversible as they alter how the body *reads* a person's DNA sequence; they are not changes to the *actual* DNA. Research is ongoing, so hopefully we will have the answers in years to come.

Dioxin

There are studies proposing environmental factors can increase the risk of endometriosis. Dioxin is a chemical compound found in the environment that results from natural or industrial processes; for example, it can be a by-product of manufacturing herbicides. More than 90% of human exposure to dioxin is estimated to come from our food and water.[31] Unfortunately, dioxin has been linked to several diseases, including endometriosis. Laboratory tests on dioxin exposure showed it led to endometriosis in primates,[32] with the severity and incidence of the disease positively related to the level of dose exposed to. This signifies the greater exposure the monkeys had to dioxin, the more severe their endometriosis. Although there is not enough solid or credible data to support that this is the same for humans, The World Health Organisation declared that dioxin can disrupt our endocrine system and immune response.[33] This valuable information supports the idea that we should minimise dioxin exposure to reduce the possible implications for our health. The lack of conclusive answers on whether environmental factors like toxins can cause endometriosis will *always* exist, as studies determining whether this is true in humans are deemed unethical. In part 3, we will discuss other toxins to avoid.

What Does Not Cause Endometriosis?

There is no scientific evidence linking abortion or douching to developing endometriosis. Individuals do not bring this disease on themselves through their lifestyle choices or things they have done.

9

What Are the Stages of Endometriosis?

Endometriosis is classified into stages or categories based on the type of endo a person has, the amount present, where they have it, and the depth of the lesions. Several classification systems exist that focus on different aspects of the disease, whether the symptoms experienced or the organs affected, but none are universally accepted. The American Society for Reproductive Medicine (ASRM) classification is the most widely used, as detailed shortly. This uses a point system, qualifying individuals into one of four stages. For example, a deep ovarian endometrioma larger than 3cm scores 20 points, making it stage 3.

Staging does not indicate the level of pain, symptoms, or impact on fertility. There should be no judgement on yourself or someone else based on stages as you may experience more symptoms at a mild level of the disease than someone with a moderate level, and vice versa. Endometriosis is generally considered a progressive disease. It used to be thought endo would advance in a similar way to cancer, causing a person to move from stage 1 to stage 4, however, this isn't clear. It's not evident if superficial endometriosis progresses to deep endometriosis or if it progresses in every person.[2] Despite this knowledge gap, it's still logical to think of endometriosis as progressive as when left untreated it can continue to grow, causing more significant symptoms. This is also due to the invasive nature of some phenotypes and the development of scar tissue. In some individuals, the disease persists at stage 1 or 2, and minimal lesions can sometimes resolve on their own.[3] The concept of having surgery to treat mild disease to prevent the development of advanced endometriosis is not proven. This is due to the different pathways that endometriosis phenotypes develop, which are not even fully understood. Furthermore, recurrence after surgical treatments tends to reappear in the same location.[4] Despite these ambiguities, health committees still agree that early detection and treatment is a priority to prevent further issues arising. The ASRM system is not the only methodology utilised, there is no gold standard for which staging system to use. The ASRM system doesn't represent every factor of the disease, namely symptoms or impact on fertility. More importantly, it doesn't describe deep endometriosis in areas outside of the reproductive system such as the rectovaginal septum, bowel, ureters, and bladder, nor whether adenomyosis is present. Other systems may be used for different purposes: The ENZIAN classification was developed to grade deep endometriosis, while the Endometriosis Fertility Index (EFI) was created to predict the spontaneous pregnancy rate in patients after surgery.

Stage 1 or Minimal (1 to 5 points)	Few small implants Superficial implants on the surface of organs or tissue lining your pelvis Little to no scar tissue
Stage 2 or Mild (6 to 15 points)	More implants than stage 1 Deeper in the tissue May be some scar tissue
Stage 3 or Moderate (16 to 30 points)	Many deep implants and multiple superficial implants Small cysts on one or both ovaries Thick of filmy bands of scar tissue called adhesions
Stage 4 or Severe (30 to 54 points)	Most widespread Numerous deep implants and superficial implants Significant scarring with thick adhesions Large cysts on one or both ovaries

Revised American Society for Reproductive Medicine (rASRM)[1]

10

What Are the Symptoms of Endometriosis

Endometriosis is a highly individualised disease. While a broad spectrum of potential symptoms exists, each person experiences a unique range with varying severity. This comes down to a variety of factors including, but not limited to, the different phenotypes, the various locations lesions grow, the quantity, whether they've invaded healthy tissues, and the presence of adhesions. Some people have no symptoms but may be diagnosed if facing fertility issues, whilst others suffer from severe life-altering symptoms. Remember, the stage of endometriosis doesn't always correspond to the gravity of the symptoms, and scientists are not exactly sure why. Pain, however, *typically* correlates with the site of disease and type of lesion. The long list of possible symptoms can complicate diagnosis. Many are nonspecific, meaning they don't point towards a specific disease. Some symptoms are similar to other conditions, resulting in individuals being misdiagnosed, commonly with IBS. There can also be situations where the predominant symptom a person struggles with misguides diagnosis. For instance, pain might be more severe somewhere outside the pelvis, such as in the legs. Or a person might believe their pelvic pain is 'normal' but visit the doctors for other symptoms, which wouldn't signal endometriosis to a doctor. As the pill can help treat symptoms, some may only start to feel the effects of the disease after coming off the pill. Listed below are symptoms that commonly occur but to different degrees. You may not have realised some of these are symptoms, so it may provide validation and help you to understand your body and why they exist. Hopefully, doctors will soon recognise these as symptoms to help guide earlier diagnoses.

Pain

Have you ever heard that the body cannot remember pain? Pain is ambiguous and inherently subjective, making it hard for people to imagine or comprehend what someone is feeling without feeling it themselves. Even if someone previously experienced a similar pain, they may rely on the memory of how they felt emotionally. Endo Warriors have devised creative ways to articulate their pain, providing a visual for others to understand what they are feeling. Common descriptions include barbed wire or knife-life sensations. Endometriosis pain can manifest in various regions of the body. It may exhibit patterns correlating with the menstrual cycle, such as before or during your period. Alternatively, some pain can be constant or perhaps appear to be sporadic. People might faint or vomit due to pain, or their suffering can become so unbearable that it necessitates a trip to A&E. It's essential to recognise that the broad spectrum of pain types and locations means the following list may not include them all.

Endometriosis can lead to cross-organ sensitisation, meaning irritation of one organ prompts referred pain felt elsewhere. The widespread experience of pain may be attributed to the complex interplay of the nervous system or possible comorbidities. Chronic pain is defined as lasting over twelve weeks, so a lot of endo pain falls in this category. It can stimulate feelings of being overwhelmed or overstimulated, increase your sensitivity, or cause disengagement from activities formally loved. So often, chronic pain can change a person's personality. If you know someone experiencing chronic pain of any kind, be empathetic to the fact they may not be themselves.

Painful Periods

In case you encounter the term 'dysmenorrhea' on your medical notes, this means painful periods. Dysmenorrhea can start before your period and persist till the end; it may be accompanied by pain in other places, such as your back. A variety of mechanisms can cause painful periods. For example, in response to prostaglandin release during menstruation, the uterine muscle contracts to help move blood to the vaginal opening. This process sometimes causes discomfort or pain. However, this can be exacerbated in endometriosis by factors such as *excess* prostaglandin release leading to intense uterine contractions, the presence of adhesions, nerve involvement, or lesions bleeding, causing irritation and inflammation. When contractions are uncoordinated, they can spasm the pelvic floor muscles, causing additional pain. Pelvic pain coinciding with the menstrual cycle means a symptom we commonly see is 'bad or painful periods', despite there being more to the story. It's important to know that period pain severe enough to disrupt your daily activities or unresponsive to painkillers is not normal and should prompt a discussion with your doctor.

Pelvic Pain

Pelvic pain may be constant, intermittent, or intensified in correlation with menstruation. Pain can vary in sensation, ranging from horrible period-like cramps to a dull, heavy, dragging feeling. At other times, it may feel sharp and stabbing. Pain may be widespread throughout the pelvis or feel deeply located in an area like the groin or hip. It may or may not respond to medications like paracetamol. Multiple factors, such as inflammation, scar tissue, large ovarian cysts, nerve involvement, or pelvic floor dysfunction, can cause pelvic pain.

Painful Sex

The medical term for painful intercourse is dyspareunia, which can occur during or after penetrative sex. Pain ranges from mild cramps to severe aches to stabbing sensations. It may occur instantly or after a few hours (or possibly even longer) — sometimes lasting days. There are several reasons for dyspareunia; the type and location of endometriosis, the presence of adhesions, or distortion in pelvic anatomy can all contribute to sexual dysfunction. Sex can move or pull on tissue or adhesions, causing pain to be felt in the vagina, abdomen, or behind the cervix. Pelvic floor spasms can also narrow the vagina, making penetration more difficult. Pain triggers will vary; some find deep penetration or quick thrusting stimulates pain, whilst for others, any penetration will cause discomfort, including putting in a tampon. Vulvodynia can also occur, which is characterised by pain in the vulva (external area of female genitals) upon any form of touch to the area, or it can occur spontaneously without touch. Painful sex can lead to feelings of isolation, emotional distress, and decreased confidence levels, but remember you are not alone, as two-thirds of women with endometriosis experience sexual dysfunction.[1] Considering the prevalence of endo, many others in the world will share similar experiences. Painful sex can cause fear avoidance or reluctance to engage in sexual activity due to the potential discomfort it can cause. In relationships, this can create challenges if sex becomes a topic of stress. However, some may find it brings them closer to their partner as through open and honest communication, they navigate these challenges, allowing them to find ways to maintain intimacy in the relationship that is satisfactory for both partners. After dealing with the trauma of painful sex, some may choose to avoid relationships altogether. This can be a complex issue to deal with as we all want our sex lives to be fun, enjoyable and a way to connect to our partner. If you are struggling with this, you are not the only one. Finding a supportive partner who can help you through your fears is intrinsic to a healthy relationship. Whether painful sex is a new or existing symptom or even something of the past, some treatments and tips can help, which are discussed throughout Part 3.

Back Pain

Back pain can be caused by adhesions, inflammation, endometriomas, pelvic floor dysfunction, or nerve involvement, such as lesions growing near or on a nerve, causing irritation and referred pain. Endometriomas are likely to cause back pain the larger they grow. Chronic pain conditions frequently lead to muscle tension as the body attempts to compensate with changes in posture or movement to alleviate pain. As the muscles in the back are heavily involved in posture and supporting the spine, this type of pain is common. Endo back pain may be gnawing or dull — inconsistent or chronic. For some, it can make sitting down difficult. If you notice you have poor posture when sitting, walking, or carrying out household activities like washing the dishes, this can perpetuate pain. We are all guilty of poor posture, but always try to maintain good posture as much as possible. Shall we all have a posture check?

Leg, Buttocks, and Feet Pain

Pain radiating to the buttocks, down the legs, or into the feet can feel similar to a leg cramp or have a throbbing or stabbing sensation. It may worsen from doing activities or being on your feet all day, affecting your ability to walk or stand. It can be caused by nerve involvement, such as lesions growing near or on the sciatic nerve, which runs from the lower back through the hips and down to your feet, or the obturator nerve in the thigh. Inflammation, adhesion, and poor posture can also stimulate leg pain, or an ovarian cyst. If the latter is the cause, pain may occur on the same side. Pain may also be felt in the anus.

Joint Pain

Joint pain includes the knees, hips, hands, feet, lower back, or spine and can affect one or more joints at a time. It is described as throbbing, aching, sore, and burning. Knee pain can make it hard to stand up without support, whilst others struggle to get out of bed from multiple joints hurting at once. Joint pain might stem from inflammation, heightened pain mechanisms associated with endometriosis, or lesions on the sciatic nerve.

Ovulation Pain

Ovulation pain, called mittelschmerz, is a normal phenomenon affecting 40% of women of reproductive age. It's typically felt in the ovary developing the follicle but is more commonly felt on the right side between days 7 and 24 of the cycle.[2] You may not feel it every month. The pain may feel sharp or like a dull ache and can last from a few minutes to several days. Other associated symptoms include nausea or diarrhoea. Despite some healthy individuals experiencing this, endometriosis might enhance this. This can be attributed to pre-existing compromised and inflamed tissues in the ovary or fallopian tubes, caused by cysts, adhesions, or lesions.

Headaches and Migraines

Those with endometriosis are more likely to suffer headaches or migraines, sometimes associated with nausea, discomfort from bright lights, or aversion to sound. Menstrual migraines (meaning they onset with your period) are seen in 65% of people with endometriosis,[3] although the cause of this increased risk is not clear. Suggestions include genetics, inflammation, or a hormone imbalance.[4] Migraines can also be triggered by a drop in oestrogen levels, which naturally occurs around menstruation, or as a side effect of the inflammatory prostaglandins that are released to help your uterus contract.

Vaginal Bleeding

Unusual bleeding includes heavier, irregular, or prolonged periods, bleeding between periods, and bleeding from sex. Heavy or prolonged periods are called menorrhagia. With endometriosis, periods can go beyond seven days or are heavy enough to necessitate changing tampons or pads every couple of hours. Period blood may be darker, sometimes appearing black, indicating old blood has been trapped in the body. Periods may also have heavy clotting. You might experience spotting in between periods or tinted discharge. Bleeding during or after sex may be caused by pre-existing tenderness or inflammation in the uterine tissue, so penetration irritates this area, causing it to bleed, sometimes lasting several days after sex. Bleeding can occur when you least expect it, so carrying sanitary products and an extra pair of knickers can help alleviate any stress. Abnormal bleeding can aid diagnosis, so recording days that you bleed can help indicate to clinicians there is a problem. Tracking your bleeding also helps to determine any patterns that may not be apparent at first. Bleeding after sex is a common symptom of cervical cancer or STIs, so if you experience this, these conditions must always be ruled out first.

Rectal Bleeding

Although rare, rectal bleeding can occur with bowel endometriosis, specifically if lesions grow through the rectal wall. This may be accompanied with diarrhoea or constipation.

Gastrointestinal Symptoms

90% of people report gastrointestinal symptoms, including painful bowel movements, diarrhoea, constipation, nausea, vomiting, gas, acid reflux, heartburn, dietary intolerance, and bloating.[5] It's believed to result from the close proximity of the reproductive organs to the bowels, with inflammation in the area contributing to these symptoms. Endometriosis or adhesions on the bowel, rectum, rectovaginal septum, or in some rare cases, the stomach, can cause GI symptoms. However, these symptoms are prevalent across all types of endo, so do not necessarily indicate bowel involvement. Additionally, pelvic floor dysfunction can contribute to gastrointestinal issues. These symptoms may be chronic, intermittent, or cyclical, often flaring up during menstruation. You may be diagnosed with IBS before endometriosis, we will delve more into this in Chapter 22.

Bloating

Severe abdominal bloating, often referred to as 'endo belly', is a common complaint, with 83% of women reporting bloating as a symptom.[5] It can be painful or uncomfortable and may flare up after eating or during your period. Many people feel they look pregnant and find clothes don't fit them as well. It may be helpful to wear loose clothing to ensure you feel comfortable and to prevent irritation. There are a handful of reasons for endo belly, ranging from inflammation to having a large cyst. The level of bloating may be cyclical, influenced by your menstrual cycle, and may last a couple of weeks or feel permanent. Abdominal bloating, accompanied by nausea and sexual dysfunction, is thought to be a strong indicator of rectovaginal endometriosis.[6]

Painful Bowel Movements, Diarrhoea, Constipation

Painful bowel movements are often described as shooting, sharp, searing, and intense. It's the type of pain that could make one understand how "Elvis died on the toilet". Yes, the pain can be that awful. Some people experience rectal bleeding with defecation. Constipation and diarrhoea can sometimes occur alongside your menstrual cycle.

Gas, Heartburn, Acid Reflux, GERD

A less recognised symptom is gas or experiencing an uncomfortable feeling after eating that may be relieved by belching or flatulence. Heartburn or acid reflux can also occur, whereby stomach acid flows into the oesophagus or mouth. These can be nasty symptoms to deal with. They may affect appetite or cause sore throats and hoarseness due to the acid. It's not entirely clear what causes this and it's likely multifactorial, but it may be exacerbated by inflammation, hormones, or bloating on the lower end of the GI tract, causing upward pressure. Depending on the cause, surgery for bowel endo may improve these symptoms, as well as hormonal treatments or physiotherapy.

Nausea and Vomiting

Nausea and vomiting can be a side effect of intense pain, sometimes experienced during menstruation when severe menstrual cramps are present. However, for many, nausea is not triggered by pain. Instead, it's a chronic or cyclical symptom that can be invasive, making it hard to function. It's unclear why it occurs, but it can stem from factors like inflammation or lesions growing near or on your bowel.[7] A ruptured or twisted ovarian cyst can also induce intense pain, nausea, or vomiting — this includes endometriomas but also follicular cysts.

Urinary System

Bladder symptoms include frequent urination, pain during or after, bladder urgency, pain when the bladder is full, blood in the urine, flank pain around the kidney, or not being able to make it in time. It may feel like a UTI, but often, this is not caused by an infection. In rare cases, urinary symptoms are caused by lesions on the bladder, ureters, or kidneys. However, this is not guaranteed as these symptoms affect many people without endo in these locations. Chronic bladder pain can be caused by interstitial cystitis, a condition described in more detail in Chapter 22.

Fatigue

Fatigue is seen in the majority of people with endometriosis. One study highlighted it affects 51% of women,[8] whilst another reported 1 in 3 people with chronic fatigue syndrome has endometriosis.[9] Fatigue differs from general feelings of tiredness, which are expected after a day's work or a bad night's sleep. Fatigue is the constant feeling of exhaustion that makes it difficult to fulfil work or social commitments. It may feel like an awful hangover that never goes. You may feel drained or weak, impacting your desire to cook, clean, wash your hair, or brush your teeth. Tiredness is often not relieved by sleep and may worsen with your period. This is a particularly horrible symptom as it's hard to manage, and it can feel like you are constantly battling the need to sleep. There are many reasons why endometriosis causes fatigue. Chronic pain and disrupted sleep from this can impact a person's energy levels. Then, it's possible that the immune response, wherein various inflammatory chemicals are secreted to try and eliminate or deal with the disease, exhausts the body, as it requires more energy to carry out these processes. Other factors to consider are persistent bleeding (including prolonged or very heavy periods) as this can lead to iron deficiency, which commonly causes fatigue. Endometriosis can also cause frequent diarrhoea, leaving the body without enough time to absorb nutrients, as the bowel movement moves too fast within the GI tract. Diarrhoeal symptoms can therefore cause malabsorption of nutrients needed for vitality and energy. Chronic or frequent diarrhoea can also lead to dehydration which is capable of provoking fatigue.

Anxiety and Depression

Those with endometriosis have been shown to suffer from increased rates of anxiety and depression. One study noted that 29% of patients with endometriosis had moderate to severe anxiety, and 15% experienced depression.[10] Whilst an analysis of 4,619 women with endo found 68% of them had psychological stress such as anxiety or depression.[11] Anxiety can be felt in many ways, such as feeling overly or inappropriately nervous, fearing the worst, or having a sense of dread. Depression can feel like all-consuming sadness or hopelessness. Both can have a significant impact on a person's life. Endometriosis' ability to affect mood can result from obvious factors such as chronic pain, concerns over health or fertility, impact on relationships and sex life, struggles with work, or feelings of being unsupported by those around them. These factors would naturally impact a person's mood, potentially causing depression or anxiety. However, there is more to this story, with many factors at play. The relationship between endometriosis and its psychological effect is discussed in Chapter 22.

Allergies, Intolerances or Sensitivities

Allergic or non-allergic food intolerances or sensitivities are caused by immune dysregulation. They cause many symptoms, including rashes, flushing, diarrhoea, bloating, gas, and stomach pain. Those with endometriosis are thought to be at a higher risk of developing these conditions which will be discussed in greater detail in Chapter 22.

Fertility

Fertility is often discussed, so it's important to clarify that an endometriosis diagnosis does not equal infertility, although the relationship between the two is not fully established. Causes for the connection include possible damage to the ovaries or fallopian tubes, inflammation, an altered immune system, hormonal changes, impaired egg implantation, or altered egg quality. Some stats say 30-50% of women who have endometriosis are infertile, or infertile women have endometriosis in 25-50% of cases.[12] However, these figures are from 1938! Fertility treatments and early diagnosis of endometriosis have come a long way since then. More research must be carried out in this area for more robust statistics. It's important to remember that the majority of people with endometriosis who are trying for a baby will conceive naturally and spontaneously — if they wish. More information on fertility in Chapter 23.

11

What Is a Flare-Up?

Endometriosis is experienced differently, so whether you have had medical treatment or not, you may become accustomed to specific symptoms occurring chronically or cyclically. A flare-up (as seen with other chronic diseases) means symptoms change or intensify, or new, less common symptoms arise. They can be unpredictable, come on suddenly, and last for varying amounts of time — but will eventually subside. Endo flares typically involve pain, including a change in the pain level, type, or location. For example, someone who often experiences chronic dull pain in their groin may feel sharp stabbing pain or pain down their legs during a flare. It's different for every person, and each flare may differ from the next. Pain may be felt in areas of the body that are not normal for the individual. Symptoms other than pain might include fatigue, nausea, depression, bowel changes, belching, painful sex, brain fog, fever, and everyone's favourite... endo-belly. Flare-ups can be debilitating, so go easy on yourself and let yourself rest.

The cause of a flare-up varies and will occur more or less frequently for different people. As endometriosis is an inflammatory disease, symptoms may worsen when the body becomes inflamed, making inflammatory triggers a likely culprit, but this isn't yet proven. Some inflammation is un-avoidable, such as from hormonal fluctuations during the menstrual cycle or physical activity. Lifestyle factors also contribute to inflammation and are capable of triggering a flare, such as high stress, lack of sleep, excessive alcohol or caffeine, or consumption of inflammatory foods. While some factors may be beyond our control, others can be managed. It's beneficial to monitor potential triggers to identify if they are problematic for you so that you can attempt to reduce or avoid these in your life. Reducing exposure to inflammatory stimuli whilst incorporating inflammation-reducing strategies can be a great way to lessen the frequency or severity of flares. There are many ways to be proactive in doing this, as discussed in Part 3.

My flares almost feel like the flu — my whole body aches, including my knees and knuckles. I get exhausted, my body feels heavy, and I get a low-grade fever. My way to cope is to get into bed, lie down, and rest. My family hates the words I use to describe the pain, so I apologise in advance. To me, it feels like I am rotting. It's the only way I can describe the bone-deep, hot, almost numbing pain. Numbing pain is an oxymoron, so that might not make sense, but that's how it feels. I also have flares where I simply get endo-belly and sore knees. One time, I even had a flare because I wore jeans that were too tight around my stomach to work, and it left me crawling into bed as soon as I got home, bawling in pain. I have realised that during times of high stress, my period may be more painful that month or sporadic pelvic pain may increase.

12

Bowel Endometriosis

Bowel Endometriosis affects between 3.8% to 37% of women. Tissue can be found in all areas of the bowel, including the appendix, but it's less common on the small bowel.[1] Bowel endo involves superficial lesions on the surface or deep lesions penetrating through the bowel wall. As lesions vary in location, size, and depth of infiltration of the bowel wall, the symptoms experienced and the extent to which they impact quality of life will differ. There can be changes to the anatomy and physiology of the bowels due to the lesions, but also from inflammation or adhesions. Although many people with endo complain of gastrointestinal symptoms, only a smaller amount of those will have bowel endo. The commonness of these symptoms is possibly due to the inflammatory nature of the disease in the dense, enclosed location of the pelvis. Symptoms of bowel endometriosis often resemble IBS, including diarrhoea, constipation, bloating, painful defecation, mucus in stools, and deep pelvic pain during sex; however, some people have no symptoms. Larger or invasive nodules usually cause a wider array and increased severity of symptoms, like bleeding from your anus during your period.[1] You may also experience nausea, gas, and heartburn. All symptoms can flare up during your period or in line with your menstrual cycle. Surgery is usually required to diagnose bowel endo. Although, doctors can investigate its likelihood through various tests, including a pelvic exam, transvaginal ultrasound, MRI and

CT scans, or colonoscopies. Medical imaging is better at detecting this type of endometriosis than other types, so you may receive a diagnosis through imaging depending on your practitioner's experience and whether the effects are visible. However, as nearly 80% of endometriosis cases present with superficial disease, most patients will not have their endo detected with any form of preoperative diagnostic test. Due to the difficulty in gauging the presence of endo without surgery, individuals who have sought medical attention for their symptoms often have normal test results, leaving their doctor to diagnose them with IBS as they cannot find anything wrong with them.

Surgery is a treatment option for bowel endo, but due to the risks like damaging the bowel, some people choose to explore alternative treatments, including hormonal therapies like the Mirena® coil, to determine if they can alleviate symptoms and enhance quality of life without surgery. It's unclear whether hormonal therapies can prevent the progression of endometriosis, so patients should be monitored periodically by their hospital with repeated imaging techniques to determine the status of the tissue and whether it is growing or remitting. Doctors will aim to prevent extensive fibrosis or thickening of the bowel lumen* as this makes the bowels smaller on the inside, so will likely cause greater issues and symptoms. Complications can include blockages, which occur if changes prevent the bowels from being emptied sufficiently. For many, surgery will help improve pain, gastrointestinal symptoms, and fertility. However, this should only be carried out by highly skilled surgeons with experience treating bowel endo. If you are based in Britain, see Part 2 for more information on accredited Endometriosis Centres. Surgery techniques may range from shaving lesions off to a large-scale bowel resection. Depending on a case-by-case basis, the risks of surgery will vary, and your doctor will go through these with you at your appointment. Treatment options are outlined further in Part 3.

*Lumen – is the space inside the bowel tube, think of it as the hole inside a water slide.

13

Rectovaginal Endometriosis

Rectovaginal endometriosis is one of the most severe and painful forms of the disease, occurring when lesions grow in the tissues between the vagina and the rectum called the rectovaginal septum. Occurrence in this location is less prevalent than the ovaries, uterus, or abdominal wall. The statistics are not completely understood due to a lack of reliable data, but it's estimated to affect between 4 to 37% of patients.[1] Rectovaginal endometriosis involves Deep Infiltrating Endometriosis (DIE) lesions, which are particularly aggressive and invade the surrounding tissues. These lesions are thought to respond to hormonal changes that occur during the menstrual cycle, potentially causing inflammation and pain, and with time, scar tissue (fibrosis) can form. Nearby organs like the vagina can suffer damage, and the Pouch of Douglas (POD) may become obliterated, which means the space is sealed with endometriosis and fibrosis, which alters its primary functions of allowing pelvic organs to move smoothly.[2]

If you've heard of the terms 'pouch of Douglas', 'recto-uterine pouch' or 'cul-de-sac' from doctors or in medical notes, you may be wondering, *like I was*, what this is. Whichever name is used, it means the same thing and describes the small area behind the uterus. I have included a diagram as it's easier to understand with a visual guide. In the pouch of Douglas, there is a thin bag-shaped membrane lining the area. The invasive DIE lesions penetrate this membrane, growing down into the rectovaginal septum. This can be understood as the septum we have in our nose, separating our nostrils; however, in this instance, the tissue separates our rectum and our vagina. Having endometriosis in this area is likely to cause painful sex, particularly severe stabbing pain from deep penetration, as it pulls or irritates the nearby lesions and scar tissue. For the same reason, it can cause excruciating pain when going to the toilet, particularly during your period when there is increased inflammation. As the stool exits the bowel, it can cause intense contractions. If deep endometriosis infiltrates the bowel or rectum, it can cause a thickening of the lumen and blockages, as well as localised inflammation, often leading to pain and other gastrointestinal issues. Due to the invasive nature of DIE lesions, the resulting inflammation, adhesions, and scarring can cause anatomic distortion of the organs in the pelvis and restricted organ mobility (an obliterated POD). For example, it may displace the rectum from its original location. These kinds of lesions are strongly associated with severe pelvic pain.[3] Symptoms associated with rectovaginal involvement may intensify during menstruation and can include the following:

- Difficult or painful bowel movements (*often described as sharp, searing pain due to scar tissue in the area*)
- Abdominal bloating (*sometimes due to difficulty in passing stools, causing a build-up of faeces and gas in the bowel, or from fluid retention*)
- Constipation or diarrhoea
- Painful or heavy periods
- Pain during sex
- Rectal bleeding
- Nausea

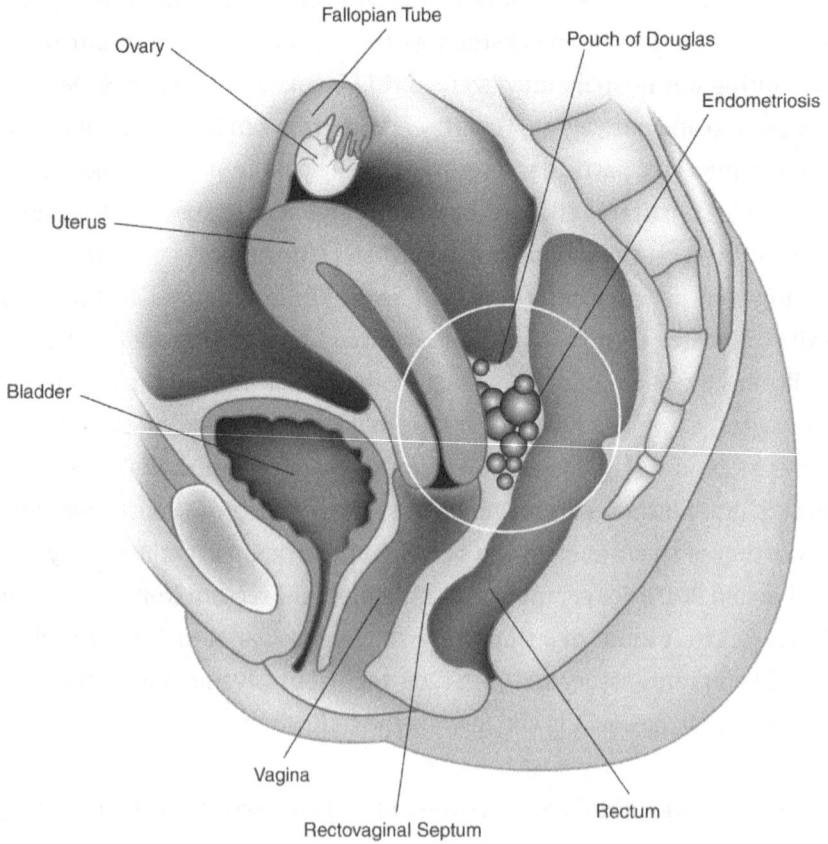

As these symptoms are frequently seen in other conditions, you may have been sent for tests to determine the likelihood of other diseases before receiving your diagnosis, or perhaps you received a misdiagnosis. Conditions with a symptom overlap include IBS, IBD, or a rectal tumour. Surgery is often beneficial in treating rectovaginal endometriosis as it can restore the functionality of the organs and correct the location of any that are displaced, whilst also removing lesions or scar tissue. This can reduce inflammation and ensure organs function the way they are meant to. Reassuringly, surgery has been shown to improve symptoms in up to 70% of patients, including sexual function, pain reduction, and improvements in fertility rates.[4] Speaking from experience, my surgery to treat rectovaginal endometriosis was life-changing. Due to the complex and invasive nature of this type of endo, it requires a highly skilled surgeon and a multidisciplinary team. There are increased risks with this surgery, and potential complications include damage to organs, a temporary stoma, or damage to the ureters (which will require temporary stents to allow healing). Although risks should be considered when deciding to have any surgery, these are typically small, with just a 6.8% risk of experiencing *any* complication.[5] Always speak to your surgeon to understand the risks involved and their likelihood before choosing surgery. It's critical your surgeon is experienced in treating this type of endo. If you live in Britain, seek treatment at an Endometriosis Centre.

No staging system sufficiently covers all aspects of the disease, and the rASRM staging system discussed earlier doesn't encompass the complexity of DIE lesions such as rectovaginal endometriosis. Therefore, other classification systems, such as ENZIAN, may be used to describe the location and depth of this type. Rectovaginal endometriosis is stage 4 according to Kirtners classification system.[4] Specialised surgical treatment is discussed in Part 3.

14

Extragenital Endometriosis

When lesions are located outside the reproductive organs, it's called extragenital endometriosis. The most common extragenital area is the bowel.[1] Lesions have also been found in the brain, lung, diaphragm, kidney, spleen, gallbladder, nose, breasts, and nervous system — although some of these are extremely rare.[2] Each location manifests differently, so can produce a wide range of possible symptoms. A person may have specific symptoms for extragenital endometriosis, as well as classic endometriosis symptoms if tissue is present on the reproductive organs. Diagnosing uncommon types is challenging; however, heightened awareness contributes to advancements in medical imaging training, facilitating the detection of these unusual forms. It also enables healthcare professionals to better comprehend and identify the symptoms associated with these types in affected patients.

Urinary Tract Endometriosis

Urinary tract endometriosis is uncommon affecting 1% of cases, although rates are higher in those with DIE lesions. It's the second most common location of extragenital endometriosis.[3] The most prevalent part of the urinary tract affected is the bladder, which can be asymptomatic or instead provoke painful urination, an urgent or frequent need to urinate, blood-stained urine, and pain in the pelvis or on one side of the back. Lesions may be superficial, residing on the surface of an organ, or a deep lesion may grow into the lining of the bladder or invade the ureters. Ureters are different to the urethra; they are tubes allowing urine to drain from the kidney to the bladder. Endometriosis on the ureters can cause blockages affecting the urine flow, which will impact the kidneys as urine cannot sufficiently flow out and away from them.

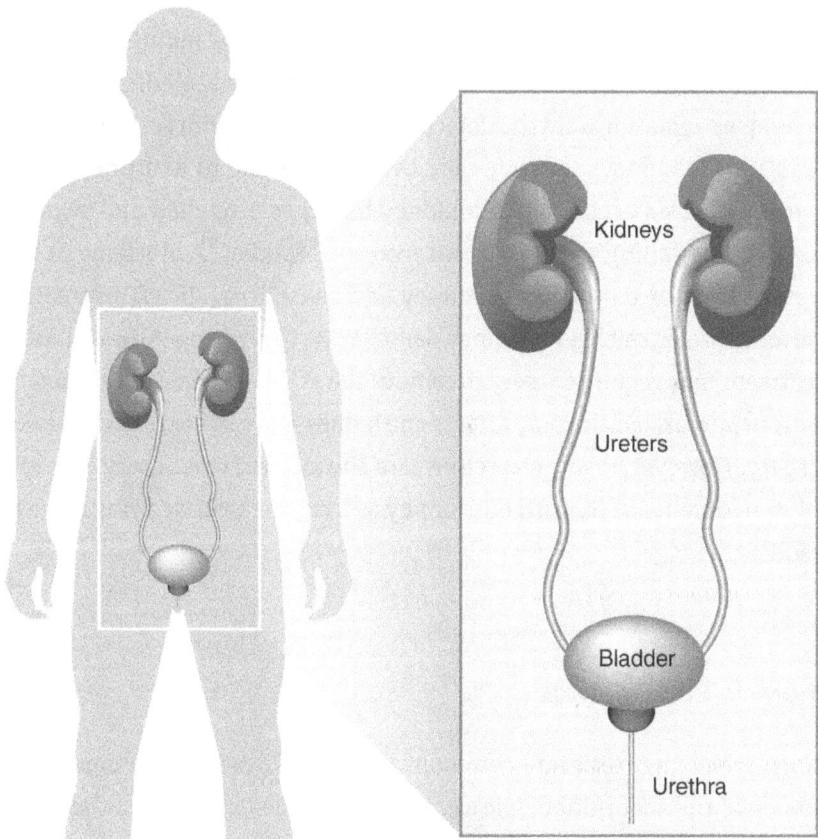

Kidneys

Ureters

Bladder

Urethra

Renal Endometriosis

Renal endometriosis affecting the kidneys is extremely rare and only occasionally reported. Of the 1% of people affected with urinary tract endometriosis, less than 1% of that group has endo affecting the kidney and urethra.[4] It can affect one or both kidneys. Symptoms usually materialise as flank pain, high blood pressure, and blood in urine. If a blockage prevents proper urine expulsion from the body, it can lead to fevers or recurrent Urinary Tract Infections (UTI). In some cases, renal endometriosis can be asymptomatic, meaning no symptoms are present to indicate an issue. In unfortunate instances where renal endometriosis goes undetected, it can lead to loss of kidney function or renal failure over time.[5] Both of which are serious life-threatening conditions. Medical imaging techniques sometimes aid the detection of renal endo with scans revealing a cyst in the kidneys, or they may be enlarged due to hydronephrosis. Hydronephrosis occurs when a kidney becomes stretched and swollen due to urine failing to drain down into the bladder. A blockage in the urinary tract or a cyst in the kidney can cause this. If left untreated, hydronephrosis can lead to kidney damage due to scarring. Although rare, treatment may require surgery to remove the affected kidney. Fortunately, hydronephrosis usually only affects one kidney and can be treated without surgery. However, if surgical removal of the kidney is necessary, you can still function healthily with one kidney as long as the underlying issue is resolved.

Thoracic Endometriosis

Thoracic endometriosis is uncommon, although it's the most common type outside of the abdominopelvic cavity, whereby lesions grow in the chest cavity, such as on or near the diagram or lungs.[6] Thoracic endometriosis can cause bleeding into the pleural cavity, the space in the chest that holds the lungs. Symptoms to look out for include shortness of breath, chest pain, shoulder pain, and coughing up blood, or it can be asymptomatic (with no symptoms).[7] Endometriosis in this location, like all others, can occur by itself, but it's typically found in individuals with pelvic endo. Statistically, classic endometriosis symptoms are felt 5-7 years prior to developing thoracic endo symptoms, meaning the average age of diagnosis is higher, but it's not clear yet if this is due to a lack of understanding of its prevalence or standard diagnostic treatments.[6] A thoracoscopy may be used for diagnosis whereby a thin camera is inserted through the chest to inspect the area. Thoracic endometriosis can be life-threatening as it's capable of causing a spontaneous collapsed lung around the time of your period. If you watch Grey's Anatomy, you may recognise the medical term for a collapsed lung, a pneumothorax, as it often comes up on the show. Treatment can include medication, surgery, or frequently both.

Cerebral Endometriosis

Cerebral Endometriosis is extremely rare, only being reported a handful of times in medical history. Symptoms include seizures and headaches, which may or may not align with the menstrual cycle.

* * *

It's essential not to worry about endometriosis spreading to areas such as the brain or kidney, as they are extremely rare. It's reassuring to consider that 1 in 10 females have endometriosis, making it a widespread disease, yet only a handful of cases are seen in rare locations, validating it's not a likely outcome for most people. Nonetheless, it's helpful to know and understand the symptoms so that you are better informed about how the disease can manifest and how it affects others in the community. Even though it is not something you should be worried about, if you are ever in doubt or have concerns, please seek medical advice.

15

Tilted Uterus

The uterus can be found in a few different arrangements. The typical arrangement is for it to be anteverted, so the top of the uterus to tilt towards the stomach, as seen in the diagram on the next page. However, it can be retroverted (also called a tilted or tipped uterus), so the uterus tilts backwards towards the rectum rather than forward towards the stomach. This is a normal genetic variation seen in 1 in 5 females.[1] Many people don't even know they have a tilted uterus, as in most cases, it doesn't cause any symptoms or issues. For others, there may be discomfort during penetrative sex (particularly deep thrusting), difficulty inserting tampons, or gastrointestinal symptoms, such as painful bowel movements. A retroflexed or anteflexed uterus describes a uterus that points towards the rectum or stomach respectively, but the top part of the uterus, called the fundus, is bent. This can cause issues depending on the location; if it's bent inwards towards the rectum, it can cause pain whilst defecating, whereas if it folds into the bladder, it can provoke frequent urination.

Anteverted	Retroverted	Retroverted Retroflexed	Anteverted Retroflexed
(Normal)	*(Normal)*	*(Normal)*	*(Normal or Abnormal)*

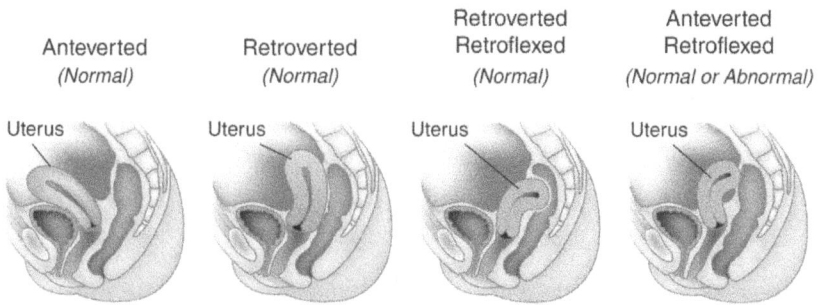

These are normal anatomical variations and are nothing to worry about. The cause for a tilted uterus to occur later in life can include pregnancy, caesarean labour, fibroids, adhesions, menopause, as well as endometriosis. A tilted pelvis resulting from endo is likely due to adhesions joining the uterus to another location in the pelvis then distorting the anatomy, or from inflammation. As adhesions are often seen in this disease, an anteverted uterus can be pulled back towards the rectum, resulting in an anteverted retroflexed uterus. This abnormality can be seen on ultrasound or MRI and can help highlight to clinicians the presence of endometriosis when used in combination with symptoms. Statistically, a retroverted uterus is more common in individuals with endometriosis.[2] However, this can also be mistaken for what is actually an anteverted retroflexed uterus. Though this is nothing to worry about, being told you have a uterus in a different location can be alarming, causing you unnecessary worry. The terms aren't intuitively understood, so it's good to know what the doctors are saying. If you are worried about a tilted uterus affecting fertility, you will be happy to hear, generally, the position of your uterus has no impact on fertility, whether spontaneous pregnancy or using IVF.[3] Nor should it impair your ability to grow a baby to full term and deliver it naturally as your uterus changes position throughout pregnancy anyway.

16

Frozen Pelvis

The term 'frozen pelvis' is an awful name that provokes a semi-accurate description and image of the condition. It's sometimes called end-stage endometriosis. It's the most extensive presentation of the disease and may develop in people with stage 4 endometriosis who have formed a substantial amount of dense adhesions. This is due to DIE, the most invasive phenotype, growing into organs, causing extensive inflammation and scar tissue. It's important to know it's not common, nor is it an eventual step everyone will get to, even if you have severe endometriosis. Remember, each person's experience is different, so don't worry about your disease progressing and causing yourself excessive stress. Understanding what to look out for can help you access timely treatment, but this information should not overburden you.

Adhesions 'glue' organs in the pelvis together or to the lining of the abdomen; they can also wrap around organs. In earlier stages of endometriosis, adhesions may be described as filmy, meaning they are thin, slightly stretchy or broken easily. However, in later stages and frozen pelvis, adhesions are thick and fibrous, meaning they tightly connect tissues and are more difficult to remove.[1] Although adhesions are seen at all stages, in frozen pelvis, there are so many thick adhesions that they create a web-like structure, distorting the anatomy whilst decreasing mobility and function. The lesions may extend deep into tissues, affecting the nerves, ligaments, lymph nodes, and muscles. As the lesions grow deeper, they cause soft tissue to thicken and harden due to scarring (fibrosis). This can cause hardened organs to fix to pelvic bones, making a person immobile.[2]

Symptoms

As you can imagine, there can be life-altering side effects from a frozen pelvis, although some people may only be diagnosed due to troubles with pregnancy. Despite this being the most aggressive form of the disease and fertility issues may be experienced, it's still possible to get pregnant. However, surgery and IVF may be required to achieve this.[3]

Symptoms will vary but can include:

Pain in Pelvis
May be extreme and chronic.
Can stem from inflammation or adhesions preventing organs from moving correctly, creating painful organ dysfunction.
Adhesions may pull on nerves, triggering pain.
As adhesions have a blood and nerve supply, they can cause pain, particularly when stimulated, such as being pulled on.[4]

Severe and Significant Change in Bowel Habits
Constipation, diarrhoea, painful bowel movements, or bloating.
Caused by inflammation, or adhesions obstructing bowels.

Frequent Urination
Can persist day and night, affecting sleep.
May stem from obstructed ureters or reduced bladder capacity.

Flank Pain
Pain around the abdomen and back.
Typically, only on one side as caused by an obstructed ureter.[2]

Severe Leg Pain Around Menstruation

Radiating pain due to involvement or sensitisation of the sciatic nerve, *which runs down your leg*, or the pudendal nerve, *the main nerve in the pelvis.*[2]

Difficulty Crossing Your Legs or Sitting Down

Extensive adhesions deep in the pelvis or around the tailbone can make it harder to move.[2]

What Is the Cause of Frozen Pelvis?

Frozen pelvis is primarily caused by extensive adhesions, resulting from lesions progressively shedding, stimulating inflammation and the subsequent gradual formation of scar tissue in the pelvis. Additionally, a leaking or ruptured endometrioma may cause the accumulation of debris, instigating scar tissue that glues pelvic organs in place. Frozen pelvis can be initiated by other conditions:

Infections that cause adhesions, such as PID
Past pelvic or abdominal surgeries
Benign (noncancerous) or malignant (cancerous) growths
Radiation therapy to the pelvic area

How Is Frozen Pelvis Diagnosed?

Frozen pelvis can be diagnosed without surgery through a pelvic examination. A clinician uses their hands to assess the pelvis and abdomen during this examination. If they detect a firmly fixed uterus, it can suggest the possibility of a frozen pelvis, though a fixed uterus alone doesn't always connote this condition. Additional diagnostic tools include a transvaginal ultrasound and a rectovaginal exam to determine the spread of abnormal tissue. Pelvic examinations may be painful due to the pulling of adhesions or pelvic organs losing their flexibility. To obtain a clearer understanding of the extent of the disease, an MRI with contrast may be performed to detect the amount of tissue affected and assess the involvement of other organs such as kidneys, ureter, and bladder.

How Is It Treated?

Treatment for a frozen pelvis requires surgery, usually advanced laparoscopy. Due to the complex anatomy, distortion, and likely involvement of multiple organs, a highly specialist team is often necessary to perform this operation. However, caution is still advised, as surgery can cause more adhesions.

17

Adenomyosis

Many people have both endometriosis and adenomyosis, although you can have one without the other.[1] Adenomyosis, pronounced **add-en-ow-my-ow-sis** is a benign disorder similar to endometriosis; however, in this condition, endometrial tissue grows strictly within the muscle of the womb called the myometrium. It's like endometriosis in that it responds to cyclical hormonal changes and is oestrogen-dependent, requiring the hormone to grow.[2] As tissue continues to shed and expand, it can cause the uterus to enlarge, growing bigger, sometimes two to three times its original size. It may be confused on scans by medical professionals as fibroids, particularly if they have not had much experience with adenomyosis. This disease may affect up to 20% of the female population[3] (although statistics are hard to quantify). It's typically seen at the later end of reproductive years, around 40-50 years of age, although it has been found as young as 16.[4] The cause or reason for developing adenomyosis is unknown. Risk factors often mentioned include increased oestrogen exposure and prior uterine surgery.[5] High oestrogen exposure includes starting periods at an earlier age and having shorter menstrual cycles. The evidence supporting whether prior uterine surgery (such as a caesarean section or surgery to treat fibroids) increases your risk is inconsistent. The idea is based on the notion that endometrial cells may be moved during surgery, allowing the direct invasion of the cells into the myometrium. Whilst some studies suggest a positive risk of this occurring, other papers do not.[6] Uterine inflammation related to childbirth is also suggested as a promoting factor.[7]

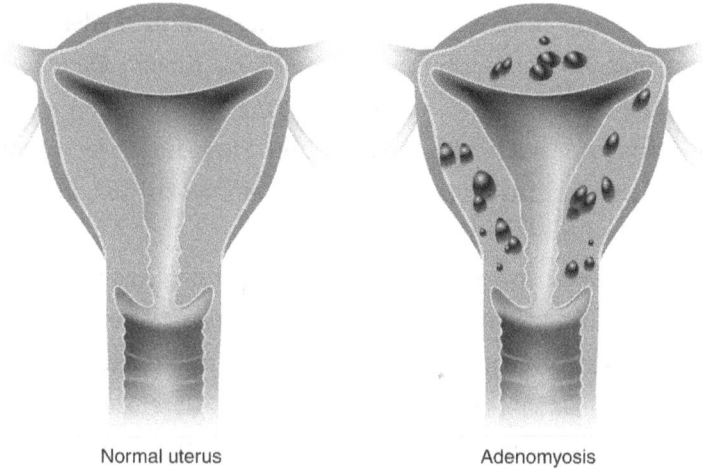

Normal uterus   Adenomyosis

Around 1 in 3 women with adenomyosis are asymptomatic.[8] Individuals that do experience symptoms often find they cease after menopause, likely because the diseased tissue uses circulating oestrogen in the body to grow, so when oestrogen levels drop during menopause, there is a reduction in the growth of adenomyosis. The symptoms are similar to endometriosis and include:

- Very heavy menstrual bleeding and clotting (menorrhagia)
- Severe cramps during periods (dysmenorrhea)
- Enlarged uterus
- Painful sex (dyspareunia)
- Chronic pelvic pain
- Abdominal bloating, or a sensation of heaviness
- Anaemia or low iron stores

Like endometriosis, adenomyosis is hard to diagnose, but we are seeing significant improvements. Along with symptoms, a doctor may carry out a physical examination to ascertain if there is a tender, bulky uterus. If adenomyosis is suspected, patients will be offered a transvaginal ultrasound as it can be diagnosed this way. However, considerable training is required to recognise the ultrasound pattern of adenomyosis.[9] Therefore, diagnosis may occur through an MRI, although adenomyosis is not always detectable by MRI, so receiving a negative result on scans does not definitively rule out having the condition. There have been significant advances in using ultrasound to diagnose adenomyosis, so hopefully this will become the norm in the future.

A definitive diagnosis requires a biopsy and histological analysis, where a tissue sample is taken and examined in a laboratory to confirm the type. Due to the risks involved in surgery, a biopsy will only be taken if you have a hysterectomy — *the surgical removal of the uterus.* Therefore, adenomyosis is usually diagnosed through medical imaging in cases where it's visible, whilst possibly ruling out other conditions with similar symptoms. A hysterectomy can cure adenomyosis because it removes all the tissue, and lesions cannot grow in the uterus if there is no uterus. This is a life-changing operation, so for many, it will not be a desired treatment choice. Furthermore, as many individuals have both adenomyosis and endometriosis, it may not treat the endo symptoms. Other treatments available include hormone therapy and anti-inflammatory medication to help relieve the pain and control heavy bleeding. There are different types of hysterectomy procedures, outlined in Part 3, explaining the different effects on the body and potential benefits to help you make an informed decision.

18

Biochemistry of Endometriosis

The biochemistry of endometriosis encompasses the physiological changes that occur within the body that may contribute to, indicate, or result from the disease. Biochemical alterations can often be detected through blood and urine tests. Understanding biochemistry helps scientific researchers understand diseases or create drugs. For doctors, it can guide potential biomarkers to help support the diagnostic process or provide insight into associated health issues. It's crucial to differentiate between biomarkers that merely complement the diagnostic process from those that directly confirm the presence of endometriosis. Biomarkers and biochemical tests <u>cannot</u> yet diagnose this disease, nor are they suggestive that a person has endometriosis when used in isolation. Scientists are trying to find out if there are any, or if a combination of biomarkers can be used to non-invasively detect endo. However, due to the complex inflammatory processes, different stages and phenotypes, *among many other variable factors*, this poses a difficult challenge. Currently, no established biomarkers are incorporated into diagnostic protocols, and routine biochemical testing is not standard practice for endometriosis. Diagnosis typically necessitates surgical intervention if imaging tests are negative and the patient feels it is essential for them to try.

Hormones and Endometriosis

Endometriosis is oestrogen-dependent, meaning lesions utilise oestrogen to implant and grow. This hormone stimulates the growth and thickening of the endometriosis, leading to inflammation and the formation of lesions. To survive and grow, lesions require oxygen and nutrients, which are provided through the formation of new blood capillaries via a process called angiogenesis, which sprout out from existing blood vessels in nearby areas.[1] Oestrogen has a role in controlling and regulating angiogenesis occurring in the body.[2] Endometriosis lesions can also produce oestrogen themselves through an enzyme called aromatase.[3] This creates a positive feedback loop with inflammation: inflammation in the lesions stimulates oestrogen production, and higher oestrogen levels cause greater inflammation.[4] This vicious cycle perpetuates the disease. Furthermore, endometriosis tissue has more than 100 times more oestrogen receptors than normal endometrial tissue, causing greater sensitivity to oestrogen present in the body.[5] This abnormality is often accompanied by a deficiency in progesterone receptors in the tissue. This imbalance can lead to progesterone resistance, meaning the tissues are less responsive to progesterone, impairing the ability of the hormone to perform its functions effectively. Progesterone has anti-inflammatory properties and opposes many of the effects of oestrogen, so it could inhibit endometriosis growth and the formation of blood vessels and nerves if it were able to carry out its duties.[6] Instead, its impaired function causes symptoms like inflammation and pain to persist, allowing the inflammatory process of the disease to continue.[7] Several theories attempt to explain the cause of progesterone resistance, including being born with it, inflammation, oxidative stress, or epigenetics.[7] As the source has yet to be agreed upon in the science community, it needs to be clarified if progesterone resistance is a cause or consequence of endometriosis.

Although hormones are not tested to confirm the presence of endometriosis, they may be measured to determine disease risk. Elevated oestrogen levels may indicate presence of the disease if used in combination with an individual's symptoms, as it highlights an imbalance in female hormones. Low progesterone levels may suggest an underlying issue with the reproductive system. However, hormone testing is not generally used in diagnosis because not every person with endo will exhibit altered hormone levels. Furthermore, hormone levels fluctuate through your menstrual cycle, making them unreliable as standalone indicators of the disease.

CA125

CA125 is a cancer marker used to help determine if a person has ovarian cancer. However, many conditions cause an increase in CA125 in the blood, including endometriosis. Therefore, testing positive for CA125 does not mean you have cancer. CA125 is a protein that grows on cells and can increase when there is inflammation in the body, which is why it's often seen in endometriosis.[8] Levels of CA125 typically increase with the severity of the disease and can be indicative of the type of endo, lesion size, and adhesion score.[9] Nonetheless, CA125 levels can vary naturally due to factors such as age, race, lifestyle habits, or rise and fluctuate during your menstrual cycle,[8] or pregnancy.[10] Although CA125 is reportedly the top-ranking blood biomarker we have, due to the lack of consistency and inability to diagnose or rule out endo, it's not a good marker nor routinely tested for diagnosis.[11]

Iron Deficiency

Iron is an essential micronutrient needed to maintain many normal bodily functions. When referring to micronutrients, the word 'essential' means the body cannot make them. As such, the body is unable to produce iron, necessitating intake through the diet by eating foods containing it, like meat or spinach. The term 'micronutrient' means that although the nutrient is required, we need a much smaller controlled amount in the body, *a micro amount*. It's not a case of thinking '*the more the merrier*' when it comes to iron. Iron has many roles in maintaining our health. It assists haemoglobin production, which comprises the majority of our red blood cells. Haemoglobin transports oxygen from the lungs to various parts of the body whilst removing carbon dioxide. Another crucial role of iron is its involvement in regulating energy production. It's used for oxidative phosphorylation, breaking down carbohydrates and fat, then turning them into ATP (adenosine triphosphate) — some of you might remember that term from school. ATP describes the body's preferred energy source, which is needed to move and function. Iron deficiency hinders haemoglobin formation, which reduces oxygen supply to organs and muscles. This impairs oxidative phosphorylation and ATP production, ultimately causing exhaustion. Moreover, iron deficiency compromises the immune system, hindering its ability to mount a proper response, which can undermine our overall health.

Now we've clarified the importance of iron for the body, let's break down iron deficiency and how it occurs. After iron has carried out its functions, any surplus is stored for when it's needed in the future. However, iron is lost when we bleed, whether through injury, cutting ourselves, or through menstruation. If we lose more iron than is consumed in our diet, the nutrient levels are depleted. Iron is primarily found in the blood but is stored as ferritin and hemosiderin in the bone marrow, spleen, and liver. The body taps into these stores to produce red cells for our blood, so if iron stores drop significantly enough, it results in an iron deficiency, which is detected through blood tests indicating low ferritin levels. In the early stages of deficiency, our stores should still meet the demands of red cell production; however, if iron levels are not replenished, this capability will start to suffer, gradually diminishing. When the stores are exhausted, and the body cannot generate any more haemoglobin, red cell production is drastically reduced, leading to anaemia developing. Anaemia indicates the blood has an inadequate amount of red blood cells, haemoglobin, or both. This is the most common nutritional deficiency globally, affecting two billion people.[12]

Iron levels are complex as the amount consumed and the amount the body absorbs can differ. This might sound strange, but it comes down to a variety of reasons, including your diet as a whole. Also, the amount of iron you need varies throughout life, such as when you are growing, pregnant, or breastfeeding. Females have higher requirements than males due to losses in menstrual bleeding. If you suffer from heavy or prolonged periods, you could be at increased risk of iron deficiency. Across the board, iron deficiency is a larger issue for females than males due to needing a higher intake. The National Diet and Nutritional Survey in the UK reported a substantial number of females aged 11–49 years have a dietary intake less than the recommended amount,[13] and 12–25% of these women have iron deficiency, whilst 5% have iron deficiency anaemia.[14] This ultimately means having a lack of energy, which leads to poor cognitive function, capable of causing issues with work and school performance, particularly if it involves physical labour.

A common symptom of endometriosis is heavy or prolonged bleeding, putting individuals at higher risk of iron deficiency and anaemia. A study on 200 patients monitored over ten years showed that haemoglobin and haematocrit were significantly lower in stage 3 and 4 endometriosis, compared to stage 1 and 2.[15] This might be due to greater blood loss, dysfunctional iron metabolism, or inflammation. This study suggests that deficiency can correlate with the stage of the disease. However, the issue with studies on this topic is that iron deficiency is prevalent, so trying to determine patterns with the disease is problematic as other factors, such as poor dietary intake, could actually be the cause. Also, the results might vary depending on the day of the menstrual cycle, so it's hard to figure out the degree to which iron deficiency and endometriosis are related. A symptom of anaemia is fatigue, which is commonly seen in endometriosis, particularly around the time of menstruation. If you also experience dizziness, lightheadedness, shortness of breath, or fainting, this could be a sign of anaemia. Your doctor can detect this with a simple blood test. Other symptoms may include headaches, depression, increased infections, and decreased mental function. The most common cause of anaemia is nutritional iron deficiency.

Due to the high frequency of this condition, even if you don't have an iron deficiency or anaemia, it's crucial to consider iron sources in your diet. Ensuring your body receives adequate iron will maintain blood levels, thus supporting energy production and optimal immune system function. Fatigue from inflammation and pain can already be exhausting, so taking proactive steps can avoid an additional layer to the problem. Moreover, we already recognise that the immune system is dysfunctional in conditions like endometriosis, so preventing further issues is essential. Being mindful of iron intake benefits overall health maintenance, providing a holistic approach to wellbeing. Many females have insufficient iron levels, so please consult a doctor if you need advice on whether you need to increase your iron sources or take a supplement. It's important to stress that you should not start dousing your body with iron supplements. Please stick to the recommended amount on the packaging because excessive iron in the body is toxic. Iron overload is suggested to be associated with the development of endo, meaning the body storing too much iron can have a detrimental impact. This idea is supported by 21 studies where iron overload was found in the abdominal cavity in those with endometriosis.[16] Iron overload is toxic and can lead to oxidative stress and inflammation, which may promote endometriosis growth.[17] In Part 3, we discuss ways of managing iron levels.

19

Microbiology

Microbiology is the study of microscopic organisms, including bacteria, viruses, and parasites, examining their interactions with humans, animals, and the environment. In recent years, technological advancements have allowed scientists to make notable breakthroughs in microbiology. An improved understanding of the human microbiome — *the collection of microorganisms that live on and inside our bodies,* has led to significant developments in medicine. The human microbiome plays a crucial role in maintaining our health and preventing disease. You've probably heard about this in the media through the promotion of gut health, probiotics, and prebiotics.

Everyone harbours trillions of diverse microbes in their body, creating an individualised population differing from one person to the next. Your population is determined by the type of microorganisms and the amount of each. Our microbiota changes throughout life depending on what we have been exposed to, as the gut is impacted by factors such as diet, antibiotics, and air pollution. Microbes are *so* important for health that a possible cause of the dramatic increases in metabolic, immune, and cognitive diseases, such as allergies and obesity, may stem from a loss of microbial diversity seen in urban areas.[1] Even factors such as the mode of childbirth can affect your microbial diversity. Infants born via vaginal birth, rather than through caesarean, are exposed to a greater variety of bacteria from the mother's vagina, meaning caesarean-born children can be at increased risk of chronic immune disorders such as asthma and inflammatory bowel disease.[2] To alleviate this, techniques like vaginal seeding aim to restore microbes by applying vaginal fluids to newborns delivered caesarean.[3]

Researchers have been correlating trends in health and disease with specific types of microbes. There are good types, such as *Lactobacillus acidophilus*, a strain found to have several gastrointestinal benefits.[4] Whereas bad bacteria can stimulate health issues, for example *Helicobacter pylori* can cause gastritis and peptic ulcer disease.[5] When there is an imbalance of beneficial and harmful bacteria, it's called dysbiosis. For optimal health, individuals should strive to cultivate a diverse array of good bacteria. A healthy microbiota protects against the colonisation of disease-causing pathogenic bacteria in the body, which ultimately keeps us healthy.[4] If you are wondering how this relates to endometriosis, well dysbiosis in the gut and reproductive tract can impact immune function, promote chronic inflammation, and cause compromised immune surveillance. Immunosurveillance is a mechanism in the body that should recognise endometriosis lesions and destroy them. Issues with immunosurveillance likely contribute to the development and progression of endometriosis and adhesions.[6] Studies support that this is worthy of attention as differences have been found in the microbiomes of women with and without endometriosis in the gut, vagina, womb, peritoneum, and faeces.[6,7] Those with endometriosis could have higher amounts of harmful bacteria across various areas of the body named *Proteobacteria, Enterobacteriaceae, Streptococcus spp. and Escherichia coli*,[8] as well as lower amounts of good types, such as *Lactobacillus*.[9] *Lactobacilli* dominance is generally considered a hallmark of a healthy vagina due to its well-established role in maintaining a healthy reproductive tract and preventing the establishment of infection-causing pathogens. Unfortunately, *Lactobacilli* can be lost through menstruation as blood binds to the microbe before being expelled from the vagina. Frequent or heavy bleeding can lead to more significant *Lactobacilli* losses, putting those with endo at risk of dysbiosis and vaginal infections.

Dysbiosis in the gut can also affect oestrogen metabolism.[10] A healthy gut microbiome minimises the amount of oestrogen reabsorbed into the bloodstream, ensuring any excess amounts of the hormone are removed in our urine and stools.[11] This process is managed by the oestrobolome, which is the name for a collection of gut bacteria that metabolises and regulates the body's circulating oestrogen through the secretion of an enzyme called β-glucuronidase which changes oestrogens into their active forms.[11] Gut dysbiosis can, therefore, lead to oestrogen dominance.[11] Women with endometriosis sometimes have higher amounts of beta-glucuronidase-producing bacteria.[6] When imbalance occurs, a rise in beta-glucuronidase allows excess amounts of activated oestrogen to be absorbed from the gut and into the bloodstream, causing hormonal imbalance and oestrogen dominance.[12] This means our gut affects the amount of oestrogen in our body, which could contribute to the development of endometriosis since it depends on this hormone for survival.

There also seems to be a link between the level of dysbiosis and the severity of the disease or symptoms.[13] Due to the two-way relationship between oestrogen and the microbiome, evidence suggests changes in the microbiome can contribute to the development of endometriosis by altering the immune response or disrupting the normal balance of hormones and other chemicals in the body. For instance, certain bacteria produce chemicals that can trigger inflammation. Unfortunately, a rise in inflammation stemming from our gut microbiota or endometriosis can alter our inflammatory immune cells in the peritoneum, promoting the growth of endo tissue.[14] In comparison, a healthy microbiota can help regulate factors that maintain a normal peritoneal environment, supporting the clearance of cells, which could prohibit the formation of endometriosis.[6] Due to this research, the 'bacterial contamination hypothesis' was theorised in 2018, suggesting bacteria could activate a pro-inflammatory response, allowing cell adhesion to the peritoneum, thus facilitating the growth of endometriosis.[15] These studies led to research on treating endometriosis using antibiotics, probiotics, and prebiotics,[16] and identified that *Lactobacillus* successfully reduced pain.[17] Furthermore, broad-spectrum antibiotics were tested on mice showing reduced endometriosis lesion size and inflammatory markers.[18] Despite positive results, all the research on endometriosis and the microbiome is typically small and, therefore, insufficient to determine if it can effectively treat humans. There is also some deviation in results, meaning more research is needed to understand why there are differences, and like everything with this disease, it confirms there is no one-size-fits-all approach. Not everyone with endometriosis will have the same microbiome, nor will the same treatment work for everyone. Research must determine which bacteria are over and underrepresented in patients, where they are located, and if they can be treated. For example, a *fusobacterium* infection has been highlighted as facilitating the development of endometriosis, and a small study in Japan found it was more common in women with the disease.[19] Then, a mouse study highlighted this bacterium increased the number and size of endometriosis lesions, but antibiotic treatment helped to reduce or even prevent the disease establishing.[20]

Women with endometriosis have a substantially higher risk of developing IBS or IBD.[21] Microbiome research might be able to identify if there's a common cause for both endo and bowel conditions. If the microbiome explains the established connection, it could lead to therapies being developed to prevent and treat both.

While the relationship between the microbiome and endometriosis is still being studied, these findings suggest interventions aimed at restoring a healthy microbiome, such as probiotics, may have potential in the treatment or prevention of endometriosis.

20

The Nervous System

The nervous system is essentially our electrical wiring system, whereby signals are sent along nerves to transmit messages across the body, allowing us to function, move, breathe, think, and feel. Very important right? Although the human body has one nervous system, there are different categories of nervous systems, including:

Central Nervous System/ Peripheral Nervous System
Somatic/ Autonomic
Sympathetic Nervous System/ Parasympathetic/ Enteric Nervous System

The nervous system allows us to feel pain by sending signals to the brain and letting us know something is wrong. Imagine if you didn't register your hand was resting on a piping hot stove and burning your skin. The nervous system is an incredible survival mechanism. In endometriosis, it's believed that over time, pelvic lesions can cause inflammation of the pelvic nerves.[1] This sometimes leads to peripheral sensitisation, characterised by heightened sensitivity of the nerves, which lowers your pain threshold, making you more susceptible to experiencing an elevated pain response due to the nerves' heightened responsiveness. This can cause chronic pain and other localised issues. Unfortunately, heightened pain doesn't always remain in the location of the lesions because nerves talk to each other, so sensitisation throughout the entire nervous system is possible. Repeated stimulation to other nerves can cause a muscle memory-like response, leading to central sensitisation. This occurs in two forms: one is having nerve hypersensitivity provoking an enhanced pain response, and the other is experiencing a pain response to something that shouldn't be painful. Central sensitisation affects individuals differently; possible symptoms include joint pain, fatigue, and cognitive difficulties. Moreover, it can trigger conditions such as IBS, painful bladder syndrome, chronic fatigue syndrome, fibromyalgia, migraines or tension headaches, anxiety or panic attacks, and depression. These are common conditions; some are more pronounced in females, occasionally due to changes in the nervous system.

Furthermore, our thoughts, emotions, and the world around us con-tribute to our experience of pain.[2] This means stress (in its many forms) can alter how we perceive pain and threats. The lower our tolerance to threats, including the threat of pain, the more we trigger nervous system reactions. Once a repeating pattern of a nerve pathway occurs, individuals may experience sensitisation, meaning symptoms are felt without an apparent threat. This can range from feeling pain for no reason to having panic attacks with no threat. Finding ways to calm down the nervous system is often an important step in recovery and something we delve into in Part 3.

21

Endometriosis Brain

Endometriosis brain is a term coined to describe the structural and functional changes in the brain that occur in some individuals.[1] Research shows endo can cause changes in the brain, including electrical properties and gene expression alterations.[2] These changes can progress to increased pain sensitisation and changes in emotion, leading to mood disorders like anxiety and depression. The management and treatment of endometriosis often deals with the lesions and how to prevent their spread and development through surgery or hormone medication. The focus on what can be seen with our eyes, or your surgeon's eyes to be more exact, means the brain is often forgotten. Thankfully, this is changing with research being undertaken in this area. This work is crucial as approximately one-third of women with endometriosis have psychological disorders, [1] whilst brain fog or a lack of mental clarity is also commonly reported. Brain fog describes a group of symptoms that prohibit your ability to think clearly, making it harder to concentrate or remember information with ease.

So, what changes are seen in the brain? Well, one study trying to determine the cause of chronic pelvic pain found women who had this (with or without endometriosis) had less grey matter volume in brain regions involved in pain perception, compared to those who didn't experience chronic pelvic pain.[3] This change is not directly related to endometriosis, as not all individuals experience pelvic pain, and women in the study who *did* have endometriosis but did *not* have pelvic pain didn't show any decreased grey matter. This shows experiencing pelvic pain is more likely to lead to changes in the brain, but not that endo is a direct cause. Pelvic pain, a symptom shared with a handful of other diseases, seems to change grey matter volume. As such, it would seem important to resolve chronic pelvic pain as soon as you can.

Another study induced endometriosis in mice and then observed changes in several gene expressions, presented in areas of the brain known to be involved with anxiety and pain.[2] This alteration suggests endo may modify how the brain functions, leading to pain sensitisation, anxiety, and depression. It's important to note that these studies represent initial exploration into this area, and further research is needed to understand the relationship between endometriosis and the brain fully. These findings, however, do indicate the condition can involve a complex neurological component.

22

Comorbidities

A comorbidity is a medical term for a patient having more than one condition at the same time. The conditions might not directly cause each other, but having one can increase the risk of developing another due to shared risk factors. They are 'co'-morbidities because they describe conditions that frequently 'co'-exist. These may develop randomly or, more likely, through shared genetic, environmental, or behavioural risk factors. This typically occurs with chronic diseases; for example, type 2 diabetes is a common comorbidity to heart disease, meaning the longer a person has diabetes, the greater the risk of developing heart disease. In this instance, high glucose in the blood damages tissues in the body, leading to the comorbidity. Plus, the conditions share risk factors making a person susceptible to both conditions, such as obesity, diet, and lack of exercise. It's beneficial for doctors and patients to understand or be aware of possible comorbidities of diseases to ensure early detection, optimal management, or where possible, prevention. Individuals with endometriosis are at higher risk of developing certain diseases or conditions. Awareness is important as it's easy to blame all your symptoms on endometriosis, particularly as it's a disorder that can affect multiple organ systems all at once. This chapter was included so that you have the knowledge to advocate for your health and seek treatment if needed. Some comorbidities are more prevalent than others, but we'll explain what they are and their symptoms. If any resonate with you or you are concerned, speak with your health provider as each comorbidity benefits from separate treatment and management. Not everyone develops comorbidities (the same way some people do not experience endo symptoms), whilst others may deal with several disorders that develop slowly over the years. The frequency of comorbidities might result from the inflammatory processes, the physiological changes in the body, an altered immune system, or potentially the shared environmental toxins that trigger endometriosis and other diseases. For example, a notable toxin is dioxin. As discussed earlier, it was shown to induce endometriosis in monkeys, but dioxin can also cause problems with the immune system. Each condition will have separate reasons for why they develop alongside endometriosis, but for many, the underlying mechanisms as to why both evolve still need to be clarified with more research. This section was not included to create fear or distress as many will not ever develop any of these conditions, but for those who do, it can be helpful to understand the cause and effect of what is happening in your body. It may shed some light on issues you have been experiencing or give you knowledge on what to look out for in the future.

Irritable Bowel Syndrome (IBS)

IBS is a condition affecting the digestive system, capable of causing the following symptoms:

- Changes in the frequency of bowel movements
- Abdominal pain
- Bloating
- Constipation or diarrhoea
- Lethargy

- Nausea
- Backache

IBS is a functional bowel disorder, signifying no structural or chemical abnormalities can be detected with blood tests or medical imaging. Instead, it's considered a disorder of the brain-gut interaction, meaning there is an alteration in the gut or central nervous system in how it processes gut pain information.[1] Because of this, no diagnostic test can confirm its presence, so if your doctor suspects IBS, they will diagnose you based on symptoms. Tests may be performed to rule out other diseases, such as Irritable Bowel Disease (IBD), due to symptoms that overlap with IBS. If all tests come back negative and you have the symptom profile, you will be diagnosed with IBS. Around 90% of people with endometriosis have gastrointestinal symptoms, and approximately 21% are diagnosed with IBS, so it's fairly common.[2] Diagnosis of IBS sometimes occurs prior to an endometriosis diagnosis, in some cases, this is a misdiagnosis to explain endo symptoms. However, individuals can still have IBS, and the two conditions can exacerbate each other's symptoms. As both conditions are poorly understood, the reason for this is not entirely clear; it may be due to dysbiosis (imbalance in the microbiome) or low-grade inflammation in the bowel. Although IBS has no cure, individualised treatment and medication can be used, such as laxatives, antidiarrheals, antibiotic therapy to treat bacterial overgrowth, or even probiotics to improve symptoms. Dietary advice is often provided for IBS, such as cutting out wheat and FODMAP foods to see if that can help.

Crohn's Disease (CD)

Crohn's disease is an Inflammatory Bowel Disease (IBD). It's characterised by inflammation and ulceration of the Gastrointestinal (GI) tract and can affect any part ranging from the mouth to the bowel to the anus. Crohn's is prone to chronically relapsing and remitting, meaning it will clear up, then relapse, causing signs and symptoms again. These can be life-altering and include:

- Diarrhoea
- Ulcers
- Weight loss
- Blood in faeces
- Stomach cramps
- Fistulae (*an abnormal connection between two body parts, often resulting in a flow of fluid between the areas*)

Various factors like stress, diet, and medications can cause flare-ups. As it's inflammatory, it can be managed with an anti-inflammatory diet and by avoiding problematic foods, such as a high intake of omega-6, animal fat, and sugar. Crohn's has a strong association with family history; the highest risk is with 1st-degree family relatives such as a mother or brother, partly due to genetic susceptibility. The relationship between endometriosis and IBD (which includes both Crohn's and ulcerative colitis) varies significantly in studies. Epidemiological studies provide a 2% increased risk compared to a nationwide Danish cohort study reporting a 50% increase.[3] The reasons for shared susceptibility may include the inflammatory nature of the diseases and the release of free radicals or other chronic immune responses. It's suggested the oral contraceptive pill[4] and NSAIDS (but not aspirin)[5] have an association with causing IBD, which many people with endo use to manage symptoms. Therefore, susceptibility may be increased this way.

Ulcerative Colitis (UC)

Ulcerative colitis, another form of IBD, describes inflammation causing ulcers or sores. The inflammation starts in the anus and may extend up the large colon consistently, meaning it doesn't skip areas and start forming somewhere else like it can with Crohn's. There are a few different subtypes of colitis, however, the symptoms often overlap, including:

· Diarrhoea
· Rectal bleeding
· Cramping
· Weight loss
· Fatigue
· Abdominal or rectal pain

In UC, decreased mucus is secreted into the large intestine. This mucus protects the body against pathogens, so when there is less mucus, the body increases inflammation to protect against pathogens instead. Unfortunately, chronic inflammation in the bowel often leads to ulcers in the large intestine. Like Crohn's, people with UC will experience flare-ups, and symptoms may include mouth ulcers, swollen joints, and irritated eyes. Cigarette smoking has a negative association with UC, meaning it may provide a protection factor in the development and progression of UC and is less common in smokers than non-smokers.[6] It's suggested smoking increases bowel mucus, which may provide a protective barrier. Despite this, no one is advising you to start smoking to avoid UC, as on the other hand, smoking simultaneously increases the risk of Crohn's and certain bowel cancers. Like Crohn's, UC can have a severe impact on your lifestyle or lead to life-threatening complications.

Fibromyalgia

Fibromyalgia is a condition characterised by chronic, widespread pain that can affect any part of the body, although the muscles, ligaments, and tendons, such as arms, legs, and back, are primarily affected. Pain is often described as aching, burning, or throbbing. Other common symptoms include:

- Mental and physical fatigue that cannot be restored by sleep
- Sleep disturbances
- Memory loss or forgetfulness
- Depression
- Anxiety

These symptoms cannot be explained by any structural causes; there is no damage to tissues in the body to explain the pain experienced, nor is it an inflammatory condition. Therefore, the exact cause of fibromyalgia is not yet fully understood, but it's believed to be a result of abnormalities in the way the brain and spinal cord process pain signals. It's often described as a disorder of pain regulation due to central sensitisation. This means changes in the body cause highly sensitive pain receptors. Several factors are considered potential causes of fibromyalgia, including genetic predisposition, stressors, or personal experiences.[1] Personal experiences encompass stress and distress, particularly experiences that caused mental or physical trauma. This can stem from a variety of reasons resulting from one or several traumatic events. Such events may alter a person's ability to cope with stress through the dysregulation of stress mechanisms[7] or induce anxiety or depression. Treatment usually includes a combination of methods; medication can be provided to improve sleep and pain, whilst holistic treatment includes vitamin D supplementation and acupuncture.[1] This condition affects females more than males and can develop at any age, although it's primarily diagnosed in middle-aged females.[8] Women with endometriosis have a higher risk of developing fibromyalgia,[9] perhaps due to the chronic pain and fatigue associated with both disorders. As fibromyalgia is often thought to result from stress or trauma, it's possible living with endometriosis, particularly if experiencing severe symptoms, can cause changes leading to central sensitisation, and therefore fibromyalgia. There may also be shared risk factors causing the development of both diseases separately. It's important to note that fibromyalgia and endometriosis are distinct conditions. If you are experiencing chronic pain or other symptoms, speak with a healthcare provider to receive an accurate diagnosis and appropriate treatment. The positive news is that researchers are working on finding new and effective therapies due to an improved understanding of the condition. It is suggested fibromyalgia symptoms may be caused by antibodies increasing the pain-sensing nerves, so soon, symptoms may be treatable with treatments reducing these antibodies.[10]

Chronic Fatigue Syndrome (CFS)

Chronic Fatigue Syndrome (CFS) or Myalgic Encephalomyelitis (ME) is a complex and debilitating disorder characterised by extreme fatigue that doesn't improve with rest or sleep but isn't caused by an underlying medical or psychological condition. Individuals with the disorder struggle with daily life activities, getting up in the morning, and can experience problems with thinking, memory, and concentration. Other possible symptoms include:

- Muscle and joint pain
- Headaches
- Flu-like symptoms
- Sore throat
- Dizziness
- Gastrointestinal problems
- Sensitivity to light and sound

Symptoms can vary day-to-day or be intensified by physical or mental activity. This condition can affect anyone, but it's most common in women.[11] It's considered a nervous system disorder related to hypersensitivity of the central nervous system. This may be surprising to you as many think it's a psychological or behavioural disorder. A functional MRI scan has been tested on individuals with CFS, showing lower blood flow to the brain, supporting that abnormalities exist in the central nervous system.[1] The exact cause is unknown, but it's believed to be triggered by a combination of factors like viral infections, immune system dysfunction, hormonal imbalances, and possibly genetics.[12] Individuals with endometriosis have a higher risk of developing this condition, with one study suggesting 1 in 3 people with CFS has endo, however, this was a small study on 36 women.[13] Whilst endometriosis and CFS are two distinct conditions, extreme fatigue can be experienced with both, and endometriosis can worsen CFS. Additionally, some symptoms of CFS, such as muscle and joint pain or cognitive impairment, can be present in endometriosis. Both are complex conditions that are difficult to diagnose and treat. If you experience symptoms suggestive of CFS, speak with a doctor to receive an accurate diagnosis and treatment.

Interstitial Cystitis

Interstitial Cystitis (IC), also called painful bladder syndrome, is a chronic condition characterised by pain and discomfort in the bladder and pelvic area. Symptoms vary but include:

- Increased frequency and urgency to urinate
- Nocturia (waking up in the night to pee)
- Difficulty urinating
- Urine may contain blood
- Burning sensation when urinating
- Intense pain, which may be felt when the bladder is filling up

IC can also cause painful sex due to the close location of the bladder to the vagina and the tenderness in this area. Symptoms may come and go, lasting days, weeks, or months at a time, with flare-ups possibly triggered by the menstrual cycle or dietary changes. Anyone can get IC, but like CFS and fibromyalgia, it predominantly occurs in females over the age of 30. It's a poorly understood condition and difficult to diagnose. No single test can diagnose it. Instead, it's a diagnosis of exclusion after ruling out other conditions with similar symptoms. Although symptoms can be comparable to a UTI, UC is not caused by an infection. The exact cause is unclear, but it's believed to be multifactorial, meaning several factors contribute to its development. Factors include underlying abnormalities or damage to the protective bladder lining, allowing urine to irritate the bladder and surrounding nerves, possibly leading to inflammation, scarring, and reduced bladder capacity. Additionally, dysfunction in the immune system is likely, possibly involving an autoimmune reaction,[1] causing the recruitment of mast cells, which release histamine upon activation. This stimulates an exaggerated inflammatory response, creating an environment where the immune system mistakenly attacks its own bladder tissue, a further cause of pain. Due to the role of mast immune cells, food or drink that are high in histamine may exacerbate symptoms while reducing histamine intake can help manage symptoms in certain individuals. Histamine will be discussed further in the 'Allergies' section. Individuals with IC may experience problems with the pelvic floor muscles used to control urination becoming tense and tight, preventing proper functioning. Furthermore, there may be a neurological involvement, leading to nerve dysfunction in the bladder, causing abnormal sensations and pain. IC can have a significant impact on everyday life, including work, mental health, and relationships. However, when a diagnosis is confirmed, various treatments are available to improve a person's quality of life.

Individuals with endometriosis are more likely to develop IC. A review found a whopping 80% of people with chronic pelvic pain were found to have both conditions, and more people have both conditions than each separately.[14] Although figures will always vary depending on what study you read, there is not a huge variation, and the relationship between the two is undeniable. Due to symptom overlap, many people with endometriosis experience urinary pain and bladder issues but don't have IC. If you have been treated for endometriosis but have persistent bladder pain, or if you have new bladder symptoms lasting longer than six weeks, please talk to your doctor. Note: there is a strong correlation between individuals with

IC also having SIBO — treatment for SIBO can often improve IC symptoms.

Small Intestinal Bacterial Overgrowth (SIBO)

Small Intestinal Bacterial Overgrowth (SIBO) occurs from an abnormal increase in bacteria in the small intestine, whilst the body's mechanisms that maintain the balance of the gut flora are compromised. Unlike the large bowel, the small intestine is relatively sterile, designed primarily for digesting food and absorbing nutrients. When bacteria typically found in the large intestine are present in the small intestine, they feed on the nutrients meant for your body, leading to insufficient nutrient absorption and potentially malnutrition; this can result in weight loss and osteoporosis. The specific type of bacteria found overgrowing in the GI tract determines the symptoms, as each bacterium feeds on different products, such as carbohydrates or bile salts, producing various effects.[15] Symptoms of SIBO include:

- Pain
- Diarrhoea or Constipation
- Gas
- Bloating
- Cramps
- Indigestion

Though not entirely understood, it's believed that changes in the gut immune function and physical abnormalities in the GI tract, such as a blockage, may increase the risk of developing SIBO.[15] Once SIBO occurs, bacterial overgrowth may trigger an inflammatory response, causing further symptoms. SIBO is associated with conditions such as IBS and Coeliac disease.[16] As mentioned earlier, around 20% of individuals with endometriosis are diagnosed with IBS, and SIBO is found in up to 38% of people with IBS,[17] possibly explaining the shared relationship. Endometriosis is also linked to gut dysbiosis, and changes in the structure of the bowel from lesions, adhesions, or surgery are possible. Adhesions can pull on the intestines, impairing normal peristalsis, which is the wave-like motion that allows faeces to move through your bowel, causing it to slow down and bacteria to fester. If you have symptoms of SIBO, seek a doctor's advice as treatments are available. Diagnosis may involve a breath test and an endoscopy. Treatment typically includes antibiotics to treat the bacterial overgrowth, whilst nutritional support for those with deficiencies can include supplements. If required and where possible, your doctor will seek to treat the underlying cause. If you have factors which increase the risk of SIBO, a doctor may look at effectively managing those to limit the risk.

Polycystic Ovary Syndrome (PCOS)

Polycystic Ovary Syndrome (PCOS) is one of the most common endocrine disorders affecting females of reproductive age. It's a hormone condition affecting how your ovaries work. Although the name suggests the presence of cysts, these are actually small fluid-filled sacs more accurately described as follicles, which are normal structures in an ovary that contain developing eggs. In PCOS, these follicles do not mature properly, leading to multiple immature follicles within the ovaries. Even then, not everyone with PCOS will have these 'cysts'. To be diagnosed with PCOS, you must meet the Rotterdam Criteria, which includes having 2 out of 3 of the following[18]:

1. Irregular menstrual cycle or no menstruation.
2. Clinical signs of hyperandrogenism such as acne, dark hair on the face, chest or neck called hirsutism, and/or biochemical signs of hyperandrogenism such as elevated levels of testosterone.
3. Polycystic ovaries, defined as 12 or more follicles in one or both ovaries, usually detected on a ultrasound scan

If a scan shows multiple follicles, similar to the appearance of polycystic ovaries, but you don't meet either of the other criteria, then you do not have the syndrome. You can have polycystic ovaries without the hormonal disorder aspect. Other than the symptoms above, PCOS may contribute to mood swings, weight gain, and infertility. Signs and symptoms may vary over time but can become more prominent with age. The exact cause of PCOS is unknown, but no single factor is responsible for the abnormalities. It's believed to be related to a combination of genetic and environmental factors. Hyperandrogenism is the state of excess production of the male hormone testosterone and is a cardinal feature in how the disorder develops. Furthermore, around 35-80% of people with PCOS have insulin resistance.[19] This is when the body's cells do not respond properly to insulin, causing blood sugar levels to increase. Insulin resistance aggravates the hyperandrogenic state of the body and is thought to have a significant role in the development of PCOS whilst causing severe symptoms. Other potential contributing factors include inflammation, stress, and exposure to endocrine-disrupting chemicals.

Endometriosis and PCOS are common gynaecological disorders that can coexist. While the exact relationship between the two conditions is not fully understood, there is evidence suggesting they can be linked, as those with PCOS might have a higher risk of developing endometriosis.[20] This might be counterintuitive as PCOS is associated with reduced or lack of a period, whilst endometriosis is associated with longer, heavier periods. PCOS is related to excess testosterone, while endometriosis shows oestrogen dominance. Despite these differences, both are prone to chronic inflammation and hormonal imbalances. The coexistence of PCOS and endometriosis can have significant implications on reproductive health. Individuals with both conditions may experience more severe menstrual pain, heavier bleeding, and a higher risk of infertility. Treatment options for PCOS and endometriosis can involve a combination of hormonal therapies, lifestyle changes, pain management, and assisted reproductive technologies (where required). It can also be valuable to consider your insulin levels and how to manage them.

Cancer

Endometriosis is a non-malignant condition, meaning it's not cancerous. You may have read that having endometriosis increases the risk of
developing certain types of cancer. This is a pretty terrifying thing to read
and creates a lot of fear; however, you'll be glad to know the associated
risks are small. Below are cancers which have been mentioned to have
a relationship with endometriosis. We are here to give you the facts, so
whilst some may have an increased risk, the overall risk of developing
cancer is relatively low. Most people do not develop cancer relating to
endometriosis, and routine screening for cancer is not recommended in
individuals who do not possess any other risk factors. Those with a family
history of cancer or who carry specific genes such as BRCA1 or BRCA2 may
benefit from more frequent screening or other risk-reducing strategies.
If you have any concerns, discuss your individual risk of cancer with your
doctor.

Ovarian Cancer

In the UK, the average lifetime risk of developing ovarian cancer is 2%,[21]
which, compared to breast cancer at 14%,[22] is relatively low. In fact,
the risk is lower than several types, including uterine, colon and lung
cancers.[23] When it comes to endometriosis, a slight percentage increase has
been reported in ovarian cancer cases. A study also found endometriosis
is observed in 4-29% of patients with ovarian cancer, [24] validating the
need to be aware of this relationship so that you can seek medical help
if symptoms arise. However, finding consistent statistics is challenging
due to a lack of accurate data, and the risks vary by country. The type of
ovarian cancer that seems to be most reported is ovarian clear-cell and
endometrioid carcinoma. These cancers tend to have a good prognosis
because they're frequently detected at an earlier stage than other types
of ovarian cancer.[25] There is also some evidence suggesting there are

better survival rates in patients with endometriosis and ovarian cancer compared to ovarian cancer patients without endometriosis.[23] This is a strange statistic to consider. It may again come down to the type of cancer or because the age of diagnosis is relatively younger in those with endometriosis, or perhaps it's because it gets picked up earlier at routine testing for endo.

So, what causes the increased risk? Well, endometriosis shares similar features with cancer, particularly Deep Infiltrating Endometriosis (DIE). A gene-sequencing study on DIE lesions showed that 26% of them have somatic driver mutations, meaning they had DNA changes that make them more likely to become cancer cells.[26] More specifically, there may be a genetic risk, as mutations in the ARID1A gene were observed in 11% of endometriosis tissues, which is also regularly found in endometriosis-associated ovarian cancers.[27] So, what causes this? The exact relationship is not understood, but it's believed chronic inflammation and hormonal imbalances associated with endometriosis may contribute to the development of ovarian cancer. For example, a high oestrogen environment might promote tumour growth or lead to malignant transformation of endometriosis cysts. Alternatively, iron produced in the fluid of endometriomas can promote oxidative stress, which is capable of causing genetic mutations and malignant transformation.[28] It's likely a combination of gene defects, inflammation, increased oestrogen, and oxidative stress are all involved in transforming endometriomas from benign to cancerous. Other risk factors for ovarian cancer suggest being overweight, obese, or having an endometrioma over 8cm.[29] Breastfeeding or long-use of the pill reduces risk.[30] Overall, the lifetime risk of ovarian cancer is small, so you do not need to be worried. Nonetheless, it's good to know of this risk and the symptoms listed below. It can be frustrating as many of these symptoms are associated with endometriosis. If in doubt, always speak to your doctor.

- Swollen stomach
- Pain or tenderness in your tummy

- No appetite or feeling full quickly when eating
- Urgent or increased need to pee
- Losing weight without trying
- Feeling tired all the time

Cervical Cancer

Cervical Cancer is found in the cells of the cervix, which is part of the body connecting the birth canal to the uterus. It's suggested patients with endometriosis are at **decreased risk** of cervical cancer.[31] Finally, some great news. The mechanism or reason for this is unknown. However, it may be explained by cervical screening for endometriosis symptoms or reduced sexual activity due to painful sex, which in turn reduces exposure to HPV. HPV is a sexually transmitted infection that causes the majority of cervical cancers. It's important to attend your smear tests to detect any changes and prevent the development of cancer.

* * *

Cardiovascular Disease

Cardiovascular Disease (CVD) is an umbrella term for conditions affecting the heart or blood vessels. It includes conditions like coronary heart disease, angina, heart attacks, hypertension, congenital heart disease and vascular dementia. Studies suggest people with endometriosis have risk factors elevating their chances of developing CVD, such as high levels of inflammation, enhanced oxidative stress, an unfavourable cholesterol profile, and hypertension.[32] Of course, not everyone with endometriosis has hypertension or unfavourable cholesterol levels, so this isn't something you should be concerned about if you have a healthy lifestyle. CVD is a leading cause of death all over the world, so it's a condition many people will face. Lifestyle factors play a significant role in the development of CVD, with a cohort study showing that more than 80% reduction in risk can be achieved by following a healthy lifestyle, including regular exercise, good nutrition, maintaining a healthy BMI, and not smoking.[33] Due to indications that those with endometriosis may be at higher risk of developing CVD in their lifetime, it's good to be aware of lifestyle factors you can use to limit this. For some people with endo, factors such as exercising might seem overwhelming if you have fatigue or pain preventing this, however, exercise still includes going for a gentle walk. It doesn't have to be running or weightlifting in the gym. Low-impact exercise such as yoga or swimming may also be favourable — more detail in Part 3.

Allergies and Intolerances

Allergies and intolerances or sensitivities caused by immune dysregulation are a prominent issue for people with endometriosis. In fact, one study found allergies were the most reported comorbidity, with 59% of participants living with them.[34] The correlation between endometriosis and allergic manifestations includes hay fever, food allergies, sinus allergic rhinitis, and food intolerances or sensitivities.[35] We know endometriosis is associated with chronic inflammation and a dysfunctional immune system; however, the disease can alter the number and function of immune cells in our body,[36] which might explain the considerable rise in allergic responses. Mast cells are a type of immune cell that has a role in the inflammatory response and are key players in regulating allergic reactions. They are also involved in processes within endometriosis, such as angiogenesis, fibrosis and pain.[37] When scientists examined endometriosis lesions in a laboratory, they found a significant increase in the number of mast cells, as well as in the peritoneal fluid in the pelvis.[37] Mast cells are responsible for prompting allergic responses, so when they come across an allergen, they release a variety of inflammatory mediators, including histamine, into the bloodstream. If you don't know what histamine is, you may have heard of someone taking an '*anti*-histamine' to help their allergies. Histamine is the chemical responsible for the symptoms of an allergic reaction, such as sneezing, itching, and increasing blood flow to the area, thus causing inflammation, redness, or hives. Whilst mast cells are a good thing and help the immune system, excessive activation of mast cells can lead to chronic inflammation, disease progression, and pain.[37] Studies have suggested oestrogen influences mast cells, causing the cells to congregate in the endometriosis lesions. Additionally, oestrogen plays a role in activating mast cells, promoting their release of inflammatory chemicals.[37] Despite more evidence needed, it's thought mast cells have a role in the development and progression of endometriosis.

So, endometriosis is related to excess oestrogen in the body, and oestrogen stimulates mast cells — causing them to release histamine, which triggers allergy symptoms. Now... this is where it gets a little complicated: when your histamine levels rise, it stimulates the ovaries to secrete even more oestrogen.[38] Oestrogen not only stimulates mast cells, but it also down-regulates a digestive enzyme in the body called Diamine Oxidase (DAO), which is responsible for clearing the histamine we ingest through our diet.[39] This means we find ourselves in a vicious cycle, where the body is creating more oestrogen and histamine but cannot remove it as effectively. As levels of histamine in the body are high, this can lead to a heightened response to allergens, meaning the immune system creates a larger response to the allergen relative to the dose or amount of allergen exposed to. This can explain why people have allergy-like symptoms to foods, even if they don't have an allergy. It might be good to explain what the differences are...

Allergy

Allergies are when the body reacts to something harmless (like dust or pollen) with an immune response. For example, in food allergies, the body carries a type of IgE antibody for a specific food it has mistakenly classified as harmful, so it triggers the release of histamine and other chemicals when ingested or inhaled. Symptoms for allergies can be mild to moderate, including itchy eyes, rashes, hives, sneezing, abdominal pain, diarrhoea, vomiting, and swelling of the lips, face, or eyes, or it can lead to severe reactions like anaphylaxis, which includes swelling of the tongue and breathing difficulties. This can be potentially fatal, so requires urgent medical attention. If you are concerned about allergies, contact your GP for tests to be carried out. Common types of allergies include:

Seasonal Allergies (*also known as allergic rhinitis or hay fever*) – triggered by pollen from trees, grasses, or weeds. Hay fever will occur in spring or summer, depending on the specific allergen.

Animal Allergies – triggered by pet dander, saliva, or urine.

Food Allergies – triggered by specific proteins in food, such as peanuts, tree nuts, shellfish, eggs, milk, or wheat.

Insect Allergies – triggered by bee stings, mosquito bites, or bites from other insects.

Food Intolerance

Food intolerances do not involve IgE antibodies and aren't typically caused by an immune system response, as with allergies. Food intolerances arise from difficulty digesting certain foods, creating gastrointestinal symptoms such as diarrhoea, gas, stomach pain, and bloating. It can also cause a skin rash, brain fog, headaches, fatigue, and joint pain. The symptoms vary widely in severity and duration, and they may be subtler or have a delayed onset compared to allergies. Food intolerances differ from person to person. A common example is lactose intolerance, whereby the body lacks the enzyme lactase needed to break down lactose found in dairy products. Intolerances can occur with all foods, as well as additives and chemicals. Whilst food intolerances can be disruptive and distressing, they are not life-threatening and cannot cause severe allergic reactions like anaphylaxis, except intolerances to sulphite and benzoate.

Food Sensitivities

Food sensitivities differ from intolerances because they likely involve the immune system. Though unlike allergies, sensitivities are rarely severe. Instead, they are thought to be caused by the interaction of certain foods with bacteria in your gut — triggering gastrointestinal symptoms. Symptoms are similar to intolerances and can appear within minutes or may be delayed, taking days after consuming the food. Removing foods that you are sensitive to will improve any symptoms. Sensitivities can dissipate with time, so later down the line, you may be able to reintroduce these foods and enjoy them once again with no repercussions. Gluten intolerance or Non-Celiac Gluten Sensitivity (NCGS) is a common sensitivity.

Oral Allergy Syndrome

Oral Allergy Syndrome (OAS) occurs when individuals experience itching, swelling, and burning of the lips, mouth, nose, or throat when eating fruits and vegetables, typically when raw. Although in severe reactions, nausea, vomiting, itchy eyes, and asthma can be present. OAS is typically triggered by tree pollen, but it's also caused by grasses or mugwort. Around 70%

of people with an allergy to silver birch tree pollen also experience OAS when consuming foods that have come into contact with these pollens.[40] Pollen can be found on foods that grow on trees, such as apples and nuts, leading to a reaction in individuals with an allergy to tree pollen. Excitingly, cooking or heavily processing the foods may diminish these reactions, as the allergenic proteins from the pollen are broken down during the cooking process. Therefore, individuals may find they don't experience any reactions to consuming cooked or processed versions of triggering foods as the allergy is to pollen, not food. Each pollen will cause hypersensitivity to different foods.

Birch Tree Pollen	Apple, Carrot, Cherry, Hazelnut, Parsnip, Pear, Plum, Celery, Peanut, Peach, Nectarine, Walnuts, Apricot, Peach, Kiwi, and Almonds
Grass Pollen	Watermelon, Orange, Tomato, Watermelon, and White Potato
Mugwort Pollen	Broccoli, Cauliflower, Chard, Garlic, Onion, Coriander, Fennel, and Bell Pepper
Ragweed Pollen	Banana, Melon, Chamomile, Kiwi, Cucumber, Courgette, and Sunflower Seeds

Histamine Intolerance

Histamine is naturally produced by the body, but it's also found in certain foods and drinks like wine. Additionally, some foods may not contain high levels of histamine but instead stimulate the body to produce histamine. When the body has elevated histamine levels, or reduced function of Diamine Oxidase (DAO) — *an enzyme responsible for clearing histamine from the body*, it can lead to histamine intolerance. Elevated levels of histamine create allergy-like symptoms in individuals without allergies to the consumed foods. While the exact cause of histamine intolerance varies, factors such as histamine-rich foods, histamine-producing bacteria in the gut, medications inhibiting DAO activity, and genetic predispositions may contribute to its development. Symptoms can manifest, affecting various systems in the body. The most common are related to the cardiovascular system, including skin flushing, abnormal heart rhythm, sudden excessive sweating, and difficulty regulating body temperature. Other symptoms include diarrhoea, headaches, asthma, hives, and itching. Symptoms are often triggered by consuming histamine-rich foods or foods that block DAO. Dietary modifications, probiotics to support gut health, DAO enzyme supplements, or using antihistamines can help manage symptoms. Some food examples are listed.

Histamine-Rich Foods	Alcohol (especially red wine) Fermented Beverages (such as kombucha) Fermented Foods (such as sauerkraut) Dried Fruits Processed Smoke Meats Avocados
Foods that Trigger Histamine Release by the Body	Alcohol Banana Tomatoes Chocolate Citrus Fruits
DAO Blocking Foods	Alcohol Black Tea Mate Tea Green Tea Energy Drinks

Nickel Allergy

Research indicates women with endometriosis are more likely to have a nickel allergy.[41] This allergy is generally more prevalent in females than males and can develop at any age.[42] It's not entirely clear what causes this, although, exposure to nickel is known to increase occurrence. This may explain why women who have worn nickel jewellery more frequently are more susceptible compared to men. Nickel is a metal present in foods such as cocoa, chocolate, soya beans, porridge, nuts, almonds and fresh and dried legumes, broad-leafed vegetables, whole-wheat flour, soy, corn, onion, garlic, shellfish, nuts, canned food, and tea. A study exploring the effects of a low-nickel diet on women with endometriosis with gastrointestinal symptoms found a reduction in both gastrointestinal and gynaecological symptoms.[43]

* * *

Autoimmune Diseases

Autoimmune diseases are a collection of disorders where the immune system mistakenly attacks healthy tissues in the body. There are over 80 types, each affecting different tissues and presenting with distinct symptoms, treatments, and varying impacts on quality of life. Endometriosis is not classified as an autoimmune disease, but it can elevate the risk of developing certain autoimmune disorders, some of which are outlined. Of course, you may have autoimmune disorders not included here, but the frequency of these is less common. The current research is not comprehensive enough to fully understand the cause of this relationship. Is endometriosis a risk factor for developing an autoimmune disease, or vice versa? Or do they share similar risk factors that lead to a person developing both? These are good questions scientists are working to understand. Chronic inflammation may drive further pathologies or exacerbate them, potentially through alterations in the immune system. Many of these conditions primarily affect females, which may partly explain the increased risk. All the listed conditions require further research to determine how strong a risk they hold and understand the mechanisms involved to explain why individuals with endometriosis are more susceptible. To be clear, having endometriosis does not mean you will develop any of these disorders, but understanding the symptoms can mean you are better equipped to get an early diagnosis. It's noteworthy that many of these conditions predominantly affect middle-aged females, and there remains a significant gap in understanding and treatment of these conditions, underscoring historical neglect of women's health.

Eczema

Women with endometriosis have a higher risk of having eczema.[44] Eczema encompasses a group of non-contagious skin conditions characterised by dry, irritated patches of skin. Depending on the type, patches may resemble rashes or blisters or be scaly, bumpy, or raised. They can also be rough, sore, and itchy. Eczema can occur anywhere on the body and cover small or large areas. Around 10% of the worldwide population experience eczema at some point in their lifetime. It's more common in children but occurs in adults too. Eczema is a chronic condition prone to relapses and flare-ups, ranging from mild to severe. Some might experience frequent flare ups whilst others outgrow eczema experienced in childhood. The exact cause is not fully understood, but it's likely related to a combination of genetic and environmental factors. Having a family member with eczema means you are more likely to develop it due to inherited genes. People with eczema have a defective skin barrier, making it dry and unable to retain moisture, rendering it more vulnerable to irritants, allergens, and bacteria. This can trigger an immune response, leading to inflammation and itching. Eczema can also be triggered by food allergies or hormonal changes like menstruation or pregnancy. Contact dermatitis occurs when external irritants trigger eczema. Irritants vary for each person but commonly include metals, fragrances, or detergents like washing up liquid or bubble baths. There's no cure for eczema, but various treatment options can help manage symptoms. Topical treatments such as moisturisers, corticosteroids, and calcineurin inhibitors can reduce inflammation and relieve itching. In severe cases, oral medications like antihistamines, antibiotics, or immunomodulators may be prescribed. You could also try identifying any personal triggers. In some cases, light therapy or biologic drugs may be recommended.

Rheumatoid Arthritis (RA)

Endometriosis can cause an increased risk of developing Rheumatoid Arthritis (RA), a chronic inflammatory disease primarily affecting the joints. In RA, the immune system attacks the lining of the joints, causing pain, swelling, warmth, and stiffness, typically in the hands, wrists, and feet. Other symptoms include fatigue and weight loss. Over time, persistent inflammation and immune activity can damage the joints, cartilage, and nearby bone. RA is a systemic disease affecting more than just the joints; it can cause inflammation and damage in other areas of the body, such as skin, eyes, lungs, heart, and blood vessels. Unpredictable flare-ups can occur, causing an increase in pain and fatigue. RA affects around 1% of the population worldwide. The exact cause is unknown, but it's believed to be a combination of genetic and environmental factors, with a higher prevalence in females and those with a family history of the condition. Diagnosis involves blood tests for specific antibodies, and treatment typically combines anti-inflammatory medication, exercise, and lifestyle changes to manage the symptoms, reduce flares, and prevent long-term joint damage. Disease-Modifying Antirheumatic Drugs (DMARDs) are used to slow down the progression of the disease and prevent joint damage, whilst biologic DMARDs target specific components of the immune system to reduce inflammation. Physical therapy and exercise can help improve joint function and flexibility, and assistive devices, such as braces or crutches, can support weakened joints. Lifestyle changes, such as maintaining a healthy weight, avoiding smoking, and reducing stress, can also help manage symptoms. Surgery is sometimes needed to repair or replace damaged joints.

The increased risk of RA in individuals with endometriosis may be attributed to shared genetic factors associated with both disorders.[45] Chronic inflammation and immune dysregulation from endometriosis may contribute to the development of RA later in life, making it critical to reduce inflammation as soon as possible with lifestyle tactics. Interestingly, clinical trials are currently underway to explore whether RA drugs like DMARDS can also effectively treat endometriosis.[46]

Systemic Lupus Erythematosus (SLE)

Systemic Lupus Erythematosus (SLE) is the most prevalent type of lupus and ranks among the most complex autoimmune disorders. It's a chronic condition characterised by the immune system attacking healthy tissues in the body, causing inflammation and damage to the affected organs. SLE can impact various tissues such as joints, skin, brain, lungs, kidneys, and blood vessels, with the severity ranging from mild to life-threatening depending on the organs affected. Signs and symptoms can vary widely and include:

- Butterfly rash across the nose
- Pain or swelling of the joints
- Fatigue
- Mouth ulcers
- Fever
- Sun sensitivity

Symptoms are contingent upon the tissues affected by lupus, which can lead to more severe complications. Flare-ups, alternating with periods of remission where no symptoms are experienced for years, are common. The cause is unknown, but lupus is believed to stem from environmental, genetic, and hormonal factors. Triggers can exacerbate lupus symptoms, including exposure to sunlight, certain medications, infections, and stress. Lupus is notably more prevalent in African, Asian, Caribbean, and Hispanic individuals than in Caucasians.[47] Despite this, it's not considered a hereditary disease as no single or group of genes have been identified. While there is no cure, medical interventions and lifestyle changes can help manage the symptoms and control the disease.

There is a significant association between endometriosis and lupus; having either one increases the risk of developing the other.[48] One possible explanation is both conditions involve an abnormal immune response. Once again, more research is needed to understand the underlying mechanisms and triggers for the relationship between the diseases. One study suggested individuals with deep endometriosis may have a higher susceptibility to autoimmune diseases due to having greater antinuclear antibodies, which attack the body's healthy cells.[49] Please remember this does not imply a direct causal relationship, so it doesn't mean you will get lupus. This complex topic needs more wide-scale research with large patient numbers, including whether specific treatments can reduce the risk of the comorbid disease developing and whether hormone medications or surgery for endometriosis can reduce the risk of lupus. One study showed positive results for people with lupus being treated with hydroxychloroquine, highlighting a possible way of reducing the risk of individuals developing endometriosis.[50] Hydroxychloroquine is a medicinal drug that can help with lupus by decreasing immune system activity.

* * *

Anxiety and Depression

We touched earlier on the issue of anxiety and depression. Even for those without a diagnosed psychiatric disorder, many people suffer from these mental health challenges, which can significantly impact their quality of life. Statistics support the gravity of this issue. In 2019, the BBC surveyed 13,500 women in the UK with endometriosis, marking the largest study of its kind.[51] Nearly all participants reported the disease severely affected their mental health, as well as their career and sex life. Heartbreakingly, around 50% of respondents stated they experienced suicidal thoughts. Another study identified women suffering from high levels of anxiety, depression, and other psychiatric disorders may endure amplified endometriosis symptoms as a result.[52] This is not a minor issue; a 'high level' of anxiety or depression indicates struggle and despair, and the consequences are evident with the detrimental level of suicidal thoughts. These studies shed light on how the psychological stress faced by those dealing with endometriosis can leak into many areas of their lives, including social interactions, work performance, and relationships. This is worthy of attention, and medical research is needed to understand the link and how to resolve it.

There is an obvious and undoubtable relationship between chronic pain, crippling fatigue, fertility issues, and their ability to contribute to mental health challenges. For instance, approximately 86% of women with endometriosis-related chronic pelvic pain reported depression.[52] However, I wanted to investigate more. Personally, I felt endometriosis directly caused my anxiety, not necessarily following the logic that the *symptoms* caused the anxiety, but the disease itself was chemically or physiologically doing something to me that caused unjustifiable anxiety and unwarranted panic attacks for the first time in my life. It's complex to determine where this issue begins. It may be a chicken or egg-type scenario: does endometriosis cause anxiety and depression, or does anxiety and depression cause endometriosis? It might seem illogical to think anxiety and depression cause endometriosis, but the initiation of endo may start when we are young due to experiences in life. Studies have indicated a relationship between endometriosis and adverse childhood experiences. In adults diagnosed with endo, 50% reported experiencing emotional neglect during childhood, while 44% reported emotional abuse, and 20% reported sexual abuse.[53] These statistics represent the specific people taking part in that study; however, if these are representative of the population, it is a significant finding: that around half of the individuals with this disease experienced trauma, whether big or small, in their childhood. Childhood maltreatment has a proven relationship in leading to a chronic inflammatory state in adulthood,[54] of which endometriosis is considered a chronic inflammatory process. Furthermore, emotional abuse or neglect in children is a risk factor for anxiety or depression later in life,[55] which is a common symptom reported in endometriosis. This suggests another explanation for the significant levels of psychological stress found in those with endometriosis, indicating the psychological stress possibly pre-existed and perhaps contributed to the development of the disease. Alternatively, it could indicate they go hand in hand; the co-occurrence is caused by childhood psychological stress, leading separately to both endometriosis and psychological disorders. These scenarios advocate there are other factors beyond simply the symptoms of endometriosis which can contribute to mental health issues.

Taking a different perspective, oxidative stress also plays a role in the development and progression of endometriosis.[56] Oxidative stress occurs when there is an imbalance between free radicals (*which can damage cells*) and antioxidants (*which neutralise free radicals and prevent cellular damage*). An imbalance of these can lead to damage to healthy cells throughout the body. Research has demonstrated a connection between oxidative stress causing anxiety and depression,[57] but to date, we cannot explain the underlying mechanisms of how this works. This implies that oxidative stress found in endometriosis could contribute to the development of anxiety and depression. Due to the role of oxidative stress, ongoing studies are investigating the use of antioxidants as a potential treatment for endometriosis. More information on antioxidants can be found in Part 3.

As described earlier, endometriosis lesions create their own nerve supply by branching off an existing nearby nerve. This process partly explains how endometriosis causes pain; the abnormal communication from endometriosis lesions to the brain via new nerve fibres influences the central nervous system, increasing pain perception.[58] Endometriosis' ability to affect the central nervous system might stimulate changes in the functioning of neurons and gene expression.[59] Repeated nerve stimulation from endometriosis lesions and inflammation can lead to central sensitisation, where a person experiences a heightened response to pain, or the brain interprets specific touch signals as painful, even in response to stimuli that shouldn't be painful. This occurs because the nerves are constantly stimulated, leading the brain to record the frequent stimulation with a stronger memory. Central sensitisation does not only affect pain perception; it can heighten all senses, including light, sound, and odour. Additionally, it's associated with causing cognitive changes such as poor concentration, poor short-term memory, and increased anxiety. A study on mice highlighted how changes in the nervous system modifying gene expression can alter brain electrophysiology, leading to both anxiety and depression. Living with chronic, severe pain in multiple areas of the body and the changes in the nervous system associated with central sensitisation can naturally lead to a fear of pain. Feeling a small amount of pain can cause catastrophising thoughts like worrying about a potential flare-up, or concerns about the pain spreading, whether it will get worse, how long it will last, and what the impact on a person's day will be. There may also be fears around pain recurring after surgery or whether the disease will progress in the future. For some, this inherent anxiety from a hyperreactive nervous system is channelled as fear of pain, but it can take many forms. Given these physical and mental health challenges, some individuals experience panic attacks centred around a loss of control. The loss of control extends beyond pain and leaks into all the other aspects that endometriosis has managed to impact: not being able to work, not being able to go to that party you had been looking forward to, being in a different career to one ever wanted, not being able to function due to relentless fatigue, not being able to have children, or not being able to eat food you love because you have developed intolerances or allergies. These are all issues individuals with endometriosis face, and all can have an incremental effect on their lives and moods. There is the possibility that changes to the body caused by endometriosis, as well as the symptoms or impact the disease has on your life, can be separate causes for anxiety, depression, and other psychiatric comorbidities.

The treatment for endometriosis may also cause psychological stress as the side effects of the contraceptive pill and other hormonal contraceptives include mood swings or disorders such as depression. If we tie back to the beginning, the BBC reported nearly 50% of women with endometriosis experienced suicidal thoughts. It's important to consider that many women (likely since their teenage years) are advised to use hormonal contraceptives such as the pill to manage symptoms and to prevent the disease from returning. Several studies have also shown hormonal contraception is positively associated with subsequence diagnoses of depression, suicidal thoughts, and suicide – especially in adolescence.[60] The use of this medication may be exacerbating certain people's mental health issues, whilst for others, it may be the primary cause. This may explain why an alarming number of people with endometriosis experience these issues. If you are suffering from these conditions and are taking hormone treatment, speak to your doctor to see if there is an alternative way to manage your symptoms (and provide birth control if you so require).

As we can see, there are multiple possible reasons why mental health conditions exist, with many more to be discussed throughout the book. The cause will vary in each person, but what's crucial is talking to someone you trust if you are struggling. Endometriosis can be very isolating because it's an invisible disease, making it hard for people to grasp if they are not adequately informed of its impact. Additionally, discussing a gynaecological disease may not be comfortable for many, especially when it affects areas of their life such as work. It's unlikely anyone wants to talk to their boss about the painful sex they had last night, resulting in them being up all night in pain, so now they're feeling exhausted and anxious from a lack of sleep, and they might also feel depressed and worn out. These sorts of scenarios can make it feel like we have to bottle things up and walk through challenges alone, which is why it's important to let you know that it doesn't have to be that way. This struggle to open up can be amplified if you've previously felt ignored or not taken seriously by doctors or labelled a hypochondriac by friends and family — all of these can have a damaging impact on self-confidence. No one wants to be the 'sick friend' constantly talking about their health problems, but sometimes we need to speak without judgement and be taken seriously. This disease can be tough. This situation can be particularly challenging for those dealing with sub or infertility, as mental health struggles can intensify. These are very personal experiences, so it can be hard to talk about or made worse if the women in their lives are having children without trouble, potentially provoking feelings of inadequacy or failure. The toll on a person's life can be immense, even if treatment received for endometriosis has alleviated physical pain, so that is no longer a key issue. Mental health issues and fertility fears are not uncommon, but having a solid network that allows you to discuss your experiences and receive support is essential, even if that means seeking help from a therapist. Healthcare systems like the NHS currently lack support for the psychological impact of the disease, instead focusing primarily on the physical side with surgery and hormone therapy. Therefore, it's often up to us to prioritise our mental health and find coping mechanisms or solutions that work. Mindfulness or yoga to calm the nervous system, whilst exercising to release those happy endorphins, and joining support groups can all help. Some may find they need to seek medication to help them. If you need to speak to a professional, talking therapy is available on the NHS and can be accessed via your GP or through self-referral in many regions. Finding what works for you should be a priority to ensure you can enjoy life. You are not alone in mental health challenges. You are important and validated here, and please know that there is always hope.

Acne

Acne, spots, or pimples are a normal part of life that most experience. Whilst acne occurs for several reasons, hormones can have an important role, which is why it's more common in stages of life when hormones change, such as through puberty, pregnancy, and menopause. Testosterone, Dehydroepiandrosterone Sulphate (SDHEA), and Dihydrotestosterone (DHT) are hormones found in both men and women. They stimulate the sebaceous glands in our body to produce sebum. When we have too much sebum, it can create blocked pores or lead to spots. Oestrogen does the opposite and can reduce the sebaceous gland size and sebum production. As all these hormones are naturally found in the body, the formation of acne can depend on the ratio of oestrogen to other hormones, particularly progesterone in the body. Therefore, many find using a hormonal contraceptive pill containing oestrogen and progestin reduces sebum production and provides clear skin. So, how does this relate to endometriosis? Acne is an inflammatory process, and as people with endometriosis have hormone imbalances and chronic inflammation, these may be potential culprits that contribute to the development of cystic acne, which is both painful and downright inconvenient. An intriguing study discovered that 20% of individuals with severe teenage acne have an increased risk of endometriosis.[61] This study suggested a genetic link between the two conditions and noted both severe acne and endometriosis tend to start at the same age. This finding resonated with me and led to an 'ah-ha' moment. I had perfect skin until I was around 16 or 17 years old when suddenly I developed severe acne...just when all my friends' skin was clearing up from their puberty-related breakouts. I could never understand why my acne started so late. The battle lasted years, requiring much dedication and money spent trying to clear. I also found it interesting that this was around the same time I started getting allergies, despite never having any before, highlighting a change in my immune system. It makes sense that endometriosis and acne may have started simultaneously, considering only six years later, I received my diagnosis.

Fibroids

Fibroids, also called uterine myomas or leiomyomas, are noncancerous growths that develop in the muscular wall of the uterus. You can have single or multiple fibroids. They vary in size; some are the size of a pea, whilst others grow to the size of a melon. As you can imagine, when they are very large or if there are several, they can cause many different horrible symptoms. That being said, the majority of people are asymptomatic, so they won't even know they have them. Fibroids are very common, affecting 70% of women across the world.[62] That's around 2 in every 3 women developing at least one fibroid in their lifetime. They can occur at any age but are most common during reproductive age, around 30-50. Statistics show a higher prevalence in those with African ancestry.[63] Other risk factors include vitamin D deficiency, hypertension, obesity, and the diet consumed in later life.[62] Individuals with endometriosis are more likely to have fibroids than those without; 26% of patients with endometriosis also have fibroids, whilst 20% of patients with fibroids also have endometriosis.[64]

Fibroids can be detected using an external or internal ultrasound scan or MRI, so they are much easier to diagnose. Both conditions can cause pelvic pain and heavy bleeding during menstruation, so it's easy to dismiss the symptoms of one as the other, but they have distinct treatment options, so it's important to distinguish between them to ensure proper diagnosis and treatment. This is particularly important if they cause severe symptoms. The combined pill or progestin treatments used for endometriosis do not typically help fibroid prevention or symptoms, although they could help reduce some of the bleeding. Fibroids can be treated with medicine to reduce heavy periods or to try and shrink them, as well as with anti-inflammatory medicine. Surgery can also be utilised where possible to remove them. The exact cause of fibroids is unclear, but they are thought to develop from abnormal growth of the smooth muscle cells in the uterus. Hormones, particularly oestrogen and progesterone, play a role in their growth, so they tend to develop during the reproductive years when hormone levels are high. Fibroids are considered oestrogen-dependent tumours, and like endometriosis tissue, have an increased amount of oestrogen receptors compared to normal uterus tissue, allowing them to use the hormone to grow.[65] As individuals with endo can have higher amounts of oestrogen in their body, the oestrogen-dominant state may be the cause for why these conditions are often observed together despite being distinct conditions. Symptoms may include:

- Heavy menstrual bleeding
- Painful periods
- Pelvic pain or pressure
- Lower back pain
- Discomfort during sex
- Frequent urination
- Constipation
- In some cases, pregnancy issues or infertility

* * *

To conclude, endometriosis is associated with various comorbidities, which can exacerbate symptoms and affect the quality of life of affected individuals. It's critical to manage these conditions to alleviate symptoms and improve overall health.

23

Fertility

We have touched on fertility, but it's an important topic deserving further insight. Infertility is a word often paired with endometriosis, leading many to immediately associate a diagnosis with a negative impact on their fertility. Some individuals will receive a diagnosis after struggling to conceive, whilst others may be suggested to have a baby as an alternative to surgery. I want to start this chapter by emphasising that people *do* get pregnant with endometriosis. Unfortunately, there is a lack of reliable statistics, making it challenging to assess the likelihood of fertility problems. However, it is suggested around 60-70% of women with endometriosis are indeed fertile and can conceive spontaneously,[1] while around half of the remaining 40-30% can get pregnant, but it may require more time or medical assistance.[2] Nevertheless, even with good statistics, it doesn't make a difference because you are not a statistic.

It's crucial to understand that for most people this condition is not a full stop on your dreams of having children. Some of us may personally know someone who conceived after a diagnosis, whilst numerous public figures with endo serve as an example, including Susan Sarandon, Padma Lakshmi, Emma Bunton, Cyndi Lauper, Tia Mowry, Monica, Halsey, Jaime King, Bethenny Frankel, and Molly-Mae Hague. These women had children despite living with the condition, each representing a different journey to motherhood. Some experienced fertility issues and sought various treatments to help them conceive, ranging from acupuncture to surgery. Jaime King said she experienced five miscarriages and an ectopic pregnancy before having her first child. On the other side, Bethany Frankel conceived naturally at 39. It should be stressed that women without this condition also experience miscarriages; this cannot be solely pinned on endometriosis. Whilst it's possible to conceive and deliver a healthy baby, being mindful that this condition has been associated with an increased risk of subfertility, so the journey may be longer or have extra hurdles along the way, can help set realistic expectations. It must also be stated that while the percentage is low, for some people in our tribe, it can indeed cause infertility or cause people to change their plans for children because the journey is too hard. Let us outline the differences between infertility and subfertility, as they are often used interchangeably, but they're not the same thing. Understanding this distinction is beneficial, especially for those who have not yet attempted to conceive so may not be familiar with the terminology. Subfertility refers to a delay in conceiving, where natural conception is still possible, but it may take longer than average. Infertility is defined as not conceiving a child after one year of regular unprotected sex. This shocked me. I believed 'infertile' meant being medically pronounced unable to have children at all. I had not realised it was based on a duration of time. While the prospect of infertility can be distressing and isn't without its own problems and psychological bearing, it's essential to recognise many fertility treatments are available to assist in conception. Many infertile couples do end up conceiving a child. Unless advised by a doctor, those who desire to have children should not rule out this possibility, assuming themselves to be infertile, as this can cause a lot of unnecessary stress. Many people have no issues having children, naturally and without medical assistance, so wasting time worrying is not of any use. Medical assistance may be needed for others and can come in many ways. The advice for those who want to start a family is to try sooner rather than later, and ideally before or around 30. I know, I know — I hate that advice too; however, this information can be important for people to be aware of, so I have to say it.

Does Stage Impact Fertility?

Stages 1 and 2 are suggested to have an easier chance of spontaneous pregnancy than stages 3 and 4, although each case is unique. For infertile individuals, surgery can improve pregnancy rates.[3] The causes of endometriosis-related infertility are complex and include both the physical impact of the disease and the systemic effects. Direct causes of endometriosis-associated infertility include lesions or adhesions interfering with reproductive organ anatomy, such as blocking a fallopian tube or altering the shape of the pelvis. There are also indirect effects on fertility, such as inflammation, immune system dysfunction, and hormonal imbalances, which can affect egg quality and maturation. Combined, this can disrupt egg fertilisation and implantation, but arguably more importantly, it can impact ovarian reserve, which is one of the main prognostic factors regarding fertility (this also relates to age). Ovarian reserve is the number of eggs you have, although no clinical tool can accurately predict this. Antral Follicle Count (AFC) and Serum Anti-Mullerian Hormone (AMH) levels are currently the most widely used to predict ovarian function. As endometriosis affects us all differently, the cause for each person's fertility issues will differ, and this can complicate clinical management as it can sometimes be hard to pinpoint the cause. For some, poor embryo quality is their primary concern, as this can be important in determining pregnancy rates. For others, issues with embryo implantation may be more prominent. Fascinatingly, if you have a compromised or removed fallopian tube, the other tube can move and collect an egg from the opposing ovary — incredible right?

There is a growing body of evidence that endometriomas have a detrimental effect on ovarian function, and the studies determining whether surgical treatment provides benefit on ovarian reserve are inconclusive.[4] One study found that 50% of women with an endometrioma were able to conceive spontaneously within 6 to 12 months after surgery, whilst another reported surgery led to a lower number of eggs retrieved for IVF in others.[5] You see, it's complicated to determine the outcome as we are all different. Methods can be utilised to assist with endometriosis-associated infertility, depending on the specific effects of the disease on the reproductive process. This is why the stage can represent the level of changes within the pelvis and help predict possible complications or successes. The Endometriosis Fertility Index (EFI) staging system uses a score to predict the chances of spontaneous pregnancy after surgical treatment. This index is a valuable tool, enabling people to make informed decisions about surgery for fertility-based reasons. It's good to remember endometriosis is not the only cause of infertility. There are various reasons why people experience infertility, and it doesn't just affect females. Around 40-50% of infertility in relationships is due to the male factor, meaning it involves issues with the penis or testicles.[6] For those affected, this is not a burden you are alone in.

How Do You Know If You Have Endometriosis-Associated Infertility?

Well, the first step is typically just to start trying. A clinician recently explained to me that when you're ready for children, you should engage in unprotected sex at least three times a week. If you want to take a more targeted approach, period tracker apps will predict when you are ovulating, which is the best time to try. You can also use ovulation strips. If you are unsuccessful in conceiving a child after 4-6 months, it's advised to schedule an appointment with your doctor to evaluate potential issues. This timeframe is shorter than the typical 12 months recommended for those without endometriosis before seeking medical advice. The UK guidelines for clinical practice state that the management of endometriosis-related subfertility should involve a multidisciplinary team, including a fertility specialist.[7] They will conduct fertility tests on you and your partner, including blood tests and semen analysis. These tests can assess ovarian reserve, which reflects the ovaries' ability to produce eggs and predict the success of hormone-based fertility treatments like

IVF. Additionally, maintaining a healthy BMI, not smoking, and limiting alcohol intake can improve fertility prospects, both naturally and with medical assistance. Treatment plans will vary, depending on the specific factors contributing to fertility issues, often beginning with medication or surgery before considering Assisted Reproductive Technology (ART) treatments.

Surgery for endometriosis-infertility can sometimes be recommended to improve the likelihood of spontaneous pregnancy, however, this is not guaranteed. The decision to undergo surgery and the level of benefit will vary on a case-by-case basis. It should be guided by the magnitude of symptoms, patient age and preferences, surgical history, ovarian reserve, estimated fertility index score, and the presence of other infertility factors.[8]

Another important aspect to consider is surgery's ability to reduce pain, particularly pain during intercourse. Trying for a baby when sex is painful, especially when advised to have frequent sex, can fill the experience with anxiety and be traumatic. If surgery can alleviate pain, it might be a worthwhile step in the process of having a child. Following surgery, attempting natural conception is typically advised for an appropriate duration, with a revisit to your doctor if unsuccessful. Sometimes, those with mild endometriosis are recommended to try for two years before considering IVF.[9] For those who continue to face challenges, ART treatments are available and recommended if there is compromised tubal function, male infertility, low fertility index score, or if other treatments have failed.[8] ART encompasses various treatments where the egg and/or sperm are manipulated to enhance fertility chances. Let's go through these treatments.

Intrauterine Insemination (IUI)

Intrauterine insemination (IUI), also called artificial insemination, involves collecting a sperm sample from the male partner or sperm donor. This sample is then washed and processed to collate a concentrated sample of healthy sperm, which is subsequently placed into the uterus via a thin tube. Timing is crucial for this procedure; it can be performed using your natural cycle, ideally just after ovulation. In cases where ovulation does not occur, fertility medication may be provided to stimulate the cycle. The insertion process is typically painless, similar to the sensation of a pap smear, and only takes ten minutes. Due to its simplicity, this method is often a first-line procedure, although the patency of the tubes should be checked first to ensure the egg has a clear path and will not be hindered by any damage or blockages to the fallopian tubes. In the UK, IUI can be recommended with ovarian stimulation for mild endometriosis as the chances of getting pregnant can improve from this method compared to trying naturally.[8] IUI can also be beneficial for couples struggling with painful sex. Access to IUI treatments through the NHS requires meeting certain criteria, and there may be a lengthy waiting list. Consequently, individuals may opt to have this procedure privately, costing between £700 to £1,600 per treatment cycle.[10] If the procedure is unsuccessful, it can be repeated with the addition of fertility medication if this wasn't used initially. If repeated attempts are unsuccessful after three months or more, IVF may be recommended.

In Vitro Fertilisation (IVF) and Intracytoplasmic Sperm Injection (ICSI)

In Vitro Fertilisation (IVF) involves retrieving sperm samples from the male partner, similar to the IUI method, however, eggs from the ovaries are also retrieved. Before the eggs are collected, a hormone called Human Chorionic Gonadotropin (hCG) is injected to help eggs mature so they are primed and ready. The eggs are then collected via a needle inserted into the follicles via the vaginal wall. Fertilisation of the eggs with sperm may occur by combining the two in a petri dish and allowing fertilisation to take place. Otherwise, Intracytoplasmic Sperm Injection (ICSI) can be used, where a single sperm is injected directly into each egg. A fertilised egg is cultivated in a lab for five to six days until it develops into a blastocyst, a ball of rapidly dividing cells — the early stages of an embryo. The best embryo is transferred into the uterus via a thin tube for the implantation and development of a foetus. This is typically painless and does not require anaesthesia or sedation. Any remaining embryos can be frozen for future use.

IVF requires hormone therapy, starting with around two weeks of daily injections to suppress the natural cycle. Subsequently, a fertility hormone called Follicle-Stimulating Hormone (FSH) is administered to stimulate the ovaries to produce multiple eggs, rather than just one. The goal is to retrieve multiple mature eggs, as a greater number of eggs to choose from increases embryo selection for treatment and successful fertilisation. You may be pleased to know that the recurrence rates of endometriosis do not increase with the use of IVF treatments.[8] Technological advancements continually improve viable embryo production within each IVF cycle. The Embryoscope™ is a piece of cutting-edge technology, allowing doctors to monitor embryo development with a camera so the best embryos are selected for transfer, reducing miscarriage rates and improving IVF success rates.

Historically, two or three embryos were transferred into the uterus simultaneously to improve pregnancy rates. However, the rate for twins or triplets was significantly higher than in natural conception, putting both the mother's and babies' health at greater risk. As a result, the guidelines have changed since 2007, shifting towards transferring a single embryo at a time to reduce these risks. Over 1 in 4 IVF births in the early 1990s were twins, which has now reduced to 1 in 20 births.[11] Don't worry, this doesn't reduce chances of pregnancy, the number of babies born from IVF continues to rise due to technological advances.

IVF may be recommended if pregnancy does not occur after 6-12 months after surgery, especially for those with stage 3 or 4 endometriosis. If an individual has fertility-compromising factors such as blocked fallopian tubes or severe scar tissue, IVF may be recommended as the immediate treatment plan. Again, this all comes down to the individual, their medical history, age, hormone tests, and their partner's fertility status, or if they are using donor sperm and eggs. While the IVF process can be a time-consuming and emotionally challenging experience, it has worked successfully for many couples, so remains a great option. Access to IVF in the NHS may be limited due to strict criteria, so some may choose private treatment. Always choose a reputable clinic with extensive experience and have a clear understanding of what is included in the cost, as this varies across clinics.

Egg Freezing

Egg freezing is considered a means to preserve fertility, whereby eggs are collected and frozen to be used in future fertility treatments. This is beneficial due to the natural decline in the quality and quantity of eggs as we age. For those who are not ready to start a family or have not found a partner, this can serve as an alternative method and backup plan. This option may be particularly desirable for members of the LBGTQ+ community who anticipate needing to use options like IVF to start their family. By freezing eggs earlier, individuals can secure the best-quality eggs for future use. The process of collecting the eggs is similar to IVF, except when the eggs are retrieved, they are not fertilised with sperm, they are frozen instead. Alternatively, you can fertilise the eggs with sperm to form oocytes before freezing them. Success rates for frozen unfertilised eggs are relatively low, with an 18% birth rate reported in the UK in 2016.[12] Frozen embryos have a higher success rate and remember, sperm can come from a donor. Technological advancements have improved over the years, and the data is gradually improving. Scientists have transitioned from slow-freezing embryos to vitrification, which prevents damage to the cells, improving the survival rates of the embryo and potential success for pregnancy. Success rates depend on the quality of the frozen eggs or embryos, emphasising the importance of freezing eggs at a younger age and in larger quantities to maximise future birth chances. Whether frozen or fresh, embryo transfer statistics show that quality matters. Higher-quality embryos are associated with a 79% live birth rate, good quality at 64%, and poor-quality embryos have the lowest birth rate of 28%.[13] For optimal eggs, it's suggested that the earlier the better, and ideally before 35 years of age. It's also important to know not all eggs survive the freezing and thawing process, and embryos may undergo changes that render them unsuitable for transfer. Additionally, while the statistics provided are overall averages, individuals with endometriosis may experience further reduced success rates due to complications associated with the condition.

Egg freezing comes at a cost and is currently unavailable on the NHS for endometriosis. A petition ran in 2022 aimed at changing this, but it only reached 41,759 signatures out of 100,000. Egg freezing costs vary, and clinics will offer different packages that are included within the price. Costs of medication, the freezing procedure, and storage need to be considered before proceeding. You may also want to factor in that one round of IVF when you are ready to get pregnant costs around £5,000. Most people can store their eggs for a maximum of 55 years for an annual storage fee. If you are considering freezing your eggs, choose an experienced clinic with high success rates, transparent pricing structures, and plan your finances accordingly.

What Happens to Your Endometriosis if You Get Pregnant?

While symptoms can worsen initially, they often improve throughout pregnancy and during breastfeeding. The myth that pregnancy cures endometriosis is sadly untrue, and symptoms may return postpartum. Some people may indeed feel 'cured', but it's not the same for everyone, so we should dispel this myth so those who continue having symptoms don't need to struggle and fight to be taken seriously. For those concerned about the risk of miscarriage, whilst this is a possibility, the overall risk does not significantly increase for those with endometriosis. The general risk of miscarriage is approximately 1 in 5 pregnancies, and those with endometriosis have a slight increase to 1 in 4. Miscarriage is sadly a common occurrence for all females. If you are worried about this, please consult your doctor for personalised guidance and support. For those struggling with infertility, it can be a difficult pill to swallow and can have a significant emotional and psychological impact. This can be devastating and feel like a bereavement, often made worse by the fact it is a hidden scar or met with societal pressures and questions.

My nurse, Orla, was a lovely woman who took care of me after my first operation. She told me with conviction that I should block out all the noise from friends, family, and the world regarding the pressures of having children and to just focus on myself because it will happen in its own time. She was speaking from her personal experience, and it was the best advice she could give because it was what had helped her. I never forgot it, so I thought I would share that with you too.

For those struggling with infertility, it's crucial to have open communication and build yourself a support network to help navigate this challenging journey and create understanding in those around you of what you are going through. Although infertility is an incredibly personal experience, it does not need to be an isolating one. Having someone to have a good cry to or discuss your fears and feelings with can help. ART is available for those open to exploring alternative paths to parenthood, and options such as fostering or adopting children who need a home can be incredibly fulfilling. I am aware my life experience to date makes it harder for me to comprehend the pain that infertility can cause. However, as a 30-year-old single woman who was diagnosed at 23 with severe endometriosis, the words often ring in my ears that I should "not wait till I am 30 to conceive". I have been bombarded with this advice throughout my research for this book. Therefore, I feel I can speak for many individuals with endometriosis who want children, that the fear of not knowing what lies before you and whether you will meet the statistic of infertility has its own psychological imprint. I worry that I am taking too long and that it may rob me of being a mother. Even so, my outlook on this topic is to try to stay positive and not let fear get involved in my day-to-day life because for all I know, I may be fine, and then I would have wasted my time and energy. If I have issues, I will deal with them when they come. Nevertheless, I am human, and the fear creeps in sometimes. Whatever phase you are in on your journey of fertility, know that you do not need to hide your emotions and that whether you decide to have children or not, there are always options. Having a surrogate, adopting a child, or using egg or sperm donors are great options, and we should not judge ourselves or others on whichever path is taken. This journey can be devastating, so we must always be sensitive to the fact people may take unordinary paths to become mothers and fathers, and they are utterly justified.

Sometimes, infertility is related to an autoimmune disorder rather than endometriosis. In such cases, getting the autoimmune disorder under control can help improve fertility. If you have a diagnosed autoimmune disorder and are experiencing fertility issues, speak to your doctor to understand if additional steps can be taken. If you don't know of any underlying conditions, it can be beneficial to be evaluated for conditions such as antiphospholipid antibody syndrome, thyroid disease, and coeliac disease, as these can increase the risk of infertility, yet treatments are available. Autoimmune disorders, particularly Crohn's, rheumatoid arthritis, and lupus, can impair fertility. Other comorbidities, such as PCOS, can also have an impact. If you feel any resonate with you, please consult your doctor for personalised advice.

24

Is Endometriosis Preventable and What Are the Risk Factors?

At present, the exact mechanisms behind the development of endometriosis remains unclear, leading to a lack of preventative measures. There are, however, notable risk factors highlighted in studies — these may stem from factors we cannot change, such as genetic predispositions, whilst other risks are linked to lifestyle factors, offering potential areas for intervention. It goes without question, you did not give yourself endometriosis. Exploring these risk factors might be valuable even if you already have endometriosis, as it's interesting to have insight into potential factors that may have contributed to the disease's development. This understanding can offer clarity or perspective on lifestyle adjustments to help manage the condition.

Family History

Having a family member with endometriosis, such as a cousin, increases the risk of endometriosis, whilst having a first-degree relative, such as a sister, most significantly increases risk. This may be due to a genetic component, shared environmental exposures or lifestyle factors, but likely a combination of both. Genes can be inherited by your mother's or fathers' line, so can come from your paternal grandmother.[1]

Early Menstruation

Starting your periods early is a risk factor, classified as before 11 years of age, although there is no correlation found between menarche before 11 and type of endometriosis.[2] It's also proposed menstruation after 14 years has a decreased risk of endometriosis.[3] I started my period around 14 or 15, which contradicts this, serving as a good reminder that all research is statistical data, not facts or rules.

Heavy Periods

Individuals who experience heavy periods lasting seven days or longer or cycles less than 27 days may be at increased risk of endometriosis.[4,5] The research on this is conflicting, with other studies stating there is no correlation. This may come down to the disease being different for everyone.

Low BMI

Body Mass Index (BMI) is calculated by comparing height and weight to determine if a person has a healthy weight. Online calculators are available to determine your BMI and health category. Traditionally, it was believed individuals with a low-normal BMI score, specifically those classified as underweight with a BMI below 18.5 are at increased risk.[6] Additionally, some studies suggest a low BMI may be associated with a higher risk of DIE lesions.[7] Conversely, research investigated whether higher body weight offered protection against endometriosis. The results indicated that being overweight or having obesity did not protect against endo and could elevate the risk.[8] Whilst fewer cases of endometriosis are observed among those with obesity compared to those who are underweight, the risk escalates again for those with obesity, likely due to the inflammatory nature of both[9] and because fat cells make their own oestrogen. Among Endo Warriors with obesity, the disease tends to manifest in more severe forms, with reduced rates found at stage 1.[10] The relationship between BMI and endometriosis risk remains inconclusive due to conflicting study results. It's evident, however, that endometriosis is not limited to those with low body weight, debunking the outdated notion it only affects 'skinny people'. Age may influence how BMI affects risk; one notable study followed over 100,000 females for 20 years and found weight at 18 years old may be key in indicating risk.[11] Those with a low-normal BMI at 18 years old were 41% more likely to develop endometriosis than those who were morbidly obese at 18. This suggests an early window of exposure may exist where low BMI has a greater impact on risk. Whilst this disease can affect anyone of any body size, it's beneficial to try maintaining a healthy BMI.

Diet & Exercise

The role of diet in endometriosis needs more research to be truly under-stood. Even so, certain foods have been suggested as possibly helping or aggravating the condition. Gluten, alcohol, caffeine, stress, and physical exercise do not have substantial evidence to say whether they contribute to the development of the disease, or not. Although, managing these factors can help alleviate symptoms. These are discussed in more detail in Part 3.

Toxins and Pollutants

There is evidence suggesting that toxins may support or facilitate the growth of endometriosis. In Part 3, we expand on this topic and how to avoid them.

* * *

To summarise, no one has caused their endometriosis, and there are no known ways to prevent this disease from occurring, especially as it likely occurs in a multitude of ways that differ from person to person.

25

Menopause

After the fertile years, typically ranging from the teenage years to the 40s, a female will enter perimenopause, although this transition can occur earlier or later. Perimenopause is the natural transition to menopause, characterised by the gradual cessation of ovarian function, leading to significant hormonal changes. During this phase, progesterone and oestrogen levels fluctuate, dropping and rising in a steady decline until they reach menopause. Perimenopause can last from a few months to around four years. The decrease in ovarian oestrogen production during perimenopause causes the symptoms we know well — hot flashes, irregular periods, night sweats, mood swings, fatigue, and vaginal dryness, among others. These symptoms vary in severity and predictability between people. Due to the erratic rise and fall of oestrogen, some experience levels that spike higher than before, which then drop severely. The high levels of oestrogen can cause bloating, breast tenderness, and heavy bleeding. Menopause is defined by the absence of menstruation, so you no longer have a period due to decreased hormone levels. The average age in the UK for menopause is 51. You are postmenopausal when you've not had a period for 12 consecutive months.

Hormone cycle throughout life

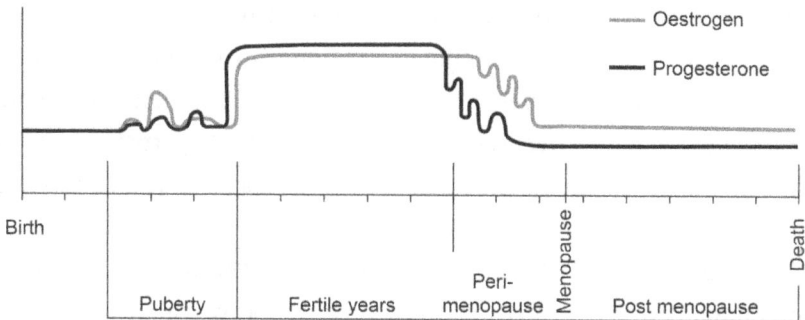

Endometriosis is an oestrogen-dependent disease, and many symptoms are often related to periods. Therefore, it's natural to presume during menopause, when oestrogen levels decrease and periods cease, the disease dies with it. But is this true? While symptoms diminish after menopause for most, some continue to experience them. The cause of this is unclear; some evidence suggests it's due to menopausal hormonal therapy feeding the disease. However, endo is also seen in menopausal individuals who do not take hormone therapy.[1] Another theory is that extra oestrogen production stems from fat and adrenal glands or excess aromatase — *the enzyme that transforms androgens into oestrogen* — stimulating problems.

Furthermore, perimenopause can sometimes be more intense, with exacerbated symptoms due to the spikes in oestrogen causing frequent or heavy periods. Treatment options are available, depending on the severity of symptoms and your medical history. Hormonal therapies like birth control pills, progestins, and oestrogen replacement therapy can be used to alleviate symptoms, although this will not be appropriate for everyone. Lifestyle changes such as exercise, a healthy diet, stress management, and getting enough sleep can also help. As the menstrual cycle declines, hormonal stimulation of endometriosis lesions decreases, so symptoms should improve. Ovulation pain should also dissipate. If symptoms persist after menopause, surgery may be necessary to address the lesions or adhesions causing discomfort. The goal of surgery is to remove the tissue while preserving the uterus and ovaries if possible. In some cases, a hysterectomy may be recommended.

Alternatively, symptoms may not improve due to a heightened sensitivity of the nervous system, developed from years of inflammation. The nervous system may retain its hyperresponsiveness to stimuli, perpetuating pain signals after menopause. Please consult your doctor if you continue to experience symptoms after menopause.

Although only reported in approximately 2-5% of cases, receiving an endometriosis diagnosis after menopause occurs is possible.[2] The cause is unclear and again may come down to HRT use, but this is not a rule. Postmenopausal endo is considered to have an even more complex pathophysiology than premenopausal endometriosis.[2] If you or someone you know starts experiencing symptoms after the menopause and you or your doctor suspect endo, you should ask for a referral to an Endometriosis Specialist Centre. If you live outside Britain, seek medical professionals with experience in this area to ensure the optimal treatment plan. Surgery to remove all tissues can sometimes be advised with postmenopausal symptomatic endometriosis due to the higher risk of malignancy with increasing age.[2]

It's important to note, pregnancy is still possible during perimenopause. Therefore, contraception should be used until menopause is confirmed if you do not wish to become pregnant.

26

Endometriosis in Infants, Children, and Adolescents

In Chapter 8, we described how foetuses' have been found with endometriosis. Although this is very rare, a handful of cases have been described in the medical literature of foetal, infant, and paediatric endometriosis. Unfortunately, there is not a lot of research on adolescent endo — *meaning diagnosis before 18 years old.* Symptoms typically include chronic pelvic pain or progressive painful sex (if sexually active).[1] Whilst in foetus', an abdominal mass may be detected via ultrasound.[2] Symptoms, just like in adults, vary, but for those who have started their period, it can cause painful menstruation as well as nausea, vomiting, diarrhoea, constipation, and changes in urination. Studies report that upon investigating chronic pelvic pain in children or adolescents, the prevalence of endometriosis is high and is considered the most common cause of chronic pelvic pain in adolescent girls.[1,3] This makes sense as it's often stated by people with endo their symptoms started in adolescence, but they were not diagnosed until later in life. Endometriosis can be found at all stages in adolescents, although it's typically diagnosed at stage 1.[3] We are not sure how long the disease takes to progress or if it advances into different types of endometriosis. Nevertheless, early diagnosis can make a huge difference to the life of someone living with a painful disease that is possibly worsening with each period. Awareness of this possibility can lead to earlier diagnosis and treatment for many, resolving pain and improving the risk of complications from disease progression, ultimately improving quality of life.[4,5] This goes to show, no one is too young to have endometriosis, and we should be aware that it doesn't just occur during reproductive age. If symptoms occur, it should be investigated by a paediatric or adolescent gynaecologist to determine if it is caused by endometriosis, particularly if the symptoms are unresponsive to the pill or NSAIDS like ibuprofen.

27

Endometriosis in Biological Males and Transgender Men

While endometriosis is typically considered a gynaecological disorder affecting biological females, it can also occur in biological males, albeit rare. Medical literature has only described around 20 cases of endometriosis in males.[1] Like in women, it's typically found in the lower abdominal wall and the lower genitourinary tract.[2] So, the disease still often includes the genitals, reproductive system, and urinary system. The main symptoms include abdominal pain and an abdominal mass, but it can also cause infertility. The most common risk factor for males developing endometriosis is having prolonged oestrogen therapy, such as for previous cancer treatment.[3,4] Due to the side effects, oestrogen therapy is seldom used today in cancer treatment. There are also reports that liver cirrhosis[5,6] chronic surgical inflammation,[7] or a combination of these may increase the possibility of males getting the disease.

Endometriosis is also pertinent for the transgender community. Transgender men who were assigned female at birth but have transitioned, have been shown in small studies to be at higher risk of developing endometriosis, likely due to testosterone therapy, which is commonly used in gender transition.[8] There is limited research in this area, but it's increasingly explored to understand how surgical and hormonal interventions impact risk and can alter the presenting symptoms. Due to these treatments, diagnosis presents unique challenges; menstruation may not occur, or individuals may have never had a period, which goes against the grain of how endometriosis typically presents itself. Common symptoms include chronic or cyclic pelvic pain and changes in menstruation. Awareness and education on this are critical to ensure everyone is acknowledged and able to receive the correct treatment.

Bizarrely, at the time of writing this book, I was unable to find published medical papers on transgender women, those who were assigned male at birth but have transitioned, and their risk of endometriosis. Considering a predominant risk factor of endometriosis in cis men is oestrogen therapy, it would be natural to presume the medical treatment provided to trans women would be capable of triggering endometriosis. While I hope this isn't the case, if it does occur, the release of medical papers will shed light on the impact, the effects, and how to recognise symptoms for these parties, which is indispensable information to have.

Many people with endo report medical gaslighting or PTSD from having their experience, symptoms, and pain invalidated. Now imagine that combined with the additional barriers that gender-diverse people can face in healthcare settings, such as discrimination and misgendering. This can cause individuals seeking help to be silenced or traumatised. This is a societal issue as well. What this information tells us is that no matter what gender you were born with and what gender you present as, anyone can get endometriosis, so don't invalidate someone's experience because their gender may not align with outdated mainstream information, as this is a form of discrimination.

II

Part Two

Understanding Diagnosis

28

How to Get Diagnosed

Getting diagnosed starts with recognising something isn't right, and the symptoms you're experiencing are not normal. Many people endure bad periods for years, sometimes since they first started, leading them to become accustomed to the effects. Symptoms can also progress; maybe your periods have become unbearable, requiring time off from school or work, or a plethora of other symptoms can evolve caused by endo wreaking havoc on the body — from chronic diarrhoea to overwhelming fatigue. If this starts happening, it's game on to seek medical help to reclaim your life and wellbeing. The first step is a trip to the doctor. If you've previously sought medical attention for symptoms commonly associated with endometriosis, such as painful periods, or if you have gone to the hospital due to pelvic pain, your medical history may provide some support for a diagnosis. In this case, you may want to book a GP appointment right away to discuss how you are feeling and what can be done. However, if you've not previously sought medical help, it's best to start recording your symptoms for at least one month before seeing a doctor. This allows you to track one or more menstrual cycles to provide your doctor with comprehensive information to support your referral. The key to getting diagnosed is asking for a referral to a gynaecologist, as they specialise in conditions affecting the female reproductive system. It's always best to start recording your symptoms from the moment you think you have endo and maintain them for as long as you need, as the more evidence you can supply your doctors with, allows them to provide a better service, ensuring you receive the best treatment plan for your needs.

Recording Periods

Several excellent period tracker apps enable you to record the days and duration of your bleeding. This insightful information allows doctors to determine your cycle length and easily detect any pattern of abnormal bleeding. You can track other symptoms on these apps, such as back pain or heaviness of your flow. For my diagnosis, I used an app to record my periods as well as days I would randomly bleed. The longer you do this, the better, as each month may be different. I had months which were a standard 28-day cycle, whilst other cycles were half this and would last for eleven days of bleeding. Getting diagnosed can be a trying experience, so this information can be extraordinarily helpful. By consistently using an app, you can establish patterns in your menstrual cycle and the app will get better at predicting your period forecast, which is particularly useful if you have irregular periods.

List and Track Symptoms

In addition to tracking periods, it's crucial to make note of any other recurring symptoms you experience and monitor these for your doctor. Symptoms may include menstrual headaches, bowel symptoms, or painful sex. It's good to note how long the symptom lasted, how mild or severe it was, if you took pain medicine, and whether that worked. You can use your phone's note app or an endo symptom tracker. Whichever method you prefer, when it comes to your doctor's appointment, summarise your record sheets by creating a concise one or two-page summary of your symptoms to print out and hand to your doctor. This provides a clear overview so the doctor doesn't need to review countless extensive tracking sheets during the appointment. While apps are helpful for recording bleeding days, provide additional details on your summary sheet, such as pain levels and the colour of your periods, so the doctor does not have to faff around on an app to find that information during the appointment. Remember, your doctor is there to help you, so make the information you present as understandable as possible to maximise the effectiveness of your appointment time. It's important to communicate if factors like your menstrual cycle trigger certain symptoms. If you have very heavy periods, you might also want to tell them how many pads you use a day and whether they are overnight pads, as this provides better insight. If your gynaecological symptoms are the most prominent issue, make this clear. Although endo has many side effects, when providing a symptom summary to your doctor, depending on your individual case, it may be best to stick to your gynaecological symptoms or those which are triggered by your menstrual cycle, such as 'painful diarrhoea on your period' to ensure they can understand why you want to see a gynaecologist.

Before seeing your GP, run through what you want to say, such as describing your symptoms and how you are feeling. Remember to address any concerns you have and request a referral. This disease involves talking about personal and intimate topics, so it's best to speak to a doctor whom you feel comfortable with so that you can talk freely and openly share your experiences. Holding back important information could limit the help your doctor can provide. You can always bring someone to the appointment if that makes you feel more comfortable. Remember, there is nothing you can say to the doctor they haven't already heard. Engaging in conversations about intimate details may initially feel unusual, but it's an experience many of us Endo Warriors share. While it's essential to express your preference for seeing a gynaecologist, consider any alternative routes your GP suggests exploring first based on your symptoms. This is what doctors are trained to do, so taking their guidance may lead to a correct diagnosis faster.

If you remember from my story, I was first referred to a colposcopy clinic due to my abnormal smear, inflamed cervix, and symptoms such as abnormal bleeding. At the time, that was the most effective route for me to take, as those issues needed to be addressed. A colposcopy clinic detects abnormal cervical cells, so in the case my symptoms were caused by cervical cancer, this needed to be resolved first. After this was ruled out but I still didn't feel any better, I returned to the GP, highlighting I still had abnormal bleeding, then I was referred to a gynaecologist. Even though you could be experiencing a wide array of symptoms, address your main issue with your doctor as this is the best way to be directed to the right place. If I had gone back to the doctor asking for help with my hip and knee pain, as well as my periods, that might not provide the doctor with the best indicator of what was wrong with me. Remember, they don't know you and what your life looks like on a day-to-day basis. You need to provide them with the information you are concerned about and what is affecting you.

Prior to attending your appointment, find out where your nearest Endometriosis Centre is. If you are lucky, it may be in your local hospital; however if not, you may need to ask your GP to make the referral there instead of a general gynaecology ward. Not every GP will be aware that these centres exist, so if they are unsure what you are asking for, kindly explain that your local hospital may have little experience treating endo, and so you want to see a specialist. If for some reason, this isn't possible or if the appointment times are too long, it's still valuable to see a general gynaecologist. If endo is visible on a scan, you can still be referred elsewhere for treatment if you request.

Before a gynaecological referral, your doctor may conduct a pelvic exam, order blood tests, or refer you for an ultrasound if they deem it necessary. This is to identify any visible, palpable abnormalities in your pelvis or cervix and to assess your overall health status. Although, remember no blood tests can diagnose endometriosis. If a general gynaecology scan did not pick up endometriosis, you can seek a second opinion with an endo specialist as they may be able to detect tissue due to receiving specialised training in imaging.

29

Endometriosis Diagnosis

The gold standard for diagnosing endometriosis is laparoscopic surgery, also known as keyhole surgery. However, ultrasound and MRI can be used by specialists to identify endometriomas and deep endometriosis. Unfortunately, many lesions, especially superficial ones, the most common subtype affecting 80% of individuals, are still difficult to detect without surgery, as they are typically not visible on scans. Even though progress has been made in recognising lesions through imaging, this requires highly specialised training. Therefore, even if an ultrasound or MRI does not show endometriosis, it doesn't rule out the condition entirely. During keyhole surgery, the surgeon visually examines the pelvic region to identify the presence of endometriosis. Tissue samples known as biopsies are taken of any abnormal tissue found and sent to a laboratory for analysis and confirmation (histology). This comprehensive approach ensures an accurate diagnosis.

As you may recall from my own story, I was diagnosed through a transvaginal ultrasound. This was a non-surgical diagnosis, but the gynaecologist determined this was my probable diagnosis due to my symptoms, ultrasound result, and her assessment. My local hospital was an accredited Endometriosis Centre with highly trained specialists within the gynaecology ward, so I was fortunate to receive an easy diagnosis. This diagnosis would later be confirmed by surgery. As endometriomas are more likely to be detected using medical imaging, the first operation is typically performed to confirm the diagnosis with a biopsy, treat the ovary, and remove any other visible endo lesions in the pelvis.

For many, diagnosis is neither easy nor quick. Statistics show endo takes around eight years on average to diagnose, and this is partly due to endometriosis being very hard to detect. Imaging can sometimes provide a diagnosis, but as it cannot rule out the disease when it fails to detect it, this is a particular problem for minimal or mild stages. As a result, many cases of endometriosis go unreported, as some people choose to avoid invasive diagnostic surgery. Remember, the stage of disease does not correlate to the level of pain experienced. Consequently, some individuals will suffer from symptoms without receiving treatment because surgery remains the only option for diagnosis, and there can be barriers to undergoing surgery, including fear, time constraints, or financial limitations.

A friend of mine went ahead with diagnostic surgery due to struggling with symptoms commonly associated with endo, only to be told afterwards that they found nothing, no endo, and no other cause. This risk needs to be weighed up by each person; some may not want unnecessary surgery, whilst for others, knowing is more important — whether they have it or not. Diagnostic surgery can be the best step for someone when medical management of their symptoms is not working and their quality of life is deteriorating. It can be an essential component to getting better. Requiring surgery for diagnosis fosters a delay in many seeking help, sometimes allowing the disease to progress further. This reaffirms the importance of research in facilitating non-invasive testing to aid the diagnostic process.

Diagnostic surgery marks many people's first experience having an operation or being put under general anaesthesia. Understandably, this can be daunting, particularly if scans fail to reveal any signs of the condition, leaving the possibility the procedure may all be for nothing. It's natural to be concerned about scars, recovery time, or needing time off work or school. It's a big moment in people's lives. The prospect of receiving a negative result can cause added stress. Many Endo Warriors have likely dealt with people making them feel like hypochondriacs or drama queens, whether that's from their parents, friends, colleagues, or even doctors. This lack of validation can make them hesitant to undergo diagnostic surgery, especially if there's a chance it may not provide an explanation for their symptoms. This fear of potential embarrassment may lead to some opting out of surgery altogether. I know of a girl who had not even visited the GP about her symptoms as she was apprehensive of being told nothing is wrong, let alone the magnitude of having surgery to provide an answer. This affirms we need to support and respect anyone who thinks they have endo and support them in their diagnosis. If surgery confirms they do not have endometriosis (or any other cause), we *still* need to provide them comfort instead of letting them feel humiliated. When someone feels so bad, it compels them to have surgery; not receiving an answer or a diagnosis can be confusing, so no one needs the added pressure of feeling embarrassed, especially as they are still left without an explanation for why they feel the way they do. Many people are not taken seriously and don't receive this support from those around them. However, we can control how *we* act, so let's promise to offer support to those around us instead of allowing others to delay their diagnosis and treatment for these types of reasons.

For those who don't have visible endo on ultrasound, other less invasive tests may be carried out to determine if there's another cause for their symptoms before having diagnostic surgery. The type of tests depends on the presenting symptoms, such as if they are gastrointestinal or urological. Suppose a person visits the doctor with painful periods, chronic diarrhoea, fatigue, and abdominal pain. In that case, it's possible they have 'normal' period pain, but their gastrointestinal symptoms are caused by IBD, so an endoscopy (a camera that photographs the GI tract) can determine this possibility. Of course, people can have both endometriosis and other conditions, but eradicating the need for surgery and providing an accurate diagnosis for another condition is sometimes the most desirable route to improving quality of life, as some people don't have symptoms from endo. If a doctor has stated there is nothing wrong with you and is reluctant to do further testing to find an answer for your symptoms, get a second opinion. We know when something is wrong with our bodies, we should trust ourselves and our instincts. I had multiple doctors' appointments to address the same issue before I was referred to a gynaecologist, not because they didn't believe me or weren't helpful, but because sometimes the process of diagnosis can be complex. We need to take our health into our own hands and continue seeking help if we need it. There is the unusual possibility that diagnostic surgery stating you don't have endo can be wrong. This may be because it's in an obscure location, the lesions were too small or microscopic, or the doctor hasn't been trained to detect the different types of endo that exist. For others who have received surgical treatment for diagnosed endo but don't feel any improvements in their symptoms, there is potential the lesions were not excised properly or are still somewhere yet to be discovered. Surgeons can also intentionally leave endometriosis behind under certain circumstances — if the risk of complications in removing it outweighs the benefits. In all these instances, if you still innately know something is wrong, seek a second appointment with a gynaecologist to explain your concerns. Requesting a referral to an Endometriosis Centre may be beneficial to ensure the best chance of an accurate diagnosis and access to highly trained surgeons.

There are several reasons why patients elect out of surgery: surgical risks, financial barriers (especially outside of the UK), or some don't feel their symptoms are bad enough to elicit having surgery. Routine screening may be provided to determine the status of their disease, allowing patients to reassess their needs over time. Another friend of mine decided against surgery for an endometrioma and bowel endo due to the risk of needing a stoma. She decided to wait and try other treatment options as she didn't feel she was at the dire point of needing surgery. Her doctors recommended a Mirena® coil, and she is monitored with various tests to track the progress of the disease. Careful monitoring empowers doctors and patients to determine the effectiveness of specific management strategies, allowing patients to continually make the best choices for their treatment. Should there be any advancements in disease, deterioration of quality of life, or circumstances in their life change, such as wanting to start a family, individuals can then seek changes in their treatment options.

Getting diagnosed can be the most pivotal moment in a person's life. It allows them to make effective choices to improve how they feel and provide the validation and reassurance they need — confirming something really was wrong and it wasn't all in their heads. Trust your doctors, but also trust your body and advocate for yourself. Receiving an incorrect diagnosis or treatment can be exhausting but there will always be a doctor out there who can help. Now, for the people who haven't got this far yet, let's explain how to get diagnosed.

30

Meeting the Gynaecologist

Once you are referred to a gynaecologist, you will receive a letter with the date and appointment time. Depending on the hospital, there may be a long referral wait but you can sometimes get an earlier appointment by monitoring for any cancellations. Whilst you wait, continue tracking symptoms so your information is up to date and record any new symptoms. The gynaecologist will have your relevant medical history, however, they will want you to tell your story and why you are there. So, before the appointment, run through everything you want to say, questions you have, and any concerns so that you're prepared when you meet the doctor. You are welcome to bring a friend or relative to an appointment with you. If you have paid for any private tests such as consultations, bloodwork, or scans, bring these with you as these may not be on your NHS file even if you have sent them to your GP for filing. If you've gone directly to a gynaecologist through private healthcare, the same applies, bring your symptom tracker, and be prepared with relevant medical records. The gynaecologist will ask questions to get a better insight into your health whilst discerning potential causes for your symptoms. They may carry out a pelvic exam which can include using their fingers to feel the inside of your vagina for any abnormalities, such as tenderness in indicative areas or nodules. If you require an ultrasound scan, this might be in the same appointment room or you will be referred to have one done elsewhere.

There is no need to feel embarrassed; these professionals do this all day, every day, and are simply getting the most accurate information for their assessment. If further testing is indicated, your gynaecologist will refer you to have these done. What happens after this depends on the outcome of your appointment. If you are referred for other tests, a second appointment may be made to discuss the results of the investigations and plan your treatment. Instead, you may be referred straight from this first appointment for surgery. Alternatively, if your doctor suspects your symptoms are unrelated to gynaecological issues and would be better addressed by a different department, you may be referred elsewhere for treatment. If your GP has referred you for an ultrasound scan instead of to a gynaecology clinic, the sonographer will send a report of your scan back to the referring doctor who will provide the results to you as sonographers are not allowed to disclose scan results directly to patients.

31

Non-Invasive Diagnostic Procedures

Let's discuss the different types of non-invasive diagnostic procedures that can be carried out prior to or instead of surgery.

External Ultrasound or Transabdominal Ultrasound

An external ultrasound is the same kind that pregnant women have. This scan requires jelly to be applied to the skin, and then a handheld probe is moved over the surface of your body, which for endo, will be the lower abdomen. This machine produces high-frequency sound waves that enter the body and bounce off different tissues, sending the information back to the ultrasound machine. This creates a black and white image of your internal structures that can be seen on a screen by your sonographer or gynaecologist. This type of scan is not typically used for endo because the images of the organs being assessed are less detailed compared to an internal scan. The probe in an internal scan is in closer proximity to the structures needed to be seen and analysed, making for clearer images and better visualisation for the sonographer. For this reason, an internal ultrasound is more commonly used, but sometimes you may have both internal and external ultrasounds. The transabdominal ultrasound will be offered when the transvaginal scan cannot be tolerated, if you deny the scan, or if you are a virgin and do not wish to have an internal scan.

Internal Ultrasound or Transvaginal Ultrasound

The UK guidelines state individuals with symptoms suggestive of en-dometriosis should be offered a transvaginal ultrasound scan. This uses the same science as an external one, but instead, the device is inserted into your vagina to provide better images of your pelvic organs like your ovaries, uterus, and bladder. Ultrasound technology is not very good at viewing your bowels as they contain gas preventing the ultrasound from generating a clear image. You will be offered a different type of scan if your bowels need to be examined. For the internal scan, you will be asked to remove the bottom half of your clothes, then when you are ready to lay on a bed and put your feet up in some stirrups. A long, thin camera wand is protected for hygiene reasons, and then coated in lubricating jelly like an abdominal scan. The probe is then gently inserted into your vagina. This can feel a little uncomfortable, but it's not typically painful, although having endometriosis can sometimes cause this scan to feel a little sore. If you are experiencing a lot of pain or tenderness on the morning of your scan you might want to take paracetamol with you just in case. This is a quick procedure, usually lasting around twenty minutes. The lights will be dimmed in the room to give the clinician a better view of the dark images on the screen, so feel free to close your eyes and relax. It's best to keep breathing normally rather than holding your breath, as this can cause you to clench up or tense, which can cause the uterus to move position, making it more challenging to obtain clear images. The sonographer may sometimes place their hands on your stomach to press or move some of your organs to help get clearer images. During this procedure, the clinician may turn the screen around to show you what they are looking at to provide you with a better understanding of any issues they see. It can be natural to worry during your appointment as sometimes there are long pauses or statements being said that you do not understand. Additionally, another clinician may be called into the room to confirm questions about the images on the screen. Please know this is all normal and does not mean you have anything scary.

During your scan, if you have any visible endo, such as an endometrioma or a large clump of tissue that is embedded in an organ suggestive of a DIE lesion, depending on the experience and confidence of your gynaecologist, they will be able to diagnose you with endo. If you are referred for an ultrasound to be carried out by a sonographer, and they detect endometriosis, they cannot give you the results. They will write their findings in a report to send back to your doctor, this should usually take between 5-10 working days. You will then be referred to a gynaecologist. Unfortunately, as the most common type of endometriosis is superficial, which often goes undetected with ultrasound, it's unlikely that this scan will be able to confirm the presence of the disease for many people. Generally, this procedure doesn't offer enough information to diagnose, but it can indicate if further diagnostic steps are required. Despite its limitations, this scan is commonly used as a first-line diagnostic tool as, in some instances, it *does* show visible endo or signs of it. For people with endometriomas or deep endo, this can provide a quick diagnosis, allowing them to have surgery to treat the disease if they desire rather than a diagnostic surgery. If an ultrasound can inform a person that they do *not* have an endometrioma or detectable deep endo, this can also be an important step, helping them consider their treatment options. The clinician can also sometimes detect here if you have adenomyosis, the sister condition to endo. Individuals with classic symptoms but a negative ultrasound scan could have superficial endo. A transvaginal ultrasound is also used to plan for surgery and to rule out other conditions with similar symptoms. It's also an easy and low-risk way to monitor endo. If you have received a negative ultrasound in the past, it can still be worth having another if you feel your symptoms have not changed or gotten worse. High-quality training and expertise can make a difference and there is continual progress in ultrasound techniques to help detect patterns of endo. Furthermore you can be referred for an advanced ultrasound with an endo specialist who can provide a second opinion. If you were discharged from the hospital based on your negative ultrasound results alone, it could also be worth a revisit to the doctor, as endometriosis cannot be excluded by ultrasound.

In some cases, a person may have a transrectal ultrasound where the probe is inserted into the rectum to get better images of specific organs, but this is far less common.

MRI

Magnetic Resonance Imaging (MRI) uses a magnetic field to analyse protons from water molecules to create images, making it particularly good at providing detailed images of the body as we are largely made up of water. MRI is particularly adept at revealing extrapelvic endometriosis in areas such as the bladder, bowel, and chest, making it a superior option when ultrasound results are inconclusive. It can show the size and growth of lesions on organs, however it's mostly beneficial for viewing DIE lesions. Your doctor may send you for an MRI to help create their surgical plan, as it offers more comprehensive information than an ultrasound. It can gauge the extent of endo in deep areas, such as within the rectovaginal septum. The information from the MRI ensures the surgical team performing your operation includes any specialists if required, such as gastrointestinal or urological surgeons who have the appropriate expertise to plan your surgery. You want to minimise the number of surgeries you have to reduce the risk of adhesions, so involving all the correct specialities to guide the surgical approach ensures the best possible outcome.

Before the scan, you may be asked to change into a hospital gown and you will need to take all your jewellery off as the room has a large, powerful magnet, and you don't want any metals flying across the room. Because of this magnet, anyone you have bought with you will be asked to wait outside. Although, you can ask for someone to come in if you are extremely claustrophobic. MRI and ultrasound machines do not release ionising radiation, so you won't have any radiation exposure during this scan. An MRI machine features a bed for you to lie on, which moves through a round doughnut-shaped hole that takes pictures of different parts of your body.

It can be quite loud, so you will be offered headphones that usually play calm relaxing music. This is also how your radiographer will communicate with you to let you know when the scan is starting, as staff will sit behind a window to take the photos. You will be able to talk back to the radiographer through the intercom at any point if you need. The room may be quite cold so they will cover you with blankets to make you feel cosy. Your doctor may request that you have an MRI with contrast, meaning a clear ink is injected during the scan to improve the visibility of internal body structures. The scan can last 15 to 90 minutes, depending on how many images are taken and if you have the injectable contrast. These images are then sent to a radiologist who is an expert in interpreting diagnostic images, so you will have to wait to hear back from your results. If this is used for a pre-operative assessment, you may wait until your pre-op appointment to hear more.

CT

A CT scan is not typically used as it doesn't provide detailed imaging of reproductive organs. It may be used to visualise endometriosis in areas such as the kidneys or ureters, and for catamenial pneumothorax, which is a collapsed lung that occurs alongside menstruation — this is often associated with thoracic endometriosis.

Bowel Investigations

Bowel investigations may be utilised for people with gastrointestinal symptoms such as diarrhoea, constipation, severe bloating, rectal bleeding, and nausea. Although these symptoms are seen with all types of endo, they are also caused by lesions that are on or have penetrated the bowel. If a patient's medical profile is suggestive of invasive bowel endometriosis through persistent gastrointestinal symptoms, they may be referred for a sigmoidoscopy or a colonoscopy. These tests also determine if there is another cause for the symptoms, such as IBD. They are both minimally invasive examinations whereby a long flexible camera is inserted into the anus and up into the colon to determine what may be causing your symptoms. The main difference between an endoscopy and a colonoscopy is the areas that they examine differ. A colonoscopy examines the entire colon, whereas a sigmoidoscopy examines the lower part. These scans can detect polyps, tumours, ulcers, haemorrhoids, strictures, and inflammation, in addition to whether the internal bowel wall has endometriosis involvement. In most cases, people with bowel endo will not have lesions penetrating through the bowel wall. Instead, they reside on the external surface. When there is bowel infiltration, in 90% of cases, it's localised on the sigmoid colon or rectum, which are the last sections of the digestive tract.[2] Bowel investigations may also be carried out so that your medical team can plan surgery, deciphering the location and extent of endo tissue. They must also determine whether the patient will need a bowel resection, which is when damaged segments of the bowel are removed due to the disease, versus a shave — where endo is sliced off the healthy tissue. Bowel investigations can also be used intermittently to monitor disease progression.

Another test that can be used is a barium enema, also called a colon X-ray, whereby liquid is injected into the rectum through a small tube covering the lining of the colon, allowing photos to be taken. X-rays are not the most effective medical imaging technique for soft tissues like the abdominal organs, but the barium coating can produce clearer images. Air is sometimes pumped into the colon for further improvement. This test helps determine if there is bowel wall involvement, detect changes or structural abnormalities in the large intestine, and identify any blockages caused by endometriosis tissue in the bowel. These procedures may be carried out during surgery once you are asleep.

Urological Investigations

Urological investigations are less common but can be conducted to assess whether endo involves the urinary system. When endometriosis lesions invade the outer lining of organs like the bladder or ureters, it can lead to various complications. Some lesions remain superficial, while others penetrate deeper. Endometriosis invading the bladder can manifest a reduced amount of urine capable of being stored, which can provoke increased frequency and urgency of urination. A range of investigations are employed to assess the extent of the condition and detect any abnormalities, including ultrasounds, MRI or CT scans, urine sample analysis, and bladder capacity tests. Additionally, a type of CT scan called a CT IVU (intravenous urography) may be conducted using a contrast medium injected into a vein to provide a comprehensive evaluation of the entire urinary system. This imaging technique can detect blockages and irregular outlines in the kidneys, ureters, and bladder, which are essential in diagnosing conditions such as hydronephrosis — characterised by kidney enlargement due to obstructed urine flow. Prompt medical attention and treatment are vital for this serious condition.

Another valuable test called a cystoscopy, involves inserting a thin camera called a cystoscope into the urethra (the hole urine comes out of) to visualise inside the bladder and ureters. If any lesions are detected, they may be removed for a biopsy. A cystoscopy helps exclude conditions like interstitial cystitis or bladder cancer, which present with similar symptoms. It is important to differentiate and rule out these conditions as they require different treatments to improve the patient's quality of life. It's important to note that a cystoscopy cannot detect endometriosis lesions on the outer surfaces of the bladder or ureters. This will require laparoscopic surgery for surgeons to be able to see, making it a common practice to conduct this investigation during a surgical procedure when the two can occur at the same time. Even if you don't have endometriosis involving the urinary system, endo located elsewhere in the pelvic region could be contributing to your symptoms, possibly due to the close proximity of these organs and the inflammation present in the area, or a large endometrioma may be compressing the ureter. By employing thorough urological investigations, healthcare professionals can gain valuable insights into the extent and impact of endometriosis on the urinary system. This knowledge is crucial for developing an effective treatment plan and improving the patient's overall wellbeing.

* * *

After any necessary diagnostic procedures, you may be offered surgery. This is a critical step for many people; however, some individuals choose to decline surgery because it's not right for them. Whatever you choose is okay. Trust your gut instincts but also consider your doctor's advice.

32

Diagnostic Surgery

If you proceed with diagnostic surgery, whether to obtain a diagnosis so you can receive further treatment for symptoms or perhaps to investigate unexplained fertility issues, let's break down what this process entails. Surgery is carried out under general anaesthesia, meaning you are put to sleep for the operation. It will be a laparoscopic surgery, which is minimally invasive, whereby small cuts are made in the abdomen rather than a large incision used for surgeries like caesarean sections. This fantastic advancement in science allows for shorter hospital stays, less pain, less bleeding, a faster recovery time, and minor scars. The aim of a diagnostic surgery is to look inside the abdominal cavity so the gynaecologist can see first-hand if the disease has manifested and where. If lesions are found, they will be biopsied, meaning removed and sent to a laboratory for analysis to confirm what they are. Endo tissue can come in many colours and appear as lesions or cysts of different sizes. Therefore, doctors may not always be able to differentiate between endometriosis and other conditions with the naked eye, so biopsies are essential for confirmation. Your surgeon should do an exploration of the abdominal cavity to confirm if lesions are present on your side wall, ovaries, uterus, and bladder, as well as in covert locations such as the pouch of Douglas. Most surgeons will be able to see and treat visible lesions at earlier stages of the disease, but some lesions may not be removable during this operation, necessitating a second surgery. Often, the first surgery is to diagnose and treat simple disease. Many gynaecologists are not qualified to treat complex disease i.e., if the disease has affected other systems in the body, such as the urinary system or if you have deep disease in difficult places to remove. Unless pre-empted with imaging that you require a complex surgery, a second operation will be required, as other specialist surgeons may be involved in planning the surgery to correctly treat those areas and reduce the risk of complications. You may also need other tests, such as an MRI, before proceeding with a second operation.

Before surgery, you will attend a pre-op appointment to have tests taken, such as heart rate, blood pressure, BMI, and blood tests, to ensure you are physically fit for having surgery and anaesthesia. Your clinician will run through your procedure at this appointment, ensuring you understand any risks and requirements. You will be provided with instructions, including when to stop eating and drinking and whether to continue taking any medications — you must follow any instructions carefully. Diagnostic laparoscopic surgery is typically a 'day surgery', meaning you arrive at the hospital in the morning, have your operation and then go home on the same day. Usually, you don't need to spend a night in the hospital, but bring a small bag of essentials like spare clothes, pyjamas, toiletries, and a phone charger. When you arrive at the hospital, you will be provided a gown and surgical stockings (a type of knee-length sock) to change into. You'll likely wait around for a while before being called for surgery, so bring a book or something to entertain yourself. When you enter the operating room, there will be lots of people who all have a role in making your surgery run smoothly and efficiently. You will meet your anaesthesiologist, who will put you to sleep through an Intravenous (IV) line in your hand and/or through a breathing mask. This feels like you are entering into a lovely, deep rest. The next thing you know, you'll be waking up in a recovery room being looked after by a nurse, and your surgery will be complete. Your nurse will ask questions such as how you feel or if you're in pain. You might feel a bit sore or nauseous, but you will mainly feel sleepy so allow yourself to rest.

During the operation, the surgeon makes a small incision in your belly button; then a tube is inserted to fill the abdomen with gas, inflating your stomach. This makes it easier for surgeons to see all your organs. Without the added gas, this area is very condensed and packed with your vital organs so this helps the surgeons move around. A camera called a laparoscope is then inserted, and the images are displayed on TV screens in the operating room for the surgeon to get a clear view of the inside of the abdomen. More incisions are cut, typically around the knicker line, where tools are inserted, such as graspers, scissors, or a cautery tool. If endometriosis is found, lesions may be treated and removed. When the surgeon has finished, the air is released, and the incisions will be sealed using either stitches, staples or glue, and dressings are applied. The duration of the operation will vary but will usually last between 30-60 minutes, depending on the procedures carried out. After your surgery, you may experience grogginess, pain, or some vaginal bleeding. Personally, I felt quite good a few hours after my first operation as the morphine was in full swing. Even if you feel fine, remember to take it easy; you have just had an operation and need to rest. As the morphine wears off, the pain may intensify. The gas used to inflate your stomach can cause discomfort or pain in the abdominal cavity, it's even commonly felt all the way up in the shoulders. Gas pain is caused by trapped air remaining in the cavity, so it needs time to resolve itself and will gradually dissipate. The day after surgery will likely be the worst as the strong pain medication has worn off, but you will increasingly feel better in the weeks to come. It's normal to feel emotional or sad in the days following anaesthesia, give yourself the grace to cry it out. Rest up, avoid exercise or stretching too much, and listen to your body. You will be given instructions on how to take care of yourself, such as how long to wait until you can shower or bathe, when to start moving, and what pain medication you can use. Typically, you will only be advised to take paracetamol as required after diagnostic surgery. You will not be able to drive for 24 hours after general anaesthesia, so make sure you have someone who can take you home and look after you. Remember to follow all the instructions provided to avoid infections and help you heal quickly.

Each person requires a different amount of time before they feel better again, but expect to give yourself a couple of weeks off to take it easy. You will feel a lot better or normal within a month. The first six weeks are when your body will be doing the most intensive amount of healing, and by three months, you should be fully healed from your surgery. Your scars will take a while to fade, but give it time and learn to love them. They are a sign of what is hopefully the beginning of your recovery, so it's good to embrace them. Your doctor will provide a follow-up appointment to discuss the outcome of your operation. If you have endometriosis, this is where any further treatment will be addressed and if relevant, your fertility options.

If you are diagnosed with endo and wonder what happens next, in Part 3, we explore treatment options available and paths you can take towards healing, from hormone therapies to lifestyle adjustments. If a second surgery is necessary with a specialised doctor better equipped to handle complex cases like yours, this is also the opportune moment to consider requesting a transfer to an Endometriosis Centre. These are specifically designed to address the unique challenges posed by endo, ensuring you receive the highest level of care and expertise. It's worth noting that diagnosing endo can be a complex task, especially for gynaecologists with limited experience in this field. The condition can manifest in various ways, making it easy to miss. Unfortunately, in some cases, even during laparoscopy, some gynaecologists fail to correctly diagnose endo, although with improved awareness, this should be decreasing. To avoid any potential misdiagnosis, make sure your surgeon is skilled, experienced, and someone whom you trust. With adolescent endometriosis, colourless lesions are more commonly found, which may go undetected by a doctor who is not sufficiently experienced, as they are incredibly subtle and easy to miss.[2] Therefore, if you or someone you know is undergoing diagnostic surgery during adolescence, seeking specialist treatment may be critical to prevent a misdiagnosis.

33

Specialist Endometriosis Centres

The British Society of Gynaecological Endoscopy (BSGE) was founded in 1989 with a clear mission to enhance surgical standards, promote training, and facilitate the exchange of valuable information on surgery techniques for gynaecological conditions. In 2003, the BSGE recognised the need for improved surgical treatment of severe endometriosis and the varying standards of surgery at the time needed to evolve towards developing specialist laparoscopic surgery techniques that could be taught and refined by gynaecologists specialising in this field. The BSGE believed rectovaginal endometriosis should only be treated by surgeons possessing the necessary surgical expertise. To ensure this, they established centres where rectovaginal endometriosis could be treated using advanced surgical techniques. These centres not only treat patients, but also collect valuable data to be shared with stakeholders to improve patient care and establish the benefits and risks associated with these treatments. These centres became the first to be accredited by the BSGE and are continually monitored for excellence. Training courses were set up to expand the centres across Britain to elevate the level of care available to patients. By 2008, consultant gynaecologists interested in endometriosis could apply to become a BSGE accredited centre. The wealth of data collected grows week by week, with more patients having surgical treatments. This data is vital for improving surgical techniques and outcomes, aiding research efforts, and inspiring new research ideas.

Fun fact, during a BSGE conference, a video of my second surgery was included in a presentation to aid surgical training for rectovaginal endometriosis. The dedication of these centres plays a pivotal role in enhancing outcomes and improving the quality of life for patients. There are over seventy accredited Endometriosis Centres offering specialised care for those with severe endo, providing a service where all lesions can be removed, wherever they are in the body. These centres boast multidisciplinary teams of gynaecologists, endometriosis clinical nurse specialists, and surgeons from various specialities, all working together to plan and execute complex surgeries. If you have undergone diagnostic surgery but require a second surgery for complex disease, I highly recommend seeking a referral to an Endometriosis Centre. It's crucial that surgeons lacking experience or expertise in treating complex cases refer patients to specialists who can provide optimal care. Nevertheless, there may be instances where we need to ensure we put ourselves in the right place to receive the best possible treatment. Remember, even if your GP is unaware of these centres, you can still request a referral. To find your nearest centre, search online at https://www.bsge.org.uk/centre/. Hopefully, some day in the future, scientists will determine less invasive methods to replace diagnostic surgery.

34

Why is Early Diagnosis Important?

As many people claim their symptoms started as teenagers, and statistics show nearly a decade-long delay in diagnosis, this raises the possibility that endometriosis develops during adolescence, even if severe effects are only noticed later in life. Early diagnosis becomes crucial because it offers the potential for treatment that can prevent the growth and spread of lesions. Beyond that, it may also avert the cascading impact that the disease can inflict upon the body. Adhesions and DIE lesions can distort the pelvic anatomy, potentially disrupting the proper functioning of your organs — causing pain, inflammation, and musculoskeletal impairments. It's also important to acknowledge the impact endometriosis can have on pelvic floor dysfunction, whereby chronic pain causes trauma to the localised muscles, causing them to tighten. Moreover, endo can induce central sensitisation and cross-sensitisation, resulting in the nervous system altering our pain perception. This can intensify pain and increase susceptibility to developing other conditions such as IBS or vulvodynia. The latter of which can profoundly affect your sex life, adding another layer of distress. Central sensitisation is also associated with conditions, such as anxiety or depression. Whilst the list of possible impacts can be disheartening, it underscores the urgency of early diagnosis and treatment. Endometriosis can wreak havoc on the body in numerous ways, and delaying diagnosis and interventions may lead to irreversible damage or necessitate costly treatments such as physiotherapy to get your body back to optimal health. Early diagnosis allows for the prevention or reduction of widespread damage, enabling people to thrive and live the life they deserve. If you or someone you know is displaying signs of endometriosis but is hesitant to seek medical help for whatever reason, it's worth reconsidering. This is especially relevant if the person has been relying on contraceptive pills for symptom management for years. Too many of us were put on the pill at a young age to mask the symptoms of a disease we didn't know we had. Whilst the pill can be a great management tool, it's not an effective form of treatment for all. Even if a person does not want or need surgery, a wide range of self-management tools and alternative treatments can be utilised, supporting individuals in effectively managing their disease and improving overall wellbeing. Before diagnosis, we often don't know what is happening to our body, but seeking help can help us get on the correct path.

III

Part Three

Understanding Management & Treatment

35

Introduction

It was important that this book not only provided education on the current understanding of endo and its effects on the body but also demonstrated ways for you to manage your disease. Part 3 covers the healing aspect and guides you through available treatment options. Online medical pages commonly state three options to treat endometriosis: pain medication, hormone treatment, and surgery. Whilst these are very important, there are a variety of other options you can utilise to help reclaim your health. You may have found this information is not clear or widely accessible. Alternatively, you may feel there is information overload available online, including misinformation, leaving you unsure of what you need to do. Everyone is entitled to share methods that work for them. However, each person has different needs and requirements from their treatment, and this might vary at different stages in their life; some may be focused on reducing symptoms, others may want to improve fertility, whilst for the majority, finding methods that make them feel in control of their health is critical. Let us be clear, there is no known cure for endometriosis to date. That doesn't mean there never will be, but it does feel we are a long way off that elusive and monumental day. Nevertheless, people living with the condition today do not have the luxury of waiting for research to confirm what they need to do. We need answers now, or in fact, most of us needed them a while ago... but we will make good with what we have. Part 3 divulges methods science or Endo Warriors have shown to help manage the condition. We will begin the way most people's journeys do, with Western medicine, discussing surgery and hormone treatments available, then expanding to alternative medicine routes and lifestyle advice involving nutrition and movement. Awareness of these methods is important to better understand how they may help you, the evidence to support them, and who they are best suited to. After utilising surgery or hormone treatments, we are kind of left to wander off into the dark to manage the disease by ourselves. I wholeheartedly thank Western medicine because it brought me back to life after my surgeries — metaphorically of course. Even so, surgery is not a cure, nor are hormone therapies. Medication can only ease the symptoms, whilst each person responds differently to surgery, with varying levels of pain reduction and improvement in quality of life after their procedure. Looking at the statistics, it's reported excisional surgery improves symptoms and pain scores in up to 60% of patients.[1] Subsequently, five years after surgery, between 40-50% of patients report a recurrence.[2] This high recurrence rate means repetitive surgery is often required in the future. Interestingly, it usually presents with the same phenotype as before, meaning if you had superficial disease, if it reoccurs, it will likely be with superficial disease.[3] To assist the physical improvements surgeons establish in our bodies by removing the endo and adhesions, we need to implement tactics to work alongside that, ensuring we take a holistic approach to our health. This is crucial as many of us don't feel 100% 'cured' from the get-go. Even if you feel cured after your surgery, it's important to incorporate other methods into your recovery plan to maintain that feeling for as long as possible. Importantly, surgery is not always utilised; sometimes it's not suitable for a person, others may opt out for personal choices, or perhaps some of you are on a long waiting list — sometimes years long. Whether or not you choose to have an operation, supplementary tools can help you manage your disease, especially as sometimes surgery cannot rectify all ways that endo has impacted your health.

As outlined in Part 1, endometriosis tissue bleeds but cannot exit the body, and the prolonged growth can have various repercussions, leaving a hidden imprint on the inside of our bodies. Distortion of organs, immune, inflammatory, and hormonal disruptions, comorbidities, and autoimmune dysfunction are all possibilities. Symptoms may be wide-ranging, affecting more than just the pelvis. It can change how our bodies work. The initial stimulation of endometriosis lesions on our nerves can induce chronic and debilitating pain or even upregulate the nervous system, facilitated by localised inflammation and nerves branching out. Sensitisation to the surrounding nerve fibres can affect organs, muscles, or other nerves, sometimes leading to other pain conditions due to peripheral sensitisation. Many organs share common nerve pathways, so the chronic remodelling of the nervous system and cross-organ sensitisation can contribute to comorbidities forming. Chronic peripheral sensitisation can overstimulate the central nervous system, which includes your brain and spinal cord, this may explain why conditions like anxiety and depression are commonly seen. This impact on the nervous system or the co-conditions that form may be what prevents people from feeling 100% better. This means surgery may not be able to rectify all the damage done. The journey for treating and healing your endo is therefore, very much one to see what works for you, your body, mind, and soul.

The toll endometriosis can have on your body did not manifest overnight, it would have taken years or decades to develop, so this needs to be taken into consideration. There are no quick fixes. Give your body patience. Look at these methods as a way of life that gives you time to heal from the multifactorial damage. This often requires a multifactorial treatment plan, looking at a handful of tools to implement to ensure your recovery gets you to where you want to be. With no cure, these techniques aim to improve your quality of life and reduce pain and inflammation, so hopefully, you can live your life how you want to. We don't just want to focus on the physical here, the psychological aspect is important in the healing process; it can be a horrible repercussion of the disease and should not be neglected. Endometriosis is difficult to treat, so although we may not be able to heal everything or have it back to the way it was before, at a minimum, we want improvements that make us happy. We will discuss ideas to optimise your health in as many ways as possible using the 'Four Pillars of Health' as a framework to hopefully subdue your endo, inflammation, and its cascading impact on the body. Each person has a different experience with individualistic ways endo has affected them. This book, nor any other product or person, will be able to give you a method that works for everyone. It doesn't exist. Part 3 breaks down various options so that you decipher what calls to you, what resonates, what is relevant, and what you can integrate into your life. Some tools are highly accessible, so you can start on them today, whilst other methods require planning. You may choose short and long-term goals or record lifestyle changes you want to build. Having a strategy to address each of your symptoms for a multi-angle approach can be effective. For example, dietary changes, exercise, or supplements may be lifestyle changes you want to incorporate, but in the short term, you realise you could benefit from physiotherapy to become realigned after finding out you have distortions in your pelvis. By providing you with the information, I hope you become an advocate for yourself and how you want to feel. Curating your toolbox can improve your symptoms, calm the nervous system, and rebuild your life to achieve your goals and wellbeing. At the end of Part 3, we unfold ongoing research to explore what potential future solutions might be available to assist in our recovery and what improvements are underway to better understand this condition.

36

Cures & Myths

Many myths, rumours, and urban legends surround endo and how it can be managed. It's important to put many of these to rest and explain the truth or the science behind them. The reason for their existence may be ignorance or because they're based on people's prior experience, so whilst there may be some truth to them, they are not fact. Starting with what we already know <u>not</u> to be accurate, we'll then explain some others in more detail.

Myths we've already dispelled
The *only* symptoms of endo are heavy or painful periods
Endometriosis is *endometrial tissue* displaced outside of the uterus
Severe period pain is *normal*
Endometriosis *only* affects the reproductive organs or pelvis
Endometriosis *always* improves after menopause
Endometriosis *always* causes pain
High oestrogen levels in the body are the *cause* of endometriosis
Endometriosis means you *will* be infertile
Douching *causes* endometriosis
Endometriosis *is only* found in older women
You *can* prevent endometriosis
Abortion *causes* endometriosis

Cure #1 - Surgery or Hormone Treatments

It's useful to know surgery and medications are not cures. Successful surgery can make someone feel so good that they feel cured, however, the possibility of relapsing and requiring another surgery, as well as other lasting side effects that surgery cannot fix, means it's not a cure. A cure means creating a complete restoration of health, making a health problem go away that is not expected to come back. Scientists need to fully understand the cause of endometriosis before being able to make a successful cure. Hormone treatments, including the pill, may assist in managing symptoms like pain or bleeding. They *may* also help prevent further growth; but they have no impact on the eradication of endo nor the long-term effect of the disease, so symptoms may return.

Cure #2 - Pregnancy

This is a confusing myth because my specialist surgeon even suggested I have a baby as a method of treatment. I will never know if it was advised due to his personal medical experience of seeing it work with other patients or because it was a more accepted notion of a cure at the time. Now, we know that pregnancy does not cure endometriosis. This may be upsetting or uplifting news to someone, depending on their circumstances. There is bitterness in the idea that a disease capable of causing infertility holds a cure, but to receive it requires fertility and having a baby. This oxymoron would be a horrible trick from Mother Nature if it were completely true. It might be relieving for individuals with infertility or those who don't want children to know they would not be cured of their pain if they had a child. Although not a cure, this myth stems from reports of people feeling their symptoms dissipate during pregnancy and continue to experience minimal or reduced symptoms after birth, or at least during breastfeeding. Symptoms can stop during pregnancy as it acts on the body the same way hormonal drug treatments do. As hormone levels in the body change with higher progesterone levels suppressing menstruation, for some, this also includes their symptoms. If someone has three or four children in a row it can feel like a decade has passed with no or very little symptoms. By which point perimenopause may be on the horizon. Pregnancy does not eradicate the disease; it suppresses symptoms, and these *may* return when your periods restart.

Cure #3 - Hysterectomy

A hysterectomy is a surgical procedure to remove the womb and sometimes the ovaries. As the ovaries produce oestrogen, and endo is dependent on this hormone, many people have this operation in the hope of curing their endo and relieving its symptoms. This is not a cure for endometriosis. A hysterectomy can only cure adenomyosis as that condition grows in the muscular wall of the uterus. If the womb is removed but you still have endo growing elsewhere, the symptoms can continue. In some cases, a hysterectomy removes the organ causing the most pain, so it can be beneficial. However, depending on where the lesions are, such as if they are primarily on the bowel, removing the womb will likely not impact the lesions causing distress. There is a risk of symptoms returning after a hysterectomy or developing endometriosis elsewhere in the body. As doctors cannot guarantee it won't come back, it's not a cure. This procedure is a huge decision, not only impacting the ability to have children, but also medication will be required for the rest of their lives. Hysterectomies are discussed in more detail in Chapter 40.

37

Pain Medications

Pain is a predominant symptom, so it's common to use medication to alleviate it. Given this reliance, I though it would be helpful to break down how medications work and what options exist. Over-the-counter drugs such as paracetamol or ibuprofen are first-line medicines that can successfully treat mild to moderate symptoms, namely painful periods, headaches, and muscle pain. Sometimes, they don't sufficiently work, so other options are available.

Paracetamol, Ibuprofen & NSAIDS

Ibuprofen is an NSAID which stands for non-steroidal anti-inflammatory drugs. This class of drugs reduce inflammation, pain, and fever. Other medications under this category include aspirin, naproxen, and mefenamic acid. These work by blocking the production of prostaglandins, which are hormone-like substances made by the body in response to injury or illness that cause inflammation and pain. NSAIDs are most effective when they are taken before prostaglandins are made, so they are best taken pre-emptively, such as before your period if you know you will be in pain. Speak to your doctor if you frequently rely on NSAIDs but are looking to get pregnant, as long-term use is associated with reduced female fertility,[1] but fear not, this is reversible on stopping use. Your doctor can advise on suitable alternatives. The difference between ibuprofen and paracetamol is that ibuprofen is anti-inflammatory whereas no one understands exactly how paracetamol works. It likely reduces signals from the brain allowing it to reduce pain and fever, making NSAIDs better suited for aches caused by inflammation. Although many endo symptoms have an inflammatory component, some prefer paracetamol for pain relief. It's processed by the liver and can be taken on an empty stomach, whereas ibuprofen is best taken with food, making it slightly less convenient. Medications called compound painkillers contain more than one active ingredient, so paracetamol and ibuprofen can be combined for targeted pain relief through different mechanisms. This is useful if you are struggling to effectively suppress your pain with either medication individually. Over-the-counter compound painkillers can be blended with codeine, which is a type of opiate to assist with more intense symptoms. These are generally safe to use, however, if you are using them frequently or for an extended period, they can have some undesirable side effects.

Opioids

Opioids block pain signals between the brain and the body. These are highly addictive because they activate the most powerful reward centres in our brain whilst administering needed pain relief, so if abused, it can lead to prescription drug addiction. Weak opioids like codeine, dihydrocodeine, and tramadol are available in their lowest doses over the counter or through prescription to treat moderate pain. Codeine can cause constipation or mild issues with the gut, so depending on your symptoms, this drug may need to be avoided. Stronger opioids, including tramadol and morphine, can be prescribed for short-term use if they are indubitably required, but it's highly unlikely you will be offered these types unless in dire need. If you are taking opioid medications daily or over ten days in a row at a time, it may be enough to cause issues, so speak to your doctor for advice.

Neuromodulators

Another form of pain medication is neuromodulators, a broad collection of drugs capable of treating endo pain by altering nerve cell communication through the central nervous system. Neurons are cells that send messages across the body, including pain signals to the brain. Neuromodulators used for managing endo pain can change the level of activity in the brain, blocking the pain messages. However, the evidence on whether these are effective is insufficient, so it's best to talk to your doctor about the latest research on these if you want to give them a go.

Medication-Free Options

Although the strategies we outline in the following chapters can help reduce bodily pain, when pain strikes, it can be a little late to think about lifestyle strategies in that moment. Having a hot bath or using a hot water bottle can help treat pain without medication, or in addition too. There are also devices on the market that use pulse therapy technology to stimulate the nerves and interrupt them, limiting pain signals being received by the brain, although their effectiveness varies for each person.

38

Hormone Treatment

Hormone treatments range from the oral contraceptive pill to hormone therapy (which is the same stuff they use when treating cancer). Endometriosis has a hormonal component being oestrogen-dependent, so hormone treatment aims to limit or stop the production of oestrogen in the body. This plays a critical role in management for many, so it's worth explaining the different types available. In those who have not yet reached menopause, oestrogen is predominantly created by the ovaries, so suppressing the normal menstrual cycle and reducing the presence of oestrogen could hypothetically hinder the growth and shedding of lesions each month. In turn, this could slow down the advancement of the disease and, in some cases, even shrink existing lesions. For many people, symptoms worsen during their period, so by influencing the menstrual cycle, these treatments often result in a notable reduction in pain. Moreover, they aim to create a hormonal environment that prevents lesions from producing or responding to oestrogen, leading to a decrease in localised inflammation, which is a crucial factor in alleviating pain. However, it's important to know that this is not guaranteed; it may only be effective at treating the symptoms, which for some is still a winning factor.

Bleeding is still experienced with some hormone treatments, like the pill where you have a cyclical bleed. This is not a menstrual period, it is a withdrawal bleed caused by the withdrawal of the hormones. This period is usually lighter and shorter as the uterus lining becomes thinner, making it less painful than a normal period (whilst hopefully reducing other endo symptoms). This could possibly assist in disease prevention by reducing the menstrual blood volume and flow, particularly if retrograde menstruation is part of the problem, as there will be a reduced chance of blood exiting into the pelvis at the risk of new endometriosis tissue forming. Despite that, these medications are not prescribed to treat endo. They are only prescribed to treat the symptoms as they have no long-term effect on the disease, and once you cease use of them, symptoms can return. Hormone treatments have no effect on scar tissue or adhesions, so they are not a form of treatment for these. Most hormone treatments reduce your chance of getting pregnant whilst using them as they are contraceptives, however, not all of them are licensed contraceptives, so other forms like condoms will still be required. Also, they are not fertility treatments as they cannot improve fertility. We'll review the various treatment options available and explain more about them and their uses. Most people find improvements in their symptoms whilst on hormone treatments, but as some can have severe side effects, they will work differently for people. Any form of hormone treatment has possible side effects, not just the heavy-duty ones; sometimes they are desirable and sometimes they are not. Please always check in with yourself when starting a new type and make sure they are working for your body and mental health. The kind you choose depends on your reason for needing them and your goals, whether for prevention, pain relief, or infertility — these factors can determine your optimal choice.

There are very few drugs licensed explicitly for treating endo. Fortunately, there's a good amount to choose from when using off-label. If you want to try something new, speak to your doctor to ensure it's the best choice for you. Hopefully, one day, a drug will be designed that can be taken long-term safely, which not only improves symptoms but actively diminishes endometriosis tissue.

Combined Oral Contraceptive Pill

The combined oral pill, or 'the pill' as it's commonly known, is a contraceptive tablet. It contains artificial versions of two hormones, oestrogen and progesterone, which, through various mechanisms, prevent the ovary from releasing an egg during ovulation, thereby inhibiting your period. The pill is taken for 21 days, then a break or inactive pills are taken for seven days to complete a natural 28-day menstrual cycle. During these seven days, a withdrawal bleed occurs mimicking your period, although it's usually lighter or shorter. This is beneficial for endometriosis, where heavy bleeding is common, plus it can reduce pain levels. Doctors may recommend taking the pill 'back-to-back', meaning you take 21 days of tablets, then start again without a break. This minimises the amount you bleed, improving symptoms associated with bleeding. Some people prefer to take three packs in a row and then take a break for a bleed to occur, as there can be progressive bloating when taken consistently — combined with endo-belly, this break can feel desperately needed. The pill is favourable as it's safe to take long-term unlike other options. It can also benefit those with acne, PCOS, and adenomyosis. It's not suitable for everyone though, such as if you're over 35 and smoke or if you have a medical history of thrombosis, heart attacks, or strokes, as it can increase the risk of blood clots. It's also unsuitable for those with certain types of migraines, lupus, or breast cancer. The pill has potential side effects, including headaches, nausea, breast tenderness, and mood swings, but this will vary between individuals. There are many different brands with varying amounts of hormones, so if the one you are on is causing undesirable side effects, you can try other types until you find one that suits you. This may involve trialling a few before finding one with minimal unwanted side effects (like excessively crying or generally feeling the blues) while giving you the desired benefits. If you suffer from severe anxiety, depression, or mental health issues or take medications for these, you may not be the best candidate for the pill.

Progestins

Progesterone is a natural hormone secreted by the ovaries after ovulation. It helps the body prepare for a potential pregnancy by maintaining the uterine lining for approximately 14 days after ovulation, creating an environment suitable for embryo implantation. Then there's progestins (the word looks similar to progesterone), which are synthetic hormones that mimic the effects of natural progesterone in the body. Although they are artificial, they behave similarly to human progesterone. As the uterine lining responds to progesterone (and oestrogen), these hormones are crucial in regulating the menstrual cycle. This is why progestin treatments can be used. The natural fluctuation of these hormones throughout the cycle can be problematic for people with endometriosis, potentially increasing the activity of lesions whilst aggravating the symptoms associated with the condition. Progestin treatments are commonly used to alleviate these symptoms and improve quality of life by partially suppressing ovulation and menstruation. You may still have a period, but these hormone treatments often result in a lighter flow and less frequent bleeding. It's worth noting some individuals with endometriosis have a condition called progesterone resistance, where the endometrium doesn't respond properly to progesterone. This can contribute to a lack of response to progestin treatments, leading to persistent symptoms despite therapy. It may also be that specific endometriosis lesions are resistant to progestin, particularly red lesions.[1] Nonetheless, progestins have shown efficacy in managing the condition and its symptoms. They can reduce pain, decrease oestrogen levels locally and in the bloodstream, down-regulate oestrogen receptors, and possibly inhibit the growth of endometriosis lesions, which rely on oestrogen.[2] Progestins may aid in reducing endometriosis-associated inflammation and promoting cell death in lesions, a process which could lead to atrophy. Moreover, they have the potential to decrease oxidative stress by minimising uterine bleeding. Different types of progestin therapies are available, and although evidence suggests they are equally effective in treating endometriosis, they have varying side effects and methods of use. This allows us to choose the treatment that suits our needs and preferences. By preventing the rapid growth of the uterine lining and endometriosis tissue, progestins might be able to hinder the development of new lesions. Since retrograde menstruation is a possible contributor to the formation of lesions, suppressing periods through progestin therapy could potentially help manage the condition or prevent further growth.

Progestin-Only Pill

When considering progestin treatments, it's essential to differentiate between combined oral pills (which contain both oestrogen and progestin) and progestin-only options which exclude oestrogen. The progestin-only option, often called 'the mini-pill', is a tablet taken at the same time, every day without a break. It's considered a slightly less effective form of contraception, though it's beneficial for those who cannot tolerate oestrogen-containing treatments, get migraines, or are over 35 and smoke.

Intrauterine System (IUS) or Intrauterine Device (IUD) - Mirena Coil or Copper Coil

Both the Intrauterine System (IUS) and Intrauterine Device (IUD) are commonly referred to as the coil. They are a small T-shaped device placed in your uterus by a healthcare professional, offering a long-term contraceptive solution that eliminates the need to remember to take a daily pill. The IUS (different to the IUD) is a plastic device that releases progestin directly into the womb. Among the various brands available, the Mirena® coil is the most used for endometriosis, which slowly releases a daily dose of progestin over five years unless you have it removed earlier. It functions as a contraceptive by inhibiting ovulation (*although not always*), thickening the cervical mucus (*making it difficult for sperm to reach an egg*), as well as thinning the lining of the womb (*making it less receptive to a fertilised egg*). The Mirena® is recommended for endo due to its effectiveness in managing heavy periods. As it reduces the thickness of the uterine lining, it can result in lighter or fewer periods; in some cases, menstruation may stop entirely. This can provide relief from PMS or period pain and potentially contribute to fibroid shrinkage. Another advantage of the IUS is progestin is released directly into the uterus, bypassing the digestive system, unlike oral contraceptives. This results in lower hormone levels detected in the blood, an amount equivalent to only taking two to three mini pills per week. Consequently, the treatment is more targeted and has fewer effects on the rest of the body.

Alternatively, the IUD, called the copper coil, is not a progestin treatment. It doesn't release hormones. Instead, copper is released into the womb. It provides contraception for 5-10 years and can be removed whenever you desire. The copper released by the IUD prevents sperm from surviving in the cervix or womb, effectively preventing pregnancy. The IUD is not usually recommended for endometriosis.

Like all forms of hormone treatment, the coil does not protect against sexually transmitted infections, so please use a condom for protection. Also, the effects of coil are reversible, so when removed, your fertility returns to normal. If you try this option, some find having the coil fitted uncomfortable or painful, so painkillers may be advised to manage any discomfort. Alternatively, the coil can be fitted during laparoscopic surgery if you wish. Initial symptoms may arise after insertion, such as mood swings, acne, headaches, nausea, or breast tenderness — these often subside after a few weeks. Taking an evening primrose oil supplement may help reduce breast tenderness. Once the coil is inserted, there is a risk of continuous or increased bleeding or spotting for up to six months. This typically transitions into lighter periods around the three-month mark. If not, speak to your doctor to discuss add-on hormones to control the bleeding in the initial months. If desired, the coil can be used during perimenopause as many find it helps manage menopausal symptoms, although it should be removed once menopause is reached.

The Contraceptive Injection: Depo-Provera®

There are a handful of contraceptive injections. In the UK, the most common is Depo-Provera®, whereby a progestin injection is given every 13 weeks, so around every three months. This makes it a convenient mid-term contraceptive option, eliminating the need to remember to take a daily pill. Depo-Provera® works as a contraceptive by suppressing ovulation, preventing your ovaries from releasing an egg, and thickening the cervical mucus, creating a barrier preventing sperm from reaching and fertilising an egg. It's highly effective when used correctly, with a 99% success rate in preventing pregnancy. However, it requires regular injections, taking your next one before the previous one expires, so if you don't remember to get your next injection, it is less effective than other methods. Once you stop the injections, it takes time for the hormone to leave the body completely. Ovulation and menstruation will not resume until the injection has fully cleared. Depending on the duration of use and how quickly a person's body metabolises the drug, it can take up to a year for fertility to return to normal after the last injection wears off. This is an important consideration for individuals planning to conceive in the near future.

Contraceptive injections like Depo-Provera® can be helpful in treating endometriosis. Reducing or even eliminating menstruation can be beneficial for those suffering from heavy or prolonged bleeding and can alleviate menstrual cramps and any associated pain. Like all other progestin treatments, this is suitable for those who cannot take oestrogen for health-related issues. It also has similar side effects, including weight gain, mood swings, and breast tenderness. Due to the potential effects on bone density, contraceptive injections may not be suitable for teenagers who have not reached peak bone mass or those with risk factors for osteoporosis (family history or certain eating disorders). This consideration should be discussed with a healthcare professional to determine the most appropriate contraceptive.

Contraceptive Implant: Nexplanon®

A contraceptive implant is a match-sized flexible plastic rod around 4 cm long placed under the skin in the upper arm by a clinician. Nexplanon® is a progestin-only implant that releases the hormone into the bloodstream slowly over three years, working as a contraceptive by preventing ovulation and thickening cervical mucus. It can be beneficial for treating heavy or prolonged periods and associated symptoms, as many people have light or no menstrual bleeding. Unlike Depo-Provera®, you don't have to schedule continual injections and unlike the coil, there is no risk of the implant falling out. This treatment allows a person to have it inserted and not think about it again, which for some, can be the swing factor in choosing this. As with all hormone treatments, there are possible side effects, including acne, headaches, nausea, breast tenderness, mood swings, or heavy or irregular bleeding. This will all depend on how your body tolerates it. The implant can be taken out at any time you wish. Your fertility will return to normal as soon as your implant is out, and it's also safe to use whilst breastfeeding, although you need to wait four weeks after giving birth.

Dienogest

Dienogest, commonly marketed under the brand name Visanne®, is a pill taken every day at the same time. It can be prescribed for the treatment of endometriosis, helping to mitigate pain and improve quality of life. Dienogest binds to progesterone receptors in various tissues, resulting in several physiological effects on the body. It can reduce the amount of menstrual bleeding and provide hormonal stability throughout the menstrual cycle. If dienogest is combined with certain oral contraceptive pills, it can suppress ovulation and therefore, work as a birth control. This reduces the production of oestradiol, which might subdue endometriosis growth.

Testosterone Derivatives

Testosterone derivatives, also known as androgenic compounds, are a class of drugs containing a synthetic version of the hormone testosterone. While not commonly prescribed as first-line treatments due to their side effects, they are sometimes used in certain cases when other treatment options have proven ineffective or intolerable. The two most used, danazol and gestrinone, are both discontinued in the UK due to adverse reactions, but they are available in the USA. Danazol and gestrinone suppress the production and activity of oestrogen, inducing a menopause-like state in the body. These drugs aim to inhibit the growth and development of endometriosis tissue, decrease associated inflammation, and alleviate symptoms. Both drugs are taken orally in tablet form. Side effects include weight gain, acne, oily skin, hair growth, mood changes, and a deepening of the voice. There can also be a risk of blood clots. All the side effects are reversible and will return to normal up to nine months after ceasing the medication. Long-term use may impact liver function and lipid profiles, necessitating regular monitoring. Testosterone derivatives are not a form of contraceptive. If you become pregnant, you should consult your doctor right away, as they shouldn't be taken when pregnant or breastfeeding.

GnRH Analogues

GnRH analogues are a second-line therapy used for endometriosis. These are heavy-duty hormone treatments, more commonly known as hormone therapy, as some are used in prostate or breast cancer treatment. They are modified synthetic versions of Gonadotropin-Releasing Hormone (GnRH), which occurs naturally in the body. These drugs bind to GnRH receptors and then through various mechanisms, suppress ovarian oestrogen production. This induces a temporary and reversible menopause state, causing endometriosis lesions to become inactive and reduce in size as they are deprived of oestrogen. All GnRH analogues are similar in what they deliver yet come in different forms and brands. For endo, they are usually prescribed in monthly injections, given in the arm, abdomen, or buttocks. Typically, you won't inject yourself; you will need to visit a doctor or nurse to receive this. For endometriosis, these drugs are only licensed to be administered for up to six months due to an increased risk of bone mineral loss or bone thinning, which is critical to prevent osteoporosis from occurring. Osteoporosis can also be caused by a lack of vitamin D and calcium, so it's worthwhile taking these as supplements whilst on these drugs to ensure your bones are getting what they need. Around the age of 30, our bones stop increasing in mass, so if your diet is insufficient in calcium, it can detrimentally take this mineral from your bones, leading to thinning. Other more frequent side effects include the classic ones we all imagine when we think of menopause: hot flushes (moments you suddenly feel very hot, sweaty, and flushed), no periods, mood swings, depression, vaginal dryness, and sleep issues, as well as headaches, weight changes, swollen ankles, dizziness, joint pain, breast changes, or tingling in hands or feet. GnRH analogues are often used in combination with add-back therapy to prevent the nasty side effects of these drugs. These are not licensed contraceptives, and if you get pregnant, there is a possibility of miscarriage or abnormalities in the baby, so non-hormonal contraception, such as a condom, is recommended. After the injections are stopped, this risk diminishes, and your fertility will not be impacted. You might be prescribed GnRH analogues prior to planned complex surgery as part of your surgical preparation or for severe symptoms when other hormone treatments are not right for you. These drugs aim to reduce menstrual bleeding and associated symptoms like pain, although they come with hefty side effects, so the benefits must outweigh these. Please speak with your doctor about any concerns to ensure they are the best choice for you. When the course of injections is finished, oestrogen levels will rise, and periods will return to normal within 6-10 weeks. The most used GnRH analogues to treat endometriosis are listed below. Drugs have multiple names, as there are the medication names and the brand names, so it can be a bit confusing, but this should make it clear:

- Leuprorelin (Prostap®, Lupron Depot®)
- Goserelin (Zoladex®)
- Nafarelin (Synarel®)
- Buserelin (Suprecur®)
- Triptorelin (Decapeptyl®)

GnRH Antagonist - Elagolix

Elagolix is a GnRH antagonist that targets the GnRH receptor similarly to GnRH analogues, such as Lupron®. However, it directly blocks the receptors, offering a more immediate and potent suppression of oestrogen. This means the initial worsening of symptoms or 'flare' that can be experienced with analogues, does not occur. Both types of drugs induce a temporary menopause-like state known as medical menopause and have similar overall results in the context of endometriosis treatment and their side effects. They can provide symptom relief for moderate to severe pain, including painful periods, painful sex, and pelvic pain. Although periods typically return to normal quicker when you cease your treatment with antagonists compared to analogues. Elagolix is a pill taken daily, which is more convenient than GnRH analogues as they require injections. Nevertheless, elagolix also cannot be taken long-term due to adverse effects, the main risk regarding bone density. Other examples of GnRH antagonist drugs used for endometriosis include linzagolix and relugolix. Brand names include Myfembree® and Orlissa®.

Hormone Replacement Therapy (HRT)

Hormone Replacement Therapy (HRT) is a treatment using low doses of synthetic oestrogen, progesterone, or tibolone. It's commonly used during natural perimenopause or menopause as a treatment to alleviate symptoms. The same use is applied when medical menopause is induced from drugs like Prostap® but is often referred to as 'add-back' medication because it adds back a small amount of oestrogen and progesterone into the body, which has otherwise been suppressed by hormone therapy. This might seem counterintuitive, but this still results in a lower amount of these hormones than what would be found naturally. The doses are carefully formulated, ensuring they are small enough to not interfere with the effectiveness of GnRH antagonists or agonists, both of which can have significant side effects due to the substantial reduction of oestrogen levels in the body. Therefore, gynaecologists recommend add-back therapy alongside hormone therapy to allow patients to benefit from suppressing their endometriosis (for symptom control or surgery) while minimising the intensity of the side effects. Although add-back therapy may not be capable of eliminating these symptoms, it can still significantly improve the quality of life for individuals on GnRH agonists/antagonists.

Additionally, you can take HRT during perimenopause to help manage bothersome symptoms, particularly if you have a family history of osteoporosis, as it can limit menopause-related bone loss. It may also be recommended after surgical menopause, whereby oestrogen levels suddenly drop after an operation, such as a hysterectomy. HRT, in this instance, helps to replace the oestrogen your ovaries made. In such cases, it manages the abrupt onset of menopausal symptoms, which can be severe. Maintaining adequate levels of oestrogen can be important for reducing the risk of health problems developing, such as heart disease, stroke, and diabetes.

HRT is administered in various forms, including tablets, patches, gels, or sprays. For endometriosis, tibolone is often prescribed as a daily tablet. If your gynaecologist did not prescribe add-back therapy and you are on

GnRH agonists/antagonists, or if you are approaching perimenopause, it's worth discussing with your healthcare provider. Remember, HRT should always be prescribed and monitored by a professional who can evaluate your condition, consider your specific needs and risks, and determine the most suitable regimen for you.

Aromatase Inhibitors (AI)

Aromatase, an enzyme found naturally in our bodies, is pivotal in trans-forming male sex hormones, like testosterone, into the female sex hormone, oestrogen. This conversion process is vital for maintaining the delicate hormonal balance in both males and females. Oestrogen is mainly synthesised in the ovaries, but also in a lesser amount in our adrenal glands and fat cells through the assistance of aromatase activity. For those of reproductive age, the ovaries are the primary source of oestrogen; however, during post-menopause, when ovarian hormone production ceases, oestrogen production shifts to fat cells and the adrenal glands. In endometriosis, aromatase activity increases as the lesions have a large amount of this enzyme in them. This is likely due to inflammation and oestrogen being linked in a positive feedback cycle, which enhances the presence of aromatase in lesions. The heightened aromatase activity allows lesions to generate their own local oestrogen, vital for growth and survival, while circumventing the need for ovarian oestradiol (a type of oestrogen).

Aromatase inhibitors are a form of hormone therapy typically used for cancer treatment and are administered in pill form. They are designed to block the pathway and inhibit the action of aromatase, suppressing oestrogen production in the body. This can stabilise endometriosis lesions, inhibiting their growth, reducing inflammation, and consequently alleviating pain. Aromatase inhibitors are not typically used as a first-line treatment for endometriosis. Instead, they are often considered for cases of severe endometriosis in instances where other treatments have proven ineffective or unsuitable. The two main aromatase inhibitor drugs used for endo are letrozole and anastrozole. They both yield similar effects; one is not better than the other, but they come with different side effects, which may react differently from person to person. Aromatase inhibitors are for individuals who have gone through natural menopause. Although they can also be used in combination with drugs that inhibit ovulation by suppressing the ovaries, such as the pill or a GnRH agonist. They should *not* be taken alone if you are premenopausal, as the ovaries are still producing oestrogen, so they can encourage the growth of ovarian cysts.

Potential side effects include hot flushes, osteoporosis, bone pain, back pain, vaginal dryness, sexual dysfunction, and nausea. These drugs are not suitable if you are pregnant. Taking extra care of your bone health is recommended by taking a vitamin D supplement at 100-1200 IU/ day and calcium if your intake is otherwise low whilst on aromatase inhibitors. It would be best if you also increased weight-bearing exercise, which requires you to be on your feet to increase your bone density. This can be low impact, like going for a brisk walk, or if you can, a more effective option is weight training.

39

Endometriosis Surgery

Surgery aims to remove endometriosis lesions, scar tissue, and adhesions, as well as restore the anatomy of organs to improve functionality and symptoms. Surgical treatments for endometriosis are typically performed laparoscopically, although occasionally larger cuts in the abdomen are required, called a laparotomy. This is a risk with all surgeries, but it is less common. Robotic-assisted surgery is also on an upward trend, whereby the surgeon uses a robotic device to carry out the operation — cool right? In Part 2, we outlined the process of standard diagnostic surgery. If surgeons need to operate on complicated or intricate areas, planned complex surgery can be required after diagnosis. Unlike hormonal treatments, surgery removes or destroys endometriosis and adhesions, which can be used to improve symptoms and fertility. While a general gynaecologist can conduct diagnostic surgery or treat mild cases of endo, for advanced stages where surgery is highly complex, or if surgery is to treat infertility, expertise from a specialised gynaecologist is required. A practitioner with relevant experience and proficiency in specialised techniques will be able to provide the most effective treatment. This is due to the risk of damaging other organs or structures in nearby affected areas and from removing scar tissue. Moreover, attaining specialists from different fields, such as urology, may be necessary. Surgery will typically last between one to two hours for mild to moderate endometriosis and up to four hours for severe or deep endometriosis. The less that symptoms are controllable with painkillers or medications, the more likely that surgery will become a desirable route. Through proper excision, endometriosis may not grow back where it has been removed (although no surgical procedure guarantees complete prevention of regrowth), so once your body has had time to heal, symptoms should improve. If they continue, endometriosis may still be present in the body, although symptoms can often be caused by something else such as persistent nerve irritation or pelvic floor spasms. Symptoms may resurface years after surgery due to incomplete removal of endometriosis or because the disease has relapsed. Therefore, while surgery may be one of the tools used for healing, understanding that it's not a quick fix guaranteed to solve all your problems is essential.

Laparoscopy Techniques

There are two main surgical techniques used to remove or destroy endo tissue, called ablation and excision. Both methods are minimally invasive, and either may be used during surgery. There is some debate on the effectiveness of ablation for long-term improvements. Some hospitals choose only to use excision as it's the gold standard of treatment for all stages, meaning it's the best treatment option on offer. Overall, the choice of surgical technique depends on the extent and location of endometriosis, the patient's preferences, and the surgeon's expertise.

Ablation

Ablation, also known as cauterisation or fulguration, is a technique used to remove endometriosis tissue by applying intense heat through diathermy or laser energy to burn off or melt away lesions. While it can provide temporary symptom relief and effectively remove visible tissue, ablation may not fully eliminate the disease. Lesions can grow deeper beneath the surface, yet ablation only targets the visible surface, potentially leaving a significant amount untreated. As a superficial procedure, ablation is not competent in treating deep endometriosis as it leaves much of the tissue behind. If any endometriosis tissue remains, symptoms may persist after surgery. The main advantage of ablation is its quick and straightforward nature, and it doesn't require additional specialised training like excision does. Even so, a higher recurrence rate of endometriosis is sometimes reported after ablation compared to excision, although this depends on a variety of factors.[1] This means it may not be an effective long-term solution as it might only provide temporary symptom improvement. If lesions reappear within the first few years after surgery, it may suggest they were incompletely removed.[2] Furthermore, ablation should only be used where it's safe to burn, making it often unsuitable for certain tissues, including the ovary, uterus, bladder, and diaphragm, due to the risks of damaging these and impairing organ function. For individuals with an endometrioma who wish to preserve fertility, ablation should be used with caution. The ovaries are delicate structures responsible for producing eggs and hormones. Ablation can damage the ovarian tissue, potentially compromising ovarian function and reducing infertility. In such cases, excision is usually recommended to preserve as much healthy ovarian tissue as possible, which is crucial for those aiming to conceive. Additionally, burning tissue during ablation can cause cell damage, which increases the risk of scar tissue and adhesions, another potential for hindering fertility. Although this is debatable as evidence suggests ablation surgery techniques still improved pregnancy rates by ~50% for mild endo cases.[3] Another drawback of ablation is that it destroys endometriosis tissue, making it difficult or impossible to obtain a biopsy for an accurate diagnosis.

While there are cases where ablation is still deemed suitable for certain lesions, it's important to consider this technique's limitations and potential drawbacks.

Excision

Excision is the recommended surgical technique for treatment. Unlike ablation techniques, which burn or destroy the surface of the lesions, excision involves cutting out the lesions alongside a small amount of healthy tissue. As this method allows the surgeon to go deeper, it's better suited for treating deep deposits of endometriosis. A key advantage of excision is that it can completely remove the disease. This provides better treatment for inflammation in the affected area and allows for organ reconstruction and restoration of functionality. Consequently, excision is often the preferred method for complex surgeries. Statistically, excision leads to better symptom improvement compared to ablation techniques, including painful periods, painful bowel movements, and chronic pelvic pain.[4] Since tissue is more likely to be fully removed, the likelihood of it growing back in the same place is reduced. This can increase the time between surgeries as it provides symptom reduction for a longer period. In fact, a study indicated that after five years of excision surgery, only 19% of patients experienced recurrent or persistent disease.[5] However, it's important to note that for any endometriosis not detected or completely removed throughout the body, there is a risk that symptoms will remain or return. Excision surgery is generally considered more favourable for individuals who wish to preserve their fertility. By precisely removing endometriosis lesions whilst preserving healthy tissue and organs, excision minimises the risk of damage to reproductive organs like the ovaries and uterus. Compared to ablation techniques, excision offers a more comprehensive and effective approach to treating endo. Excision surgery also requires specialised training and greater expertise due to its intricate nature. Surgeons who have undergone this training are more skilled at accurately identifying and removing endometriosis, which can be crucial to ensure effective surgery.

Even though it is preferable to have your surgeon operate with excision, this isn't always possible for some lesions, and ablation will therefore be used. An endo specialist will know when each method is needed.

Complex Surgery

Part 2 provided an in-depth look at diagnostic surgery and the laparoscopic procedure, so if you skipped that part but want to learn more about the basics of surgery, please revert to that chapter. Now let's focus on the post-diagnosis stage, specifically if you require complex surgery. You will need diagnostic tests beforehand, including scans such as an MRI. This helps surgeons better understand how endometriosis is affecting your body, enabling them to plan a safe and well-executed treatment and ensure the right team of professionals are in the operating room. You may have multiple tests or procedures, as most scans cannot reveal everything, and your surgeons are striving to gain the best possible understanding of what's happening inside your body before proceeding. Complex surgeries can last many hours, with surgeons working tirelessly to achieve the best outcome for their patients. They will try to minimise the need for future surgeries due to the risk of new adhesions forming, as these can lead to more pain, obstruction, or fertility issues. The success rates of complex surgery depend on many factors, including the extent of the disease, the chance of complications, and the surgeon's skills. Doctors often advise taking a hormone treatment of some kind to prolong the benefits of surgery and further manage symptoms. This is your choice; you don't have to if you do not want to. In the NHS, the Mirena® Coil is generally recommended, but you can choose any of the hormone options outlined earlier. After surgery, it will take a short while before you feel back to normal again.

Ovarian Endometrioma Surgery

Ovarian endometriomas don't typically respond to medical therapy alone (treatments like medication). If you decide to wait to operate, it's usually recommended to not wait forever because the cyst may continue to grow, rupture, or cause adhesions. These complications can lead to increased pain or a more complex surgery in the future. Surgical removal of endometriomas is the gold standard and is typically necessary, particularly if the cyst is larger than 4cm or if you are having difficulty conceiving, as removal can improve fertility rates.[1] However, it's essential to discuss your individualised risks with your doctor as surgery may reduce your ovarian reserve or, in some cases, result in the loss of an ovary, particularly if you've previously had ovarian surgery.[2] Generally, it's not recommended to have surgery before Assisted Reproductive Technology (ART) procedures as it doesn't significantly improve success rates in these cases.

Surgeons remove endometriomas through a procedure called an ovarian cystectomy. The specific technique used depends on the size and location of the cyst, as well as the surgeon's expertise and the patient's circumstances. It can be a challenging procedure as surgeons want to preserve as much of the healthy ovarian tissue as possible whilst still ensuring all the endo tissue has been removed. For treatment, cysts are drained, and the cyst wall is removed intact, preferably through excision. This ensures complete removal of the endometrioma, which is crucial for preventing recurrence, minimising the need for future ovarian surgeries that could further diminish ovarian reserve. Some surgeons advocate for excision-only techniques, whilst others opt for a combined cystectomy using both ablation and excision. Speak to your surgeon prior to surgery to understand what technique they plan to use and the reasons behind their choice. After removing the endometrioma, the surgeon will control any bleeding and ensure proper closure of the ovarian tissue.

Endometriomas are often associated with severe pain, heavy periods, and painful sex — surgery is commonly successful in being able to treat these. Depending on the size of the cyst, endometriomas can often cause uncomfortable bloating or a heavy, dragging feeling. Surgery should also minimise this as the enlarged ovary is now closer to normal size, and over time, after healing occurs, inflammation will reduce, further decreasing any bloating (a welcoming thought for many I'm sure).

Bowel Surgery

Bowel surgery for endometriosis is a complex and delicate procedure. It should be carried out at a specialist centre after presurgical mapping of the disease via MRI. It's the most common treatment option when other conservative methods, such as pain medication or hormone treatments, have failed to provide sufficient relief, particularly if you experience obstructive symptoms. Unfortunately, if left untreated, bowel endometriosis can worsen over time, making surgery a crucial intervention. It can cause a range of debilitating symptoms, including abdominal pain, bloating, constipation, diarrhoea, and rectal bleeding. In some cases, bowel movements may become extremely painful, leading to a significant decline in quality of life. Bowel surgery aims to restore normal bowel function and ease the associated discomfort. A thorough evaluation is conducted beforehand to assess the extent of endo on the bowel to better understand the disease's severity and guide the surgical approach. Prior to surgery, you may also be asked to take hormone therapy or a type of GnRH drug to put you into medical menopause, though this is typically discontinued after surgery. Bowel preparation is required just before the procedure which involves taking a laxative to empty the bowel and reduce the risk of infection — this will be taken either at home or at the hospital. There are different types of laxatives the hospital can provide; some require drinking a lot of fluid, whilst others are given in pill form. Once you are in theatre, your surgeon will get to work on removing the endometriosis tissue and adhesions. Bowel endo can cause extensive damage to the surrounding pelvic structures, so the surgeon will also work to repair these. Studies have shown there are significantly more nerve fibres found in intestinal deep endometriosis than in other DIE locations, contributing to severe pain.[1] If possible, surgeons will remove any nerve-entrapped scar tissue to provide long-term pain relief. Various surgical techniques can be used, so the extent of the disease will determine the approach chosen by your surgeon, taking into consideration the size of your lesions, how many there are, as well as the length and grade of infiltration into the bowel wall. Lesions can be superficial, found on the surface of the bowel, or deep lesions will penetrate through the wall. Superficial lesions might be shaved off so as not to damage the organ, although this could leave residual endometriosis behind. Surgeons may instead decide to excise lesions from the bowel and close any resulting hole. In more severe cases where extensive disease or damage is present, a segment or section of the bowel may need to be removed, followed by a re-anastomosis, where the two healthy ends of the bowel are re-joined. If the operation is particularly complex, open surgery may be necessary, where a larger incision is made into the abdomen, allowing surgeons more room to operate successfully. Precision and care are key during surgery to avoid complications, given the bowels' vital role in digestion and waste elimination. Sometimes, a temporary stoma is required to allow time for the bowel to heal (described later in 'Possible Complications'). Your surgeon will discuss your individualised risk of needing a stoma, although it's rare to require a permanent stoma.

These operations are long and complicated, so you will have an extended recovery time compared to diagnostic surgery, and you may spend more time in the hospital. You will have a catheter in place overnight to drain your bladder, and you may experience nausea and vomiting, but you will be provided anti-sickness medication if so. A gentle laxative may also be given to prevent constipation. The time needed for recovery varies from person to person, but you'll likely need at least a month. It's common to experience discomfort, fatigue, and bowel irregularities during the initial recovery period.

If a bowel resection is performed, you may experience Low Anterior Resection Syndrome (LARS), which involves changes in your bowel function such as urgency, frequency, incontinence, or loose stools. This is primarily due to having less space to store your stool. LARS can last 6-12 months before proper functioning is regained. This can be frustrating and horrible to deal with, but it does get better with time. Your body has gone through a lot, so be nice to yourself. Food and nutrition can be helpful tools for managing LARS and promoting bowel health during recovery. The presenting symptoms can guide nutritional choices; for those experiencing diarrhoea, more bulking foods are necessary, whereas constipation requires fibre-rich meals. Foods that many find troublesome are outlined below, although each person is different, so you should manage your diet through trial and error to find out what you individually can or cannot tolerate. Over time, you may be able to reintroduce foods that initially caused issues.

Potentially Troublesome Foods	Alcohol, Caffeine (including chocolate), Red Meat (including pork), Fried Food, Nuts, Seeds, Cabbage, Broccoli, Cauliflower, Spicy Food, Dairy, Legumes, Corn (including popcorn)

Even if you don't have a bowel resection or a colostomy bag, ensure you eat a healthy diet during recovery to help your body heal. A bowel-friendly diet can prevent constipation and improve your microbiome. The NHS recommends following a low-fibre diet for the first 4-6 weeks post-surgery, then slowly reintroducing high-fibre foods. Some examples are listed below.

High-Fibre Options	
Protein	Almonds, Beans, Lentils, Quinoa
Carbohydrates	Wholemeal Bread, Brown Pasta and Rice, Bran, Oats
Fruit	Raspberries, Dates, Blueberries
Vegetable	Asparagus, Sweetcorn, Cabbage

Low-Fibre Options	
Meat	Fish, Poultry, Ham, Bacon, Shellfish
Other Protein	Eggs, Tofu, Smooth Peanut Butter
Carbohydrates	Mashed Potatoes, White Bread, White Rice, Pasta
Dairy	Butter, Milk, Cheese
Fruit	Kiwi, Apple, Peaches, Melon, Nectarines, Papayas (all required to be peeled)
Vegetable	Carrots, Cucumber, Broccoli (no stalk), Lettuce Tomato Sauce (without skins or seeds)

Remember to stay hydrated, ideally with water, but whatever way works best for you. It can be a lot to get used to at first, but the good news is long-term outcomes are generally positive, with low recurrence rates, improved pregnancy rates, and many patients having no major complications.[2] Whilst your bowels heal, if you experience faecal incontinence, you may find carrying wet wipes or a change of underwear around with you provides some peace of mind. Overall, surgery can provide relief from symptoms and improve quality of life, though recovery often requires patience, care, and dietary adjustments.

Surgery for Rectovaginal Endometriosis

Rectovaginal endometriosis involves part of the bowel; however, it's the last section of the large intestine called the rectum, as well as the vagina in a space called the rectovaginal septum. Please read the previous chapter for more information on bowel-related surgery.

This is one of the most severe and painful forms of the disease, capable of causing distortions to the anatomy in the area. Still, surgery can be an incredible tool for treating rectovaginal endo. Due to the location, it's a challenging place to operate, so surgery should only be performed by an experienced surgeon who specialises in this area and has the appropriate expertise. BSGE Endometriosis Centres were founded on the premise that better surgical procedures were required for this type of endo. Even with their remarkable advances, this focus is still at the core of their work. If you skipped Part 2, I recommend going back to read about these centres if you are based in Britain. Various surgical techniques can be employed for rectovaginal endometriosis, depending on the severity and location of the tissue, as well as other factors individual to the patient's health status. Techniques may include excision, resection, or shaving of endometriosis lesions, along with the restoration of anatomical structures. The surgeon will determine the most appropriate approach for each case. As with any surgical procedure, there are potential risks and complications associated. Your surgeon will go through any you need to be aware of, but these typically involve bowel injury, a stoma, bladder damage, or ureteric injury. These risks are low, but this is why you will want a capable doctor to ensure you are in the best hands. You may require GnRH-based hormone therapy for around three months prior to surgery, and you will often need a bowel prep the night before. Your surgeons will use a nerve-sparing laparoscopic technique, which allows for minimal impact on your urinary and bowel function, limiting risks of bladder, rectal, or sexual dysfunction. You will likely need to stay in the hospital overnight, and you may have a catheter in for longer than diagnostic surgery. Ureteric stents will also be inserted into your ureters during the operation, described in more detail in

Chapter 41. Following the operation, you may have nausea and vomiting, but your nurse will be there to look after you. You may also experience increased pain, but you will be provided medication to ease this and a stool softener is often given to alleviate constipation. As this can be one of the most incapacitating forms of the disease, surgery can have a huge role in regaining quality of life and improving symptoms such as pain, fatigue, nausea, and heavy periods.

Urological Surgery for Urinary Tract Endometriosis

Urological surgery addresses issues in the bladder, ureters (the tube that connects the bladder to the kidneys), and the kidneys. The bladder is the most common site to be affected in the urological system, although, to be clear, endo on the bladder is relatively uncommon. Symptoms include bladder urgency or blood in the urine. As with all locations, lesions may be superficial or invade the organ's wall. It's unclear why some people get endo in these areas whilst most don't. In some cases, lesions from other locations can entangle with the urological system. For instance, the ureter, which runs down the side of the pelvis, can become compressed or pinched by an endometriosis lesion on the pelvic sidewall. If these lesions are DIE phenotypes, they can narrow the ureters, leading to kidney issues due to the flow of urine being obstructed. Interestingly, patients with a retroverted uterus are less likely to develop bladder endometriosis and if ureteral endometriosis is present, it's more commonly found on the left side due to anatomical differences in the pelvic structure.[1]

Treatment for urological endometriosis involves different approaches depending on the location and severity. A multidisciplinary team involving a gynaecologist, urologist, and sometimes a colorectal surgeon is required, who will work closely together to plan and execute your surgery. A high level of skill is required to operate on complex areas like these, ensuring they can preserve the integrity and function of your organs and tissues like the ureters, which are delicate structures. If endometriosis involves the bladder, a partial cystectomy may be necessary, whereby part of the bladder is removed to effectively eliminate the tissue. The bladder is then stitched up and restored. This can cause bladder capacity to be reduced, resulting in a need to urinate more frequently or urgently.

During gynaecological laparoscopic surgeries, a catheter is inserted into the urethra to allow urine to flow out of the body and into a bag. In most cases, the catheter is removed before a patient wakes up, but for urological surgery, it may be left in place for a few days. You may also require an x-ray of the bladder, called a cystogram, at a later date to ensure the bladder has healed. Once the catheter is removed, normal urination should resume, but if you experience any difficulties, the catheter may be reinserted to ensure proper urine flow. Sometimes, patients are required to go home with the catheter. This is a temporary measure, giving your body additional time to heal. You will be provided with care instructions by the hospital, please follow them to avoid infection. Drinking plenty of fluid is recommended to prevent bladder infections from occurring.

In addition to a catheter, narrow silicone tubes, called ureteric stents, may be placed in the ureters during surgery. These stents provide semi-rigidity to the ureters, reducing the risk of the surgeon inadvertently injuring them during the procedure. These are removed before you wake up; however, there are instances where they are left in place for a few weeks, which we discuss later. After surgery, it's normal to experience urine stained with blood, this may be alarming, but generally, it's not painful. If any issues or symptoms arise, you must communicate them to your nurse or doctor.

The success of the surgery will depend on the location and extent of the disease. Although complex surgeries carry greater risks, such as bladder damage, these occurrences are uncommon. Your surgeon will review your individualised risks and potential benefits to help you make an informed decision. Choosing the right surgeon or hospital can significantly improve your symptoms and bring an end to many of your issues. You don't need to have surgery if you have urological endo, this is your choice. However, if your symptoms include changes in pain during urination, back pressure, or any indication there is irritation to your kidneys, you should seek treatment to prevent irreparable kidney damage occurring. Damage to the urological system is often silent, so take any symptoms seriously and seek medical help if they occur, as urological endo can cause hydronephrosis or kidney failure, but surgery can limit this. Your doctor will be able to provide personalised advice and guidance.

40

Hysterectomy

A hysterectomy is a surgical procedure involving the partial or total removal of the female reproductive organs. It's the second most common surgery for women, the first being a caesarean section.[1] In the US, endometriosis pain is a leading reason for women choosing a hysterectomy as a form of treatment.[2] It's essential to understand that a hysterectomy is a non-reversible procedure, so comprehending its short and long-term effects on the body is crucial before making any decisions. Most hysterectomies are elective, meaning you must request one. Your doctor should not be proposing you have a hysterectomy as treatment for endometriosis unless there is a valid and specific reason unique to your situation. You can select the type of hysterectomy you undergo, but your doctor will offer advice based on the most appropriate option for you, your expectations, and medical history. The different types of hysterectomies are outlined on the next page.

Total Hysterectomy	• Removal of the uterus and cervix. • The most common type.
Subtotal Hysterectomy	• Removal of the uterus but the cervix remains. • Periods sometimes continue until menopause.
Total Hysterectomy with Bilateral Salpingo-Oophorectomy	• Removal of the uterus, cervix, fallopian tubes, and ovaries. • Bilateral means both sides of the uterus are operated on, so both fallopian tubes and both ovaries. • You can decide to have only one side of your ovaries and fallopian tubes removed.
Radical Hysterectomy	• Removal of the uterus, cervix, fallopian tubes, ovaries, and surrounding tissues including lymph glands and fatty tissue. • This is an extensive procedure not typically used for endo, it's primarily performed on those with cancer to ensure all of the disease is removed.

A hysterectomy is not a cure for endometriosis. It's a cure for adenomyosis because this condition has tissue invading the uterine wall. If you remove the uterus, you will be unable to regain disease in something that is no longer in the body. As there is a relationship between individuals experiencing both endometriosis and adenomyosis, having a hysterectomy for adenomyosis cannot guarantee endometriosis won't recur or develop in other parts of the body. If you choose to have a hysterectomy, it's crucial your surgeon addresses any endometriosis tissue present in the body during the same procedure. This maximises your chances of a successful surgery with notable symptom reduction and satisfaction. Nonetheless, this can be a daunting decision as there is no guarantee you will feel better.

A hysterectomy can be chosen for various reasons. Some people have had multiple surgeries that were unsuccessful in providing relief, leaving them drained after spending years in relentless excruciating pain, and the impact on their mental health, career, family life, and quality of life has reached its limit, so they see it as their only way out. Others might recognise their symptoms are specifically related to their uterus, so a hysterectomy may bring them needed relief. If a significant portion of a patient's pain is related to uterine cramping and the menstrual period itself, a hysterectomy may provide remission. Furthermore, adenomyosis and uterine fibroids may also be present, which can be a tormenting combination, so a hysterectomy becomes a last-resort treatment option when other methods have failed. Living with a life-altering disease, whereby symptoms have persisted despite surgeries, and all other treatment options have been explored with no avail, can cause profound emotional distress.

For many, a hysterectomy represents their last hope. Endo can have detrimental long-term effects on a person's wellbeing and spirit, leaving this is a drastic decision faced by many plagued by the disease. Fortunately, studies show this procedure provides improvements for women, including long-term pain reduction; however, this isn't promised.[3] A hysterectomy should never be the first treatment option or recommended for those who wish to start a family, as pregnancy is not possible without a uterus. If you are interested in having biological children through surrogacy, it may be possible to receive IVF for egg retrieval prior. Of course, adoption is always an option after this operation if you choose to have a family that way.

As with all operations, there are possible surgical risks and complications. These are rare but include heavy bleeding, infection, and damage to the bladder or bowel. The recovery process after a hysterectomy is significant. Typically, you will stay in the hospital for 3-5 days, and a full recovery can take around 6-8 weeks. The speed at which you heal can be influenced by factors such as age and overall health. During this time, it's crucial to rest and refrain from lifting anything heavy, including groceries or children. Gentle exercise can aid in the recovery process, but sexual activity should be avoided for about six weeks or until your doctor confirms it's safe. This is necessary to allow your abdominal muscles and tissues to heal properly.

All forms of hysterectomy pose the possibility of entering menopause earlier than you would have naturally. If your ovaries are removed, you can decide whether that's one or both. If both ovaries are removed, you will go through menopause immediately after the operation, called surgical menopause. This will include all the typical side effects of natural menopause, from vaginal dryness to decreased libido. Hormone Replacement Therapy (HRT) may be offered to reinstate some of the hormones lost from removing the ovaries. Typically, the lowest effective dose of oestrogen, sometimes combined with progesterone, is used to mitigate the symptoms. Natural menopause occurs over several years, whilst surgical menopause produces a sharp drop in oestrogen capable of causing severe symptoms. HRT should reduce this whilst alleviating the risks associated with premature loss of oestrogen, such as bone thinning. Your doctor will select a dose that is not high enough to stimulate endo tissue growth.

It's essential to understand that a hysterectomy has lifelong consequences for a person's health. There are increased health risks associated, ranging from obesity to dementia to heart disease. Regardless of your age, undergoing a hysterectomy is a significant decision. It can be amazing for some people and not suitable for others. Importantly, people 30 years or under are more likely to regret their decision, and this should be discussed with your doctor.[4] Endo Warriors choosing such a drastic surgery to relieve their pain underpins the importance of investment into medical research to improve the lives of those with endometriosis.

41

Surgery Care

On the day of your surgery, you will be given a robe and compression stockings to wear and a bed to relax on until you're called for your operation. Various medical professionals will come to speak to you, including surgeons, nurses, and anaesthesiologists. They will explain the procedure and ask if you have any questions. This is your opportunity to share any concerns or queries and get the answers you need so that you go into surgery feeling reassured. For example, before my first op to treat my endometrioma, I told the doctor I didn't want my ovary removed, to which he reassured me they would try and preserve the ovary as much as possible. I also inquired if the incision in my belly button would cut through the hole of my piercing, and he informed me it wouldn't (in case anyone else reading this wants to know). You could ask whether it's possible to see photos of your surgery afterwards — it's super interesting to look inside your body and see the thing that has been causing you so much pain but until now was invisible. It's good to save these in your records, alongside any doctors' letters and notes, in a folder for any future treatments you may require.

Make sure you get prepared before having any operation. There is an upcoming checklist of all the actions you might consider doing around the house or items you perhaps need to buy before heading to the hospital so that you are prepared for when you return home. I've also listed items to consider bringing to the hospital to make the best of your stay. Your hospital will provide the relevant information for your operation at your pre-op appointment, but it can be helpful to see what Endo Warriors suggest from their experiences. Before my first operation, I scoured checklists on forums to get clued up on what essentials to have, like peppermint tea or lozenges — items I never contemplated needing as I had never had an operation before. Peppermint tea can soothe gas pain resulting from having your abdomen inflated during a laparoscopic procedure. This can range from mildly uncomfortable to sharp and painful, but peppermint tea can help until it naturally dissipates with time. The lozenges are for your throat, as it may be dry and scratchy from the breathing tube inserted in your nose or throat during the operation, which maintains your breathing and oxygen levels once you are unconscious.

Although many operations are day surgeries, meaning you should be in and out of the hospital within the same day, bring an overnight bag with the bare essentials in case of any changes. Some surgeries require a longer stay at the hospital, but you will be advised of this at your pre-op appointment. Being prepared will make your recovery as smooth as possible. Find a friend or family member you trust to help and provide support, as you must have someone pick you up from the hospital and take you home in a car or taxi. You are not allowed to drive until at least 24 hours after the operation due to the anaesthesia. It would be best if you also had someone stay overnight with you after your operation. If you have children, arrange for someone to look after them for a few days; this includes doing the school run and cooking dinner. You will be exhausted from the operation and there's the inevitable pain or tenderness, so plan easy-to-cook food or pre-prepared meals that require little energy to cook and clean up after. Diet can be a valuable part of your recovery, so ensure you eat healthy nutritious meals. This is particularly important if you have bowel surgery or a bowel cleanse so we can get your gut health back to optimum. It's also good to be aware that after having general anaesthesia, you may have emotional bouts where you feel sad or need to cry. This is perfectly normal; ride the wave and speak to someone who can support you. This will pass after a short while, and your emotions will return to normal.

After Surgery

When you wake up from surgery, you will be in the recovery room. You may feel slight pain or nausea, but a medical professional will be there to look after you. Always tell someone if you are not feeling good. You will then be moved back to the ward but will likely be asleep for most of this. When you wake up properly, you may initially feel a little groggy. You will experience bleeding, but a large sanitary towel will be in place, so there's nothing to worry about. At some point, your surgeon will come and speak to you to explain their findings. You will be drowsy and may not remember all the information, but you will receive a letter from the hospital to go home with. Your surgeon may suggest a further operation if they were unable to remove all the affected tissue. During the procedure, a catheter is inserted in your bladder to collect urine and a cannula is placed in your hand to receive liquid drugs. Both will be removed when you're ready to go home. Although sometimes, particularly in the case of mild to moderate excision surgery, the catheter will be removed at the end of your operation, so you wouldn't know it had ever been there. Before being discharged, you must be able to pee normally (i.e., on the toilet without a catheter). Your nurse will not be able to let you go home otherwise. Urinary retention is common and can be caused by anaesthesia, inflammation, or medication, making it harder to pee, although this is more common in males and those who are older. Any trouble peeing should usually resolve on its own.

Recovery

After your operation, expect to have downtime for a short while. Recovery time varies depending on the person, the procedure, and if there were any complications. You may feel fine to return to work after two weeks, whilst others will need at least a month to feel normal again. Please do not push yourself to feel better sooner, it's not a race. For treatment for mild or superficial endometriosis, recovery should be quicker. As you recuperate, you will feel fatigued for the first few days and will probably be in and out of sleep. Let your body get this rest. Just because you cannot see the healing taking place inside your body doesn't mean it's not there.

Your hospital will provide after-care instructions for you to go home with. Follow these all carefully and to the letter to avoid infections occurring. You will have two or more small cuts in your abdomen or, in some cases, a larger incision; these must be kept covered and dry for a few days. You will not be able to wash, have sex, or exercise straight away, but your hospital will provide any relevant advice. You will be able to shower sooner than you can have a bath, but until you can bathe properly, wet wipes or a flannel can be used. To aid your healing, eat nutritious food, stay hydrated, and gently exercise. This is to get your body moving, limit muscle weakening, and improve circulation to prevent blood clots. The best exercise is walking a couple of times a day, and you can do small movements whilst sitting, such as moving your feet in a circle or bending your leg in and out. You should avoid heavy lifting, stretching, or intense exercise.

During recovery, have a positive outlook, believing your surgery was successful and that you are getting better each and every day. Endorsing positivity in your recovery can reduce stress, which reduces inflammation. Importantly, studies show there are many benefits of having optimism in surgery recovery, both in the short and long term. Positivity can affect how well and fast a patient recovers, reducing any possible symptoms. It's not clear as to why this works. Similarly, we don't quite understand the mechanisms of how a placebo drug works. Naturally, if you don't feel good do not ignore that, but choosing to have hope can be helpful.

Possible Complications

Infection

If you experience oozing, bleeding, or itching from your incisions, or if they are red and sore, this could indicate an infection, which is treatable with antibiotics. If you have severe pain, fever, lose your appetite, are vomiting, or feel faint or dizzy, this denotes something is wrong. In both instances, call your hospital. You will be given a leaflet with a number to call for these such cases. Your doctor may wish to see you face-to-face on the same day, and this may require a hospital readmission.

Urine Infection

If your urine is burning or stinging, or you need to pass it more often, this may indicate a urine infection. Call your doctor, as this can easily be treated with a course of antibiotics.

Deep Vein Thrombosis (DVT) or Pulmonary Embolism (PE)

Deep Vein Thrombosis (DVT) is a blood clot which most commonly forms in the leg or pelvis and poses a risk following surgery. Other contributing factors include contraceptive pill usage, smoking, or diabetes. Symptoms may manifest as swelling in the leg that is painful, hot, or difficult to bear weight on. A Pulmonary Embolism (PE) occurs when a blood clot becomes dislodged and moves through your circulation until it reaches the lungs, leading to symptoms such as coughing up blood-stained phlegm, chest pain, and breathlessness. DVT or PE can be fatal and requires urgent medical attention and a trip to your local A&E. To mitigate this risk, continue to wear compression stockings and engage in regular movement to promote circulation.

Ureteric Stents

During surgery, narrow silicone tubes called ureteric stents may be inserted into your ureters. These flexible tubes provide support to your ureters whilst aiding the surgeon in the safe removal of endometriosis. They also serve as a precautionary measure to safeguard ureters against potential damage or cuts during your procedure, ensuring that you maintain uninterrupted urine flow even if there is damage. Stents are typically removed before you wake up. However, if the ureters sustain damage during surgery, they will remain in place until the ureters heal. Between 1 to 6 weeks later, you can return to the hospital to have these removed through your urethra. This is slightly uncomfortable but should not be painful. The decision to use ureteric stents is made on a case-by-case basis, but they are often used if investigations are needed to determine the presence of endometriosis in the urinary system. It's common to have blood-stained urine (haematuria) after removing stents, but it will pass. Contact your hospital if you experience persistent or worsening haematuria or other symptoms such as difficulty urinating or a fever.

Colostomy

A colostomy involves diverting part of the colon to an opening or incision in your stomach. This opening, known as a stoma, is where a pouch or bag is attached to collect faeces. A colostomy can be temporary or permanent. If temporary, another operation will be performed at a later date to reconnect the bowel to its original location. Bowel surgery carries the risk of a colostomy in case there's damage to the bowel requiring time to heal or if a large portion of diseased tissues needs to be removed. A colostomy has unique risks, including infection, blockage, leakage, stoma prolapse, and skin problems. Following surgery to reconnect the bowel, it's crucial to monitor for signs of infection, such as a high temperature. Your hospital will provide you with all the necessary information.

Damage to Organs

One potential risk associated with surgery is organ damage. The extent and impact of this will vary on a case-by-case basis. The damage may necessitate additional surgery to correct it, while minor injuries often resolve naturally over time. The likelihood of experiencing complications is low, although your doctor will discuss the relevant risks associated with your surgery prior to it taking place.

What to Pack for the Hospital	
Bag	You may be required to put your belongings in a locker during surgery, so bring a soft cased bag that will fit.
Current Medications	Bring medications you are on or would need during an overnight stay.
Phone	To keep in contact with friends or family and provide entertainment whilst at hospital. You can play games, go on social media, or listen to music to help relax or uplift you.
Phone Charger	A portable charger is preferable in case you don't have access to a plug socket.
Dressing gown	You will be given a gown to wear on the ward; this is open-backed, meaning yes, you can see your bottom from behind. A dressing gown allows you to cover up if you need to go to the bathroom, and it's nice to feel cosy during your stay.
Slippers or Slide-on Sandals	After surgery, bending down to put shoes on will be difficult, so slip-on shoes are preferable for wearing home. You may also want to bring slippers for the ward. I opted for Birkenstocks because I could wear them on the ward and to the bathroom, as well as to and from the hospital.
Knickers	Make sure these are big and loose, a.k.a. granny style, so as not to irritate the surgical markings. Also, choose knickers in a soft, breathable material like cotton while your wounds heal.
Glasses/ Contact Lens and case	As required.
Entertainment such as a book	It can be nice to have something to keep you occupied while you wait for your operation or for overnight stays. Downloading movies or TV shows onto your phone or tablet can be a great way to pass the time.
Lozenges	Your throat may be sore from the breathing tube during surgery. Lozenges or warm tea can soothe this.

Pyjamas	Required for overnight stays, but keep it light, airy, and easy to put on. A night dress may be the best bet to avoid any pressure on your stomach. Personally, I have always stayed in my hospital gown until I am discharged.
Spare Change of Clothes	Wear comfy, loose clothes that are easy to put on after surgery, such as a dress. Do not bring tight clothes, such as jeans or leggings, as your stomach will be swollen and tender.
Hair Ties and Hairbrush	As required.
Toothbrush & Toothpaste	Or mouthwash.
Toiletries	You probably won't need any toiletries as you will be exhausted and focused on resting. But in case you want to freshen up after surgery or if you stay overnight, it may be nice to bring some essentials. Opt for travel sizes that don't take up much space.
Sanitary Towels	The hospital will provide you with sanitary towels, but these are very bulky, so you may want to change before you go home. Do not bring or use tampons.
Lip Balm	Your lips may be dry after surgery, so if this will irritate you (hands up to all my fellow lip balm addicts), I recommend being prepared.
Sleep Mask	A sleep mask can come in handy for overnight stays as the lights may be on all night or turned on very early.
Earphones or Earbuds	Earphones can help block out some of the noise from the hospital at night. If you struggle with sound while sleeping, I recommend bringing noise-cancelling earbuds.

What Not to Pack	
Valuables, Jewellery, or Large Sums of Money	You don't need any of these, and hospitals will not accept liability if anything gets lost or stolen, so you should leave anything valuable at home. The only jewellery you can wear in surgery is your wedding ring, so remove all jewellery, including body piercings, before you go.
Makeup, Nail Varnish, False Nails	You will not be able to wear any of these in surgery.
Normal Socks	You will be given long socks called compression stockings to wear to help prevent blood clots or DVT from developing. Unless it's winter or you live in a cold area, you won't need to bring socks. For longer hospital stays, you may wish to bring a change of socks; these should also be compression socks.
Snacks	You cannot eat while waiting for surgery, and when you wake up, you will be given something small to eat and drink, such as biscuits and tea. For overnight stays, you will be fed from the hospital menu, but having easy-to-eat healthy snacks such as grapes can be nice to have on hand. I know grapes are a cliche, but they are small, sweet, and hydrating. Be warned: grapes aren't suitable for individuals on a low-fibre diet post-surgery.

How to Prepare for Surgery

You should complete these tasks before your surgery, as you likely won't have the energy or motivation to do them afterwards. Preparing ahead of time will help reduce stress, allowing you to simply rest and recover after the procedure.

Paracetamol	Paracetamol can be taken to manage the pain, so get stocked up on this as you will likely need it.
Peppermint Tea	This can be helpful for relieving gas pain from laparoscopic surgery.
Ginger Tea	Helpful for alleviating nausea.
Healthy Snacks	Snacks like fruit or nuts are good for grazing on to support your body's healing process. Instead of reaching for fast food or unhealthy snacks, you should eat nutritious foods. Constipation is common after drugs like morphine, so fibre in your diet can help. However, check with your doctor to see if fibre is okay for you.
Baby Wipes	You will not be able to shower immediately, but you can wash with baby wipes or a flannel.
Easy to Cook Meals	Standing up to cook long meals will be exhausting for your body, so quick and easy options are best.
Sanitary Towels	You will likely experience some bleeding after surgery, so sanitary towels or pads are essential to remain clean and comfortable. Do not buy or use tampons during recovery.
Water and Fluid	You will need lots of fluid post-op, so if you live in a building where it is quite far or inconvenient to get water or other drinks, buy bottled water so that it will be easily accessible.
Clean Pyjamas	You will undoubtedly spend most of your recovery in pyjamas or comfy clothes, so get them washed and ready to go.
Clean Your Space	You will spend a lot of time at home after surgery, so make sure your space is clean and ready to enjoy. You will be unable to do anything strenuous for a while, such as hoovering or taking the bins out.
Clean Bed Sheets	You'll be spending a lot of time in bed, so to minimise the risk of infection, wash your bedsheets and make your bed before leaving for the hospital.

42

Do You Need Surgery?

Deciding whether to undergo surgery is a deeply personal choice, and it's valuable to weigh your options carefully. It can be a powerful tool in reducing symptoms and restoring a sense of normalcy, allowing those who have spent years in pain or not feeling quite themselves to feel healthy and fully engage in life once again. Surgery often ceases further prolonged suffering, whether that's a partial or complete remission of symptoms, so while it's not a definitive cure, for some, it can create a feeling of being cured, and that alone can be a compelling reason to consider it. Nevertheless, it's vital to recognise that surgery doesn't provide relief for everyone or address every aspect of the condition's systemic effect on the body. As a result, implementing additional strategies for a comprehensive approach to healing is necessary. It's also important to acknowledge that not everyone feels ready or willing to undergo surgery, and that's okay. Many people choose to postpone surgery until they believe it is a vital component of their treatment plan. If you're uncertain, rest assured there are alternative options that may benefit you. As previously discussed, hormone treatments may help manage symptoms, and we'll explore other lifestyle adjustments in the following chapters. Your treatment plan should be tailored to your specific needs. Factors such as the severity and impact of symptoms, your personal beliefs, age, extent of disease, and whether you want children or have fertility concerns all play a role in determining the best course of action. Just as endometriosis presents differently in each person, your treatment plan will be as unique as your condition. In many cases, your doctor will suggest using hormone treatments first, as medical therapy can sometimes manage symptoms effectively enough to eliminate the need for surgery. However, finding the right treatment might involve trial and error, as not every approach works for everyone. Whether you opt for surgery or choose to wait, it's important to have a strategy in place to address your symptoms. Without treatment, symptoms may persist or worsen over time. For example, if your scans indicate deep endometriosis, which is more aggressive and tends to invade nerves-rich areas, delaying surgery could lead to severe pain and a more complex operation down the line. Additionally, if endometriosis is growing near the vagina, it can have a significant impact on your sex life, which may be something you want to address sooner rather than later. If the condition is suspected of affecting your kidneys, surgery is strongly advised. Without intervention, this can lead to irreversible damage with devastating consequences for your overall health.

Ultimately, the decision to have surgery is entirely yours. It's not mandatory but an option to consider based on your unique circumstances. Keep in mind though, that surgery cannot guarantee lifelong resolution to your symptoms. You may need additional operations in the future, although it's also possible that one or two surgeries could be sufficient, so I don't think it is good to worry about this. It's simply useful to have realistic expectations about your treatment journey. Remember, you are not alone on this path. Take the time to discuss your options with your healthcare provider, ask questions, and consider seeking support from fellow Endo Warriors who have faced similar experiences. With a comprehensive approach and personalised treatment plan, you can reclaim control over your health and embrace a brighter future.

Before my endometriosis diagnosis, I wasn't the biggest enthusiast of Western medicine (probably immature, but I know some others out there will be in the same boat). I was drawn towards alternative and natural systems that have existed for thousands of years, such as Chinese,

Herbal, and Ayurvedic medicine. However, my perspective shifted after my surgeries and witnessing first-hand the incredible advancements in medicine. I developed a profound appreciation for the dedication of medical professionals who devote their careers to continually improving surgical techniques, surgical equipment, and knowledge to treat a wide range of diseases. I realised this was not to be dismissed. If you feel the same way, I want to reassure you that putting my health into the care of Western medicine was the best thing I ever did. While I still value alternative treatments, I now understand the importance of embracing the strengths of both approaches and utilising them when appropriate. This combination has been key to managing my health, and it may be for you too.

43

Fertility and Surgery

A burning question many will have is whether surgery improves or impairs your fertility. To shed light on this complex topic, let's examine the available research and the various factors that can influence fertility outcomes.

Understanding Fertility without Surgery

Research on the relationship between fertility and endometriosis is lacking, so the statistics and reasoning are not clear and may vary between studies or by country. One resource estimates that 60-70% of people with endo are fertile and can get pregnant spontaneously, meaning without medical assistance.[1] The degree to which endo affects fertility varies and hinges on numerous factors. These include the stage, location, and severity of endometriosis, as well as the extent of inflammation, adhesions, immune dysfunction, toxins in peritoneal fluid, or ovulatory dysfunction... among many others. Additionally, any previous treatments may play a role. Beyond endometriosis, various factors can influence fertility, such as age, overall health, BMI, diet, and lifestyle choices like smoking, vaping, and drinking.

Peritoneal Endometriosis

A 2021 study explored the impact of surgery on fertility rates in women with stage 1 or 2 endometriosis affecting the peritoneum.[2] The results were encouraging: 62% of women who had previously struggled with infertility but desired to conceive, became pregnant within five years of surgery, and the majority achieved pregnancy without Assisted Reproductive Technologies (ART) such as IVF. Moreover, 76% of the participants reported being symptom-free or experienced significant improvements from surgery. Pregnancy statistics rise even higher when you look at studies that factor in the use of ART in addition to surgical removal.[3] Therefore, even if conception does not occur naturally after surgery, the subsequent use of ART can offer an added benefit. However, it's important to note, surgery isn't always necessary; EndometriosisUK suggests that 75% of people with minimal-mild endometriosis will get pregnant without medical intervention.[4]

Endometrioma

An ovarian chocolate cyst might raise fertility concerns, and whilst surgery is available, it may not be required to achieve pregnancy, as one study showed a high pregnancy rate without it.[5] Endometriomas, however, can impact pregnancy through their inflammatory effects, diminished ovarian function, and decreased levels of Anti-Müllerian Hormone (AMH), which indicates reduced egg supply.[6] Additionally, they may hinder the success of ART procedures. The good news is surgical excision of cysts is considered an effective fertility-enhancing procedure in some cases. Nevertheless, there is an ongoing debate regarding whether surgery is the best option when fertility is desired in the near future, as cyst removal can lead to a decrease in ovarian reserve, affecting the number of follicles in the ovaries at any given time. This risk must be factored into your decision-making process, alongside your surgeon's advice, to ensure surgery aligns with your goals and needs. Moreover, different surgical techniques used to remove cysts can yield varying effects on future fertility outcomes. Advice may differ based on the size of your cyst; endometriomas greater than 5cm have been shown to significantly reduce the number of oocytes retrieved through IVF.[7] If you are planning to use ART to conceive, surgery to remove the cyst may not be recommended as it can decrease the ovarian output of eggs. However, if your cyst poses a substantial risk of rupture, will impede egg retrieval, or causes severe pain during ovarian stimulation for ART, surgery may be recommended. Despite these potential challenges, it's reassuring to know that endometriomas don't appear to cause a decrease in clinical pregnancy or live birth rates; the outcomes of IVF remain similar to those without endometriosis.[8]

Fallopian Tubes

Endometriosis and adhesions can encroach on the fallopian tubes, impairing their function or cause blockages. Leaving these issues untreated can lead to infertility, which may then necessitate treatment as natural conception isn't possible. Individuals may use ART instead, as there are techniques which bypass the fallopian tubes, opening possibilities for conception.

Deep Endometriosis

Untreated Deep Infiltrating Endometriosis (DIE) has the lowest statistical spontaneous birth rate, with one study reporting figures between 9 and 13%.[9] Of course, DIE lesions can impact various organs to varying degrees and display a range of changes to the pelvic anatomy, so they will have unique implications on fertility with each person. Additionally, hormonal and immunological functions will be impacted differently, further influencing fertility outcomes. A study tracking pregnancy rates over seven years in individuals undergoing treatment for deep colorectal endo revealed surgical treatment enhanced fertility by over 50%.[9] Notably, those who had a bowel resection instead of lesion shaving had a significant improvement in spontaneous pregnancies. Another review noted that bowel surgery also improved outcomes in IVF treatment.[10] Similar results were observed in cases of ureteral endometriosis following surgical intervention.[11,12] Despite some reports that surgery improved pregnancy rates across all types of DIE and helped improve the effectiveness of IVF or other ART methods, the ESHREs guidelines remain that there isn't enough evidence to comprehensively state that surgery for deep endo improves fertility. However, it can still represent a treatment option for symptomatic patients wishing to conceive.[13]

* * *

Surgery can play a crucial role in managing endometriosis by removing diseased tissue, reducing inflammation, and restoring organ function, all of which are vital for pregnancy. Another critical factor to consider is many of the debilitating symptoms from endo make it harder to conceive. It's not fun creating a baby when you're exhausted, in pain, or experiencing painful sex. Surgery has the potential to diminish these symptoms whilst putting you in better stead of being a parent, as symptoms like fatigue can be particularly troublesome. Remember, many people get pregnant spontaneously and reach full term without issues, whilst for others, there may be a few fences to jump before getting there. Each person's fertility needs are different and will require different strategies. There is no one-size-fits-all approach to dealing with someone's ability to conceive. If you are looking to start a family or are dealing with fertility problems, incorporate other methods outside of medical treatment to assist this. Drinking alcohol and smoking cigarettes or vapes is associated with a negative impact on fertility, so reducing or stopping these can help to improve pregnancy rates. A healthy body mass is also an important factor in fertility. A BMI below or above the normal range can cause difficulties or delays in getting pregnant. Of course, BMI is not the most helpful tool sometimes, as someone who is very athletic and has a high muscle mass will have a high BMI, but if you are aware that you are underweight or overweight, working on this may support pregnancy chances. Adjustments to BMI can be made through exercise and diet, or terms I prefer — movement and nutrition. Listed are foods that research has proposed to have an impact on fertility, whether they are beneficial or should be limited. Take from this list items you know you can enjoy and easily incorporate, and remember a healthy balanced diet is key. Don't start gorging on any foods excessively assuming they will make you fertile.

Engaging in regular exercise, adopting a healthy diet, and discussing individualised fertility plans with your healthcare provider can enhance your chances of achieving a successful pregnancy. While surgery can sometimes offer improvements for fertility, it's essential to weigh the potential risks and benefits and make informed decisions based on your consultation with your medical team.

Foods to Consume More Of:	
Monounsaturated Fats [14]	• Plant Oils (olive, peanut, and canola) • Avocados • Nuts (almonds, hazelnuts, and pecans) • Seeds (pumpkin and sesame seeds)
Non-Haem Iron[15] (iron that comes from plants can decrease risk of ovulatory infertility)	• Whole grains • Nuts • Seeds • Legumes • Leafy greens
Foods Containing Vitamin D	• Oily Fish (salmon, mackerel, anchovies, sardines and herring) • Egg Yolks • Fortified Foods e.g. cereal
Food to Consume Moderately:	
Animal Sources of Protein [16]	• Protein should be eaten daily but this can also include plant-based sources.

44

Management Outside of Surgery & Hormone Treatments

Now we've covered medical treatments for endometriosis, we'll run through additional tools and strategies you can incorporate into your life. Lifestyle options are crucial because surgery and hormone treatments have their limitations and are not capable of addressing the underlying cause of the issue. Endometriosis is complex, and the exact cause remains unknown, potentially varying among individuals due to the numerous factors to consider. Although lifestyle options aren't quick fixes (there aren't any!), they can help mitigate triggers and possibly address the cause of some of your symptoms. Taking proactive steps gives your body a fighting chance. As research continues to address the questions and uncover the answers, we should recognise the value of lifestyle changes. As aestheticians often advise, "There's no point in getting preventative Botox injections for wrinkles if you're not going to use sunscreen". This same logic applies to your endometriosis treatment. Surgery alone may not suffice without also considering supplementary factors to improve your overall health. Doctors do a lot, but they can only do so much, so greater involvement in the treatment journey from patients is required. Lifestyle changes require time, commitment, and self-assessment to monitor what works for you and what else can be tried. Ultimately, this is your life and only you can choose to make changes. Maintaining an open and positive mindset to try new tactics can make all the difference in how you feel. This section lists treatments that can complement surgery to further relieve symptoms or serve as an alternative, as surgery is not available or desired by everyone. By making the science behind these options accessible, I hope you are better informed on what remedies are available, helping you make choices.

45

The Four Pillars of Health

The four pillars of health form the foundation of a healthy lifestyle and are comprised of the following elements:

Nutrition

Movement

Sleep

Wellbeing

These modalities encompass various aspects of our lives, and with care to incorporate good habits in each of these can translate into improved physical, mental, emotional, and spiritual health. Each pillar is equally important as the next and deserves individual attention; however, they're all interconnected, so by focusing on one, you impact the others. The four pillar approach is beneficial as it prevents people from feeling overwhelmed with an abundance of ideas or the perception there is too much to change, so they don't know where to begin. Instead, it offers a structural framework, allowing you to address multiple areas of your life simultaneously with ease, knowing there are four distinct areas to focus on.

46

The Four Pillars of Health – Nutrition

Nutrition is an ideal starting point for those seeking to improve their health and pave the way for a better future. It's hard to think of a single chronic disease that isn't powerfully affected by diet. It can help heal your physical health and improve your immune system, which can, in turn, benefit your emotional and spiritual health. Our diet can be a powerful medicine or a harmful poison to our bodies. In today's world, this statement is quite apparent and doesn't need much explaining on a surface level. Obesity, type 2 diabetes, and heart disease are just a few examples of conditions in which diet plays a crucial role in the development and remission. We are surrounded by processed foods full of sugar, salt, and various chemicals at our disposal, offering convenience and satisfaction. Not only do some of these processed foods contain ingredients that are bad for our health, but a fundamental problem with these foods is they are nutritionally void, meaning we are consuming food lacking the nutrition our bodies need to function. Nutrient deficiencies can lead to other issues or diseases, which I'm sure you want to avoid. Maintaining a nutritious and balanced diet is vital for good health and disease prevention. Nutritionally-dense foods are rich in nutrients relative to their calorie content. They might contain vitamins, minerals, lean protein, complex carbohydrates, and healthy fats, without added sugars. As a rule of thumb, these are the types of foods we should focus on eating. Each mechanism within our body relies on different nutrients in varying amounts, making diet pivotal in providing our bodies with everything necessary to function like a well-oiled machine. If we run low on specific nutrients, the body manifests symptoms, ranging from dry skin to fatigue, as the body struggles or stops being able to carry out certain duties.

Diet plays a critical role in influencing the maintenance of our immune system, a complex network of organs, cells, and proteins that defend the body against external invaders and abnormal cells. It creates antibodies to remember every germ ever encountered, facilitating quicker responses from the immune system in subsequent encounters. It also safeguards against cell changes that may lead to illness, such as cancer. It has a vital role in our survival, and as our nutrition significantly impacts this system, it is essential to consider. A deficiency in a single nutrient can alter how our immune system functions. For instance, the absence of Vitamin C can hinder the formation of antibodies, posing potential problems. We aren't just referring to micronutrients here; energy derived from proteins, fats, and carbohydrates also plays a role as a strong immune system requires adequate energy. This is a newish and exciting area of science called immunometabolism, which studies the relationship between metabolism and immunology, which were once thought to be two separate and distinct disciplines. One aspect of immunometabolism to reflect on is our gut microbiome, as numerous interactions occur between molecules produced by the microbiome and our immune system. Any changes in our microbiome can significantly impact immune function and energy production.[1] These interconnected systems create overlapping networks, communicating with each other and exchanging information. The bacterium in our microbiome has a profound impact on our health, influencing our susceptibility to illness and our ability to recover. Remarkably, about 80% of our immune cells reside in our gut.[2] Mounting evidence suggests a healthy, diverse microbiome can shape an immune system that effectively defends against both external and internal threats. As diet significantly affects the composition of our gut microbiota and the immune system, it signifies the vital role nutrition plays in improving health.

So, we now understand that food holds immense importance for everyone, regardless of their health status, but how does diet relate specifically
to endo? Well, there's limited scientific research on the direct impact
of diet, so there's no scientific basis to guide us on what to eat or avoid.
But this doesn't mean you cannot still utilise food as a powerful tool to
manage your quality of life. You may hear people claiming to have the
answers on what to eat or to avoid, but be sure to understand if these
recommendations are based on personal anecdotes or scientific evidence.
Even if they are based on research, I advise you to take these with a pinch of
salt. It doesn't mean they are wrong, but their effectiveness may vary from
person to person. Also, the reductionist notion that if you eat a particular
food, it will heal you, and if you remove a certain food, it will heal you
— is problematic. A restrictive diet can put more stress on someone who
may not need to personally eliminate those specific foods. Furthermore,
when cutting out food groups, replacing the nutrients they provide with
alternative sources in the diet is crucial. This is where the philosophy of *a
little bit of everything and not too much of anything* comes from and is often
recommended. For most, this is the easiest way to ensure you attain a
broad spectrum of nutrients while minimising the risk of deficiencies. Just
like your fingerprint, your microbiome is unique. Since the microbiome
influences food digestion, immune system function, allergies, mood, and
gastrointestinal symptoms, it's essential to focus on what suits you as
an individual. What worked for someone else may not work for you, and
vice versa. While we await more research in this area, you should do a self-
study, which arguably is more important. Each one of us will have different
food preferences, allergies, sensitivities, cultural backgrounds, beliefs,
lifestyles, finances, and other health conditions that will impact our food
choices and determine what we experiment with in our self-study. If you
are curious about what we will discuss in this chapter if there's no one-size-
fits-all endo diet, we will address common myths and topics associated
with endometriosis, breaking down why they work for some people. We
will outline foods you may want to incorporate or eliminate from your
diet. I know I just mentioned eliminating foods can cause unnecessary

restrictions, but this is where your self-study comes into play. My goal is to provide data from scientific papers so that you can make informed decisions about what you want to try and then determine what works for you and what doesn't. I am not here to dictate what you eat. I'm here to give you the power of information. Sometimes, research states there is no evidence to suggest particular dietary choices are beneficial or they cannot be proven; however, if they work for you, that's the main goal to measure.

Food can be utilised both to alleviate symptoms, and as part of a long-term lifestyle strategy for overall health. For some, adopting specific dietary choices can be beneficial in managing symptoms like pain or gastrointestinal issues, ranging from nausea to diarrhoea. At a minimum, diet serves as a powerful tool to bring joy, nourish your body, and provide energy. Simultaneously, you should avoid foods that exacerbate discomfort, distress the body, or contribute to inflammation and pain. I know when you're amid gruelling endo symptoms or a flare-up, thinking about diet can feel exhausting, as can the idea of cooking. While it's acceptable to turn to processed comfort foods when you're stressed, tired, and in pain, it's crucial not to make it a routine, as it can ultimately harms your long-term health. I strongly believe that food should be fun and not a stressful burden. So, I suggest a gradual, relaxed approach to working with your diet; baby steps can be great if that works for you. Once you have decided what options you want to try, work out a plan that can be split up into weeks or months, depending on the size of the goals. For example, you might list out that the first step in your plan is to eat an extra piece of citrus fruit a day for a fortnight before trying to come up with another goal, so that you have time to make a new habit stick. Being specific can help you achieve your goals, so following the fruit example, you might decide to eat a tangerine when you get to work each day. This provides structure and routine that will make this new goal easy to achieve and maintain. It's worth noting, doctors are generally not extensively trained in nutrition. If you want individualised advice, seek a nutritionist or dietician who can work with you to ensure you meet your specific requirements.

Myth #1 - Food has No Role in Managing Endometriosis

The first myth to debunk is that *'you have no control over your disease'* and *'diet cannot help'*. Whilst yes, there is indeed limited research into this area and diet cannot cure endo, there is research we can discuss. Type 2 diabetes was once thought of as progressive and incurable; now we know remission can be achieved in some people, with diet playing a key role in this. Whilst we're not saying endometriosis can be put into remission with diet, its possible role in influencing disease severity or progression shouldn't be dismissed. Endometriosis is an oestrogen-dependent disorder, and studies on other oestrogen-dependent conditions, such as breast cancer, highlight diet has a strong effect on factors contributing to disease development. The Western Dietary Pattern was significantly associated, showing a 14% increase in the risk of oestrogen-receptor tumours.[1] Other studies demonstrate that a diet high in omega-3 or monounsaturated fats but low in omega-6 is protective against breast cancer.[2] This might seem strange as omegas are supposed to be good for us, right? Why would a diet low in omega-6 be protective against cancer? Well, this is because the ratio of omega-3 to omega-6 is important, but we'll get into that in a moment. Omega-3 fatty acids are often mentioned in endometriosis diets, and many web pages will claim you need to increase your intake, so what's the science behind this? Omega-3 has an anti-inflammatory effect on the body, and as endo is an inflammatory disorder, reducing inflammation may have a role in preventing the disease or managing it. Animal studies also show that omega-3 may be able to suppress endometriosis.[3,4] This is because omega-3 levels can influence the immune, angiogenic, and proliferative factors in the early establishment of endometriosis.[5] A Nurses Health Study in 2010 also noted that patients with a diet high in omega-3 fatty acids were 22% less likely to be diagnosed with endometriosis.[6] Then, in 2023, a study determined dietary fat may be linked to the progression and development of endo, as risk increased with higher consumption of saturated and trans fats.[7] It also concluded monounsaturated fats and omega-3 may lower risk and reduce disease severity. Several studies note that the ratio between omega-3 and omega-6 is of significance, when omega-3 intake is higher than omega-6, it can reduce pain and inflammation.[7,8] So if a low intake of omega-6 is associated with lower breast cancer risk, and a low ratio is beneficial to endo, does this mean omega-6 is bad? No, not at all; omega-6 is needed in the body and plays a crucial role in how well our cells function. The body cannot make omega-6, and a diet deficient in it will cause symptoms such as dry skin and brittle nails. We need to consume omega-6, however, *too* much can have harmful effects on the body as it's pro-inflammatory. Every person wants a diet higher in omega-3 than in omega-6. In endometriosis, a diet too high in omega-6 can increase pain symptoms, including uterine cramps, due to the pro-inflammatory compounds derived from omega-6 fatty acids.[9] These are just some highlights from studies I found, yet there is a consistent picture that diet and omega-3 have a beneficial role in the prevention and management of endo. To what extent is still debatable; we need a large, double-blind randomised placebo-controlled trial to confirm this (this is the gold standard for studies as they minimise bias that can be found in other study designs). Omega-3 supplementation may also be helpful in treating painful periods due to its anti-inflammatory properties and antioxidant properties.[10]

If you have heard of antioxidants and know they're good for you but are not entirely sure what they are, let us break it down. Antioxidants are natural substances found in food. The best sources of antioxidants come from plants which work at fighting oxidative stress. They *anti* the *oxidation* in our bodies. But what is oxidative stress? It's a condition caused by free radicals; these are unstable molecules produced in the body as a by-product of normal cellular processes. However, their production significantly increases in response to environmental toxins such as radiation, stress, alcohol consumption, tobacco smoke, UV rays, and air pollution, which can be problematic. Antioxidants interact with free radicals, neutralising and preventing them from causing damage. When there are not enough antioxidants to neutralise the free radicals in the body, it causes oxidative stress, meaning damage occurs to our cells, proteins, and DNA. The greater the amount of oxidative stress, the greater the level of damage inflicted on our cells, which, over time, can harm our organs and tissues. Oxidative stress has been linked to premature ageing and various diseases, including diabetes, cancer, and Alzheimer's. It is reported women with endo have increased systemic oxidative stress, which can affect our reproductive system[11] and have a role in the pathogenesis or progression of the disease.[12] The damage on a cellular level causes inflammation, *but* antioxidants help fight this inflammation, reducing pain and other symptoms of endometriosis. The good news is that we can get more antioxidants into our bodies with food. Fruits and vegetables are rich in antioxidants — look at the list of sources and try to incorporate these into your diet. Whilst some of the compounds in these foods can be extracted and taken as supplements, it's best to get antioxidants and nutrients from food. Whole foods come in a complete package with essential vitamins and minerals alongside important substances like fibre needed for a healthy gut. Antioxidants tend to work best in combination with other nutrients and compounds, which supplements often do not provide. Choosing the right foods means having one of nature's pre-made cocktails that nourish the body and contains nutrients that work together to provide the sustenance you need, with the added benefit of good flavour and enjoyment attached.

Antioxidant Foods (in no particular order)

Cloves, Sumac, Ceylon Cinnamon, Sorghum, Oregano, Cumin, Parsley, Basil, Sage, Mustard Seed, Turmeric, Thyme, Paprika, Ginger, Garlic, Pecan, Walnuts, Hazelnuts, Almonds, Pistachios, Red Kidney Beans, Pinto Beans, Black Beans, Chickpeas, Cacao, Dark Chocolate, Pomegranate, Cranberries, Acai Berry, Prunes, Artichoke, Apple, Red Lentils, Macadamias, Wheatgrass, Mangosteen, Goji Berries, Broccoli, Cauliflower, Oranges, Spinach, Beetroot, Figs, Cherries, Lemons, Limes, Aubergine, Pears, Tangerines, Cabbage, Grapefruit, Red Potatoes, Onions, Carrots, Grapes, Mangoes, and Kiwi.

Foods Sources of Omega-3 Fatty Acids	
Fish	Mackerel, Salmon, Seabass, Oysters, Sardines, Shrimp
Plant Sources (good for vegan and vegetarians)	Seaweed, Algae, Chia Seeds, Hemp Seeds, Flax Seed, Walnuts, Edamame, Kidney Beans
Fortified Foods	Some foods may have omega-3 added to them, which will be advertised on the food product.
Foods Sources of Omega-6 Fatty Acids	
Protein	Tofu, Chicken, Lamb, Beef
Plant Sources	Walnuts, Sunflower Seeds, Brazil Nuts, Pumpkin Seeds, Peanut Butter, Avocado
Oil	Safflower Oil, Walnut Oil, Sesame Oil

Earlier, we mentioned a study that found endometriosis risk increased with higher consumption of saturated and trans fats. Saturated fat is found in meat, dairy, and eggs, as well as coconut and palm oil. These fats occur naturally, and although they are often labelled as 'bad fat', they're not inherently harmful to us and still form part of a healthy, balanced diet. The problem is that too much of it can be bad, and Western diets are typically high in this type of fat and trans fats. Some trans fats are also found naturally in animal-based products, but these are not a cause for concern in their natural form. The trans fats we need to steer clear of are artificially made through a process called dehydrogenation, found in processed foods such as doughnuts, margarine, frozen pizza, and shop-bought baked goods like cakes, cookies, and pies. Artificial trans fats are notorious for their damage to the body, such as raising LDL (bad) cholesterol and their links to disease. Due to concerns, many countries have banned trans fats, whilst others have regulations on the maximum amount foods can have. The EU limits 2g per 100g of fat. Whilst fat is essential to consume and incredibly healthy, this study is not alone in finding a relationship between fat intake and endometriosis. A review of studies on this topic concluded a diet rich in saturated fatty acids or trans fat could have an adverse effect on the course and treatment of endometriosis due to the inflammatory processes that can occur.[13] In fact, a high intake of trans fat meant women were almost 50% more likely to have endo.[6] Red meat, a source of saturated fat, has been singled out as a risk factor for higher consumption.[14,15] This may be attributed to its ability to increase circulating oestrogen levels and reduce Sex Hormone-Binding Globulin (SHBG).[16] SHBG regulates sex hormone activity in the body, so when SHBG binds to oestrogen, it prevents tissues from using it. Elevated oestrogen levels can promote inflammation and stimulate the growth of lesions. Red meat can also raise C-Reactive Protein (CRP) levels, an inflammatory marker in the blood that doctors sometimes use to determine the presence of inflammation in the body.[17] Reducing red meat consumption might bring down oestrogen levels, helping to manage endo. If you enjoy red meat and still want to consume it as part of your diet, it may be beneficial to limit this to one serving a week because a study found those who consumed two or more servings of red meat a day have 56% higher chance of endo compared to those who consumed it once or less a week.[18] It might be good here to confirm what is meant by red meat, it includes beef, pork, lamb, veal, venison, and goat products. So, this means ham, steak, sausages, bacon, salami, or other cured meats. You should always listen to your body and what it reacts to because the research so far is inconclusive. A study in Iran found red meat was protective against endo.[19] This deviation in results may come down to the diet as a whole, lifestyle factors, or the types of red meat consumed, the fat content, whether it is organic, and how it was cooked. Therefore, if you eat red meat, aim for lean cuts.

Dairy, another source of saturated fat, is also suggested to affect oestrogen levels in the blood, but the research on dairy and endometriosis risk is contradictory. Some suggest there is no significant association, whilst others showed dairy could be protective against the condition.[20,21]

High saturated fat consumption is related to oxidative stress and inflammation. In contrast, a diet rich in antioxidants, including omega-3 (*a type of fat*), can counter oxidative stress. This can reduce inflammation (*and therefore symptoms*), as well as protect against cellular damage occurring. A healthy, balanced diet rich in vegetables, omega-3, and lean protein, whilst reducing red meat and trans fat, may decrease your risk of further aggravating endometriosis whilst serving as protection against other diseases or conditions. Most Western diets have sufficient omega-6, so the best way to improve your ratio is to focus on consuming more foods containing omega-3. Incorporating these goals into your diet can reduce circulating oestrogen and inflammation, making diet an integral component of managing your disease.

Myth #2 - You Have to Be Vegan

Myth 1 brings us nicely to our next myth, which is "You must be vegan if you have endometriosis to manage the disease". You may have heard this on social media or from Endo Warriors; you might also discern from the research in Myth 1 that managing this disease requires a plant-based diet. So...do you need to be vegan if you have endo? The short answer is no. Do some people benefit from vegan or vegetarian diets? Yes, many do. Some individuals have undertaken their self-study and found vegan or plant-based diets to be the most useful in minimising their symptoms, and perhaps feel there is research behind it that supports long-term health for their bodies. When people go vegan or plant-based, they may lower their dietary fat by reducing milk, cheese, yoghurt, chocolate, et cetera, while eating more fruit and vegetables, or plant-based proteins like beans or legumes, which all contain fibre. Of course, this is not the case for everyone, but as a general notion, this is possible. Reducing your dietary fat whilst increasing fibre intake is associated with a reduction in oestrogen circulating in the blood, which might be beneficial for endo.[1] As highlighted in Myth 1, consumption of red meat has also been associated with higher levels of oestrogen and inflammation, so there may be an argument to eliminate this from the diet. Therefore, by removing red meat and animal fat whilst increasing fibre, the vegan diet may be useful in protecting against disease and reducing inflammatory processes in the body.[2] Nevertheless, not everyone needs to be vegan; in some instances, it can be unhelpful. Please note, from now on, I will use the term 'plant-based diet', as veganism has a philosophy behind it, centred around the rejection of animals as a commodity, which is different to choosing this diet for health reasons.

Let's explain why it's not good to encourage a plant-based diet for everyone. When cutting out large food groups from the diet, the removed nutrients must be obtained elsewhere, namely protein, omega-3, vitamin B12, calcium, iodine, and iron. If you choose to adopt a plant-based diet, you need to allocate time to explore alternative sources of these nutrients and determine how you will still attain them in your new diet. That doesn't mean it's impossible, but some individuals may not have the time or knowledge to change diets whilst ensuring they attain all their nutritional requirements. Furthermore, many people who opt for a plant-based (or vegan) diet rather than a *whole-food* plant-based one end up reaching for many processed foods, which ultimately aren't good for you either as they contain lots of additives. A Whole-Food Plant-Based Diet (WFPBD) means eating foods that have been processed as little as possible, which is a better alternative. You primarily buy or eat foods as they are found in nature, then prepare them into meals at home. As someone who has explored veganism, pescetarianism, and a dairy-free diet, I know from first-hand experience that trying processed foods that meet my new dietary requirements are fun to try and sometimes super convenient. This is particularly problematic with protein sources as the food industry has created enticing versions of fake meats, which are highly processed and contain lots of added junk. Good dietary sources of plant-based protein are beans, lentils, tofu, chickpeas, quinoa, edamame, and peanuts. No matter which diet you have, always aim to consume most of your food as single-ingredient foods or whole foods that have been processed and refined as little as possible. If you are interested in trying a WFPBD but need help to ensure you are meeting your dietary requirements, you might want to use meal plans. Alternatively, the 'Daily Dozen' app has a checklist of the types of foods you should eat daily to ensure you receive all the nutrients needed for optimal health on a WFPBD. This app was based on the work of Dr Gregor, who wrote the book *How Not to Die* and can be an excellent tool to help you get started. You tick off 12 servings of foods when you have eaten them, making it easy to know what to eat. For example, you should consume one portion of berries daily, so breaking down the information this way can be insightful.

Another reason why advocating a strict "you *must* go vegan" stance is unhelpful is that some people have a history of disordered eating, so encouraging dietary restrictions can be potentially harmful rather than beneficial. There is also the concern of allergies, intolerances, or Oral Allergy Syndrome (OAS), which many people with endo have, limiting their consumption of certain fruits, vegetables, or nuts. As someone with OAS, at one point, I was a vegan who couldn't eat many foods that grew on trees and sometimes other foods like celery or carrots — quite limiting right? Individuals may already experience restrictions in what they're able to eat. In such cases, prioritising a varied diet becomes a critical factor. Hence, eliminating further foods and limiting food choices without first identifying if they are specifically problematic for them is not the most suitable option. Considering there are a multitude of personal factors at play, determining the most appropriate dietary choices requires a personalised approach. Therefore, encouraging blanket statements on eradication diets is unreasonable. We are all unique and require an individualised approach to our diet.

If you decide to go vegan, vegetarian, pescetarian, or any other type of diet, labels for dietary choices can be very helpful when informing others of the types of foods you eat or if you are in a restaurant and want to communicate your needs. However, labels can also be limiting and create added pressure or stress. It doesn't always need to be an 'all or nothing' approach, particularly if food choices are not based on moral or religious beliefs but a personal choice for our body. Some may find it advantageous to adopt a *mostly* plant-based diet while allowing flexibility on certain days, meals, or occasions where dietary rules are relaxed. Your needs and preferences may evolve over time, and it's ok to adjust your rules to align with what feels right for your body and lifestyle at any given period. Trust me, I have been there; I have changed my food choices every year or so to match what my body and spirit feel called to at that time.

With Myth 1, we described the association between saturated fat and inflammation, highlighting research suggesting that consuming large amounts may not be advisable for anyone, particularly those with endometriosis, which has an inflammatory component. Saturated fat is primarily found in animal products, and studies show that high consumption of red meat has greater endo risk, pinpointing why some people may choose to remove it altogether. Replacing red meat with other animal proteins like fish, shellfish or eggs was associated with a lower risk of endometriosis.[3] Fish and shellfish contain omega-3, particularly fatty fish such as salmon or sardines, which is great for calming inflammation. The antioxidant components protect our cells from free radicals, keeping our cells healthy and reducing the risk of disease. Remember, we cannot make omega-3, so if you don't eat fish, take an algae supplement and try to consume other plant-based sources of omega-3 to maintain this benefit. If you still want to consume meat in your diet but want to reduce red meat intake, you could swap it out for fish, shellfish, or lean poultry. It's good to think practically and how you plan to do this. If you often have a cooked breakfast on the weekend, rather than eating sausages and bacon, try salmon and eggs instead.

Dairy products such as milk, cheese, butter, and yoghurt contain saturated fat, as well as the hormones oestrogen and progesterone,[3] so does this mean dairy needs to be eliminated from our diets? Meta-analysis research conducted in 2021 suggests otherwise.[4] The study summarised the findings from other studies and found that consuming more than three portions a day of full-fat dairy was associated with a lower risk of endo, except for high butter intake, which *may* increase risk. Despite no concrete evidence that you should remove dairy to improve symptoms, anecdotal evidence suggests some people experience improvements in gastrointestinal symptoms, general wellbeing, and fatigue after eliminating or reducing their dairy intake. Given that people with endo are more likely to struggle with digestive symptoms or food intolerances, dairy sensitivity or lactose intolerance may be a reason some find benefit from removing these foods. If you are considering cutting out dairy to assess whether it can relieve any symptoms, it's advised to eliminate all types of dairy products for at least a month to allow your body time to adjust to life without it and to get a clearer understanding of whether elimination helps you. That being said, you may not need to cut out all types of dairy to experience benefits; for some, it's just fermented types such as kefir, Greek yoghurt, and cottage cheese which are problematic. After giving your body time to adjust to a dairy-free life, reintroduce one kind of dairy at a time to monitor its effect on your symptoms and whether the body tolerates it. Even if you experience a radical improvement and decide to continue without reintroducing dairy, maybe reconsider this if lactose intolerance is the underlying issue. Studies indicate avoiding all foods with lactose can decrease tolerance levels over time, whereas including them semi-regularly can improve intolerance. The good news is that going dairy-free is much more attainable than it once was, so experimenting to find what works for you doesn't need to be filled with dread. Various dairy-free milks, yoghurts, butters, ice creams, and cheese options are now available, making it easier to find substitutes while determining your long-term preferences. Be mindful of potential nutrient gaps when eliminating dairy from the diet. Dairy is a significant source of calcium, crucial for maintaining strong bones, especially for individuals who are more susceptible to osteoporosis or are on hormone therapy. To ensure adequate calcium intake, check the ingredients on your chosen dairy alternatives and opt for products fortified with calcium at a minimum. Some products may also be fortified with vitamin D, iodine, or various B vitamins to further support nutrition.

Iodine is a mineral commonly found in foods from the sea, such as fish, shellfish, and seaweed varieties, as well as dairy and, to a lesser degree, meat and plant-based sources. Our bodies require iodine to produce thyroid hormones, which are vital in controlling many bodily functions, including metabolism, and during pregnancy, to ensure the development of a healthy brain and nervous system in the foetus. Iodine deficiency occurs when the body has an inadequate intake of iodine, leading to an enlarged thyroid (known as a goitre) as the body compensates by working harder to make the hormones. If left untreated, iodine deficiency can progress to hypothyroidism, an irreversible condition that requires lifelong medication to manage. Hypothyroidism provokes symptoms like weight gain, fatigue, and sensitivity to the cold. The UK population is reportedly mildly deficient, with particular concern on women who are pregnant or of childbearing age. It's essential to ensure dietary sources of iodine to prevent this deficiency if you do not consume animal products. Luckily, you can get your hands on iodised salt; this is essentially table salt with iodine added. It's suitable for all dietary requirements, doesn't taste any different, and costs the same as other table salt brands. It's worth having in the house (even if you prefer to use sea salt), especially if you are vegan and don't eat seaweed regularly. Interestingly, seaweed is a food you could consider incorporating as it's been shown to have oestrogen-modulating activities, which can lower oestrogen levels in the blood.[6] The higher the seaweed intake, the lower the oestrogen concentrations found.[7] Whilst we await research on whether this is applicable to those with endometriosis, it may be worth exploring to observe any potential improvements, but of course, as with everything, don't overdo it.

If adopting a vegan or plant-based diet proves effective in managing your pain or gastrointestinal symptoms, that is a fantastic win. Similarly, if you have chosen a plant-based diet with the belief that it will help protect you from future endometriosis, that is commendable, as it shows your commitment to taking care of yourself and your future. Regardless of your motivations, it's crucial to ensure you meet your nutritional needs and stay flexible and open to adjustments that best serve your health. I hope that future research will provide better insight into these areas. Vegans should supplement with vitamin B12 and consume sufficient amounts of Vitamin C daily to enhance the absorption of non-haem iron derived from plant sources.

Myth #3 - You Need to Go Gluten-Free

Gluten often gets a bad reputation. I'm sure we have all heard of people avoiding gluten, but why? What is it, and should everyone avoid it? Gluten is a protein found in wheat, barley, and rye products like bread, couscous, pasta, etc. Although not inherently bad, some conditions require the avoidance of gluten, such as coeliac disease, wheat allergy, and non-coeliac gluten sensitivity. The first two are particularly troublesome and can have severe consequences for those affected if not managed. Coeliac disease is an autoimmune disorder where the body's immune system attacks itself upon exposure to gluten, releasing antibodies that cause chronic inflammation, swelling, and damage to the intestines. Wheat allergy also involves the immune system, where specific antibodies trigger a cascade of allergic reactions upon consumption of wheat. Non-coeliac gluten sensitivity is diagnosed when someone experiences symptoms similar to those of other gluten-related conditions but does not have celiac disease or a wheat allergy. Individuals diagnosed with any of the aforementioned conditions should not eat gluten. For those without gluten-related conditions, gluten is generally safe. If you can digest it without issue, it's considered harmless. Signs of potential gluten sensitivity can include bloating, diarrhoea, constipation, abdominal pain, and headaches, although these symptoms are non-specific and can be caused by a variety of reasons, including endometriosis itself. If you suspect you have an issue with gluten, consider removing it from your diet to see if there is any symptom improvement, or consult your doctor for proper testing to determine a cause. Some research suggests IBS or autoimmune conditions such as type 1 diabetes, Hashimoto's thyroiditis, and Graves disease might benefit from a low- or gluten-free diet. People with endometriosis are more prone to developing IBS and autoimmune disorders, so if you fall into this category, it may be worth experimenting with a gluten-free diet or at least trying to opt for gluten-free options where possible to minimise your intake and see if you feel any benefit.

You may be wondering if there is any research that has examined the relationship between gluten and endometriosis — there is. A study in 2012 explored whether eliminating gluten from the diet would provide any benefit to 207 patients experiencing severe endometriosis-related pain.[1] The study tracked symptoms across three categories: painful periods, non-menstrual pain, and pain during intercourse. After following a gluten-free diet for one year, 75% of participants reported significant improvement in these symptoms, while the remaining 25% saw no change. Interestingly, *all* patients experienced improvements in vitality, mental health, and general health perception, which is impressive. This study suggests that women with severe pelvic pain might benefit from a gluten-free diet and that mental health might also improve. If you try this, keeping a journal to track any changes is advised, as relying on memory to see if something is working is not very reliable. It can be hard to remember subtle shifts in symptoms over time. Similar results were found in another study, indicating that wheat avoidance showed greater improvement in overall wellbeing in comparison to those who consumed wheat.[2] Unfortunately, none of these studies explained why or how these results were achieved by so many, leaving us without a clear understanding of what occurs in the body to accomplish these results and who it is best suited for. Gluten may have inflammatory or hormone-disrupting properties, so when removed, this diminishes, but scientific evidence is not there to validate this.

On the other hand, contrasting research exists. The Nurses' Health Study II, conducted in 2022, concluded it was unlikely gluten had a role in causing endo or its associated symptoms.[3] Due to the conflicting evidence, randomised control trials are needed to assess whether dietary changes are attributable to the components itself or if there is a placebo effect, wherein individuals believe that eliminating certain foods benefits their health, so they perceive feeling better. Either way, if it ultimately improves how a person feels, the precise mechanisms don't really matter, but having robust scientific evidence would help people make more informed decisions about their diets. If you have IBS, chronic pelvic pain, gastrointestinal symptoms, or a higher risk of developing autoimmune conditions, such as having someone with celiac in your family, it may be worth trying a gluten-free diet. Despite a lack of conclusive evidence, many anecdotally report that going gluten-free improves their quality of life. If you are curious, removing gluten for a month can be worthwhile to see if it makes a difference. Like going dairy-free, experimenting with gluten-free options in this day and age does not instil the same dread it once did with a vast array of options you can incorporate.

Myth #4 - Soy is Bad for Endometriosis

When I was first diagnosed, I remember reading that you should avoid soy and soy-based products, including edamame, tofu, soy milk, miso, tempeh, soy sauce and soy nuts, on the premise that they contain naturally occurring oestrogenic compounds called isoflavones. This is not the same as the oestrogen found in the human body, but are phytoestrogens, which are molecules found in plants with a similar structure to human oestrogen. This myth may have originated from the assumption that phytoestrogens behave in the body the same way as oestrogens do. So, people with an oestrogen-dependent disease like endo should avoid these food products. While it's true that phytoestrogens are considered weak oestrogens and dock onto the same receptors in the body, activating them and, therefore, they are able to mimic the effects of human oestrogen, there's more to the story. Interestingly, by binding to these receptors, phytoestrogens may potentially prevent stronger human oestrogen binding, as they are blocked. This can result in an anti-oestrogenic effect in the body, which may be the opposite of bad for us.

There are two main types of oestrogen receptors in the body, called alpha and beta. Oestrogen we make ourselves prefers to bind to alpha receptors on our reproductive organs and tissues, whilst some phytoestrogens found in plants like soy prefer to bind to beta receptors.[1] These receptors are found in various amounts in different parts of the body. This means the effect of phytoestrogens in foods like soy depends on the type of tissue they dock to, the number of alpha and beta receptors present, and their affinity for either receptor (meaning which one they are more drawn to). Endometriosis tissue has a higher number of beta receptors, a whopping 100 times more beta receptors than normal endometrial tissue.[2] Therefore, ingesting soy products could mean additional oestrogen-like substances bind to the beta receptors on endometriosis lesions, provoking issues like inflammation and growth. On the other hand, it could mean it blocks stronger human oestrogen from binding to these receptors, which could theoretically reduce growth. Studies have shown that targeting beta receptors and treating mice with non-hormonal beta-receptor agonists resulted in complete regression of lesions in 40-75% of the mice studied.[3] This suggests focusing on beta receptors might be an effective approach to treating endometriosis. The activation or inhibition of the oestrogen receptors can induce or hamper oestrogen acting in the body, thus disrupting oestrogen signalling. Whether this is beneficial or detrimental depends on the individual, the specific tissue affected, and their health status. For example, interfering with normal oestrogen function might be advantageous for someone with breast cancer or oestrogen dominance. Disrupted oestrogen signalling is also a characteristic of endometriosis, sometimes contributing to progesterone resistance and oestrogen dominance.[4]

Endocrine systems are highly regulated networks of glands and tissues that create and release hormones directly into our bloodstream to control various bodily functions. Soy-derived isoflavones are believed to have anti-oestrogenic properties and so also act as endocrine disruptors.[1] The impact of these may lead to oestrogenic activity in low-oestrogen environments, such as in menopausal women who make lower amounts of oestrogen.[5] Although activity may be small, there is an overall increase. Whether this is good or bad varies; even though this may inherently seem bad, we need to consider the person's health status. For example, this pro-oestrogenic effect could reduce classic menopausal like hot-flushes.[6] Furthermore, phytoestrogens might have an anti-oestrogenic effect in high-oestrogen environments such as endometriosis and endometrial cancer, so they could help to restore hormone balance closer to normal.[5] It would then seem soy is a good choice to incorporate into your diet. If soy can have an anti-oestrogenic effect, it may be able to reduce the growth of lesions or limit inflammation and pain. The truth of this isn't simple to determine. Well-constructed studies need to be conducted to get conclusive information on whether soy, among other phytoestrogens, can do this. There are studies suggesting dietary isoflavones found in soy do reduce the risk of endometriosis,[7] however, other evidence also shows the opposite to be true.

Endometriosis affects more women in Asia than in any other continent in the world.[8] Soy is generally also a staple part of the Southeast Asian diet, posing the question: does this validate that high intake increases the risk of endometriosis, confirming a relationship between the two? It's currently unclear if a diet high in soy equals a greater risk of endo or if it's more nuanced. One study reported women who were regularly fed soy formula as an infant were twice as likely to have endometriosis in adulthood.[9] As phytoestrogens are oestrogenic in a non-oestrogenic environment,[10] is the associated risk in parts of the world where there's a high soy intake, actually based on women having a high intake before puberty when oestrogen levels in the body are low. This would mean the age at which you start consuming soy could play a vital role in determining risk, with high intake before puberty posing a more significant risk factor than soy intake as an adult. This possibility needs to be studied in greater detail as isoflavones have been shown to affect different populations in different ways, which need to be evaluated.[11] It's good to note that not all phytoestrogens have the same impact on endometriosis, so it's harder to differentiate how the studies carried out relate to soy products uniquely. The myth that soy is bad for us and so needs to be avoided is not proven to be true. As the research is not definitive, if you want to incorporate soy into your diet, go ahead, although it's probably best to stick to eating a sensible amount. It can be a particularly important component for vegans and vegetarians as a complete source of protein, but as always, moderation is key. Try limiting soy intake to two servings a day, such as a soy cappuccino in the morning and some edamame for lunch. Unprocessed or minimally processed soy products, like soybeans, edamame, soy milk, tofu, and tempeh, are better options to include over the highly processed forms seen in supermarkets, particularly in alternative meats. Some people may find their symptoms improve or dissipate with soy intake. There isn't much research to validate this either way, so always listen to your body.

* * *

Now that we've debunked some of the myths, what else should we consider when it comes to our diet and what other research has been conducted?

Food to Support the Microbiome

'All Disease Begins in the Gut.'
- Hippocrates, The Father of Modern Medicine

What we eat, when we eat it, and how we feel about our food is often overlooked by the medical system. There simply isn't enough time for doctors to look at this aspect of treatment with every patient, nor does every patient have access to see a dietician or nutritionist to determine if what they're eating is causing an environment in the gut fostering disease. With that in mind, I think it's best to discuss how to optimise your gut health in this book. We have discussed how the trillions of microbes comprising your microbiome can produce hormones and vitamins which significantly influence your health, mood, and energy — but what makes a healthy gut? You can take supplements, which we will get into in the next chapter. However, you should never solely rely on supplements, and they shouldn't replace taking care of your diet and what you put into your body each day. Probiotic supplements usually only contain bacteria, and although this can be very helpful, it doesn't provide the whole package. So, let's discuss dietary strategies to support our microbiome.

Fibre

Fibre is a carbohydrate found in plant-based foods like fruits, vegetables, nuts, legumes, and whole grains. It cannot be digested by the body in the same way other nutrients are, but plays an essential role in gut health. Some fibres are *fermented* by gut bacteria and other fibres may *affect* the gut microbiota. Gut microorganisms feed on fibre, so while you can take prebiotic supplements, which are essentially food for the organisms to eat, we don't want to rely on these, so fibre should come from your diet. Fortunately, this is not hard to achieve. Most of our immune system cells are found in our digestive tract, so keeping your gut healthy supports your immune system. A fibre-rich diet is believed to have many health benefits, including the prevention of diabetes, cancers, and obesity.[1] It can also increase the amount of oestrogen excreted by the body. Once the body has used oestrogen, it is broken down by the liver and should mostly exit through our urine and faeces. This is what we want to happen. However, sometimes oestrogen gets reabsorbed from the intestines back into the bloodstream — raising our oestrogen levels. By positively influencing the gut microbiota, we can decrease this reabsorption of oestrogen, lowering the amount of free oestrogen circulating in the blood,[2] which, in theory, could lower endometriosis risk.[3] Whilst several types of fibre exist, they are commonly divided into insoluble fibre and soluble fibre, making it easy to categorise the types and translate them into dietary choices. These work in tandem with your microbiome to keep your gastrointestinal system balanced, healthy, and flowing. Most foods contain both types, so you don't need to worry about which type you are getting; it's better to consider the quantity you eat and try to get more into your diet. Variety is also key here, so consume an array of fibre-rich foods because different fibres are thought to feed different bacteria, which creates healthy diversity. High-fibre foods include most plant-based foods, so getting in your 5-a-day and choosing whole grains rather than refined products like white bread is an excellent way to increase variety. It's also best to eat whole fruits and vegetables to receive your nutrients rather than drinking fruit juice, as the juicing process removes the fibrous materials. If you elevate your fibre intake significantly, you may notice an elevation in wind, bloating or discomfort. Although, this should dissipate as the gut bacteria adapt to the increased intake. You should also boost your water intake if you are increasing fibre to avoid constipation.

Soluble Fibre

Soluble fibre attracts and dissolves in water, turning into a gel during digestion. This process slows down digestion and helps regulate blood sugar levels, preventing rapid spikes. This is good for everyone, particularly those with diabetes or PCOS. Soluble fibre can also promote feelings of fullness, aiding in weight management. Examples include oat bran, barley, nuts, seeds, beans, lentils, peas, apples, blueberries, and chia seeds. Psyllium is a common supplement containing soluble fibre.

Insoluble Fibre

Insoluble fibre, or roughage, remains relatively unchanged as it passes through our gastrointestinal tract. If you have ever noticed sweetcorn in your stool, this is because it's a source of insoluble fibre. This type adds bulk to your stools and acts as a natural laxative, helping food pass through the intestines and preventing constipation. For those with bowel obstruction from endometriosis, too much insoluble fibre may cause problems by bulking the faeces, making it harder to get out. Examples include whole wheat flour, nuts, beans, cauliflower, potatoes, and green beans.

Prebiotic Foods

Prebiotics are a type of fibre that feed the bacteria in your gut. By nourishing the microbes, you help them thrive and maintain a balanced gut ecosystem. They differ from probiotics, which contain the actual microorganisms. Prebiotics are fermented rapidly, which can cause symptoms such as gas and bloating, making them unsuitable for some. If you have IBS, SIBO, FODMAP intolerance or other gastrointestinal issues, you may need to avoid prebiotic-rich foods such as garlic or onion as they can trigger pain, diarrhoea, or constipation. It's always best to listen to your body. If consuming prebiotics causes discomfort, don't put yourself through hell to get prebiotics in. Below are some prebiotic foods and their associated health benefits:

Chicory Root	Chicory Root is a historic healing plant with one of the highest contents of inulin, a type of fibre. It has been shown to increase good gut bacteria, including Bifidobacterium. Chicory Root has an anti-inflammatory and antioxidant effect and has a role in appetite regulation. [4]
Onion	Improves health of gut microbiota and can strengthen the immune system. [5]
Garlic	Promotes growth of the beneficial bacterial called Bifidobacteria. Garlic may provide protection against gastrointestinal disease. [6]
Artichoke	Artichoke also contains inulin, which increases the amount of bifidobacteria and lactobacilli in the gut. This can prevent the growth of pathogenic disease-causing bacteria. [7]

Dandelion Greens	Dandelion Greens are the leaves that grow on dandelions and can be cooked or eaten raw. It is amazing to think, that a plant many people associate as a weed has been linked to numerous health benefits. It contains a high amount of inulin and can stimulate the immune system. Dandelion greens contain taraxasterol, which has antimicrobial activity against Staphylococcus Aureus, which can cause a wide array of clinical diseases.[8]

Eat Bacteria

A key aspect of maintaining a healthy gut is consuming foods that facilitate the growth of beneficial bacteria, creating an environment that cultivates a thriving microbiome to provide numerous health benefits. But how do we introduce good bacteria into our bodies? Food and supplements are the primary sources. While many foods naturally contain bacteria, some have higher concentrations of either beneficial or harmful types. For instance, salmonella is a harmful bacterium that can contaminate animal products, which is why we must sufficiently cook meat to ensure any existing salmonella is killed by the cooking process. On the other hand, fermented foods are rich in beneficial bacteria. Fermentation is a process where sugars are broken down by yeast or bacteria, giving these foods a distinctive bitter or sharp taste. Examples include yoghurt, kimchi, sauerkraut, miso, kombucha, tempeh, and some cheeses such as gouda. These foods often contain live, active cultures of bacteria that are good for our health. Naturally, the types vary between foods, but a good bacteria called *lactobacilli* is commonly found in some of these. Eating these foods improves the microbiome by stimulating the growth of good bacteria while minimising the growth of harmful, pathogen-causing bacteria. When incorporating fermented foods into your diet, please be mindful of added sugars. Products like yoghurts and kombucha drinks often contain high amounts of added free sugar, which can be detrimental to your health. It's best to opt for plain or unsweetened versions and, if needed, add natural sweeteners like fruit or honey, which is often a better alternative to the sugar the manufacturers add.

Sugar

When we talk about 'free sugar', we're referring to sugars added to foods, not those naturally found within the structure of whole foods like fruit. Even though honey, syrups, and fruit juice may be natural, they are also classified as free sugars because their sugars are not inside cells. Free sugar, particularly when consumed in excess, is harmful to our health. It's recommended that no more than 5% of our daily calories come from free sugar. Yet only 13% of adults meet this target, with children often consuming the highest amounts, primarily through sugary drinks.[9] Excessive sugar intake contributes to tooth decay, easy consumption of too many calories, obesity, and type 2 diabetes. It's also linked to inflammation and the development of chronic, metabolic, and autoimmune diseases.[10] The exception here is honey, which, when consumed in moderation, can exert anti-inflammatory effects, lower bad cholesterol, and potentially aid in preventing cardiovascular and metabolic diseases.[11] Not all honeys are the same though; the best varieties are raw, manuka, and dark honey, as these typically retain a greater amount of beneficial nutrients. Sugar is thought to have a detrimental impact on the microbiome, reducing the population of beneficial bacteria, which then shakes up the balance between the good and bad, leading to pro-inflammatory properties and metabolic dysregulation.[12] The Western diet is notoriously high in sugar, even hidden in foods we consider savoury, like condiments, sauces, and ready-made meals, making it challenging to reduce sugar intake. However, cutting back can bring significant benefits, especially in reducing inflammation, which is valuable for endometriosis. If you are having a flare or are having a bad period, it can be easy to reach for sugary or convenience foods, but they can make symptoms worse. Sugar is highly addictive and more rewarding to the body than drugs like cocaine.[13] Reducing your intake can be tough, but it's important to be aware of this and feel proud of any efforts in cutting back. If you have a high sugar intake, baby steps with a gradual reduction may be more manageable than going cold turkey, depending on your personality and level of addiction. The most effective way to reduce sugar intake is to remove sugary drinks from your diet, like fizzy drinks and sweetened tea or coffee. This step may be very challenging, but it's the easiest way to remove excess sugar from your diet. Be cautious if you drink alcohol with mixers such as lemonade or cola; this can be a quick slide into overdoing the sugar intake. Spirits mixed with soda or tonic water is a better alternative, and you could still flavour it with lemon or lime. If you don't drink sugar-sweetened drinks but know you consume high amounts of sugar from other types of food like sweets, cakes, chocolate, pastries, crisps, dried fruits, or ready-made meals, make appropriate ways to combat your intake that suit you and your lifestyle.

Overall, diet greatly impacts our microbiome and gut health, signifying it has a notable role in our immune system and inflammation levels because remember, 80% of our immune cells live in our gut. Taking care of your gut can determine whether you get sick, how quickly you recover, and help prevent future diseases. As evidence exists postulating the microbiome is impacted by endometriosis or our microbiome may contribute to the development and progression of the disease, taking care of our gut is therefore of the utmost importance. One thing that can set your microbiome back is antibiotics, so if you need to take them, it's essential when you've completed your course of medicine, to add back good bacteria through probiotics or diet. Poor bacterial health in the colon is a physical stressor on the body and can exacerbate inflammatory conditions and oestrogen signalling.[14] Stress and depression can also alter the microbiome through stress hormones, inflammation, and other processes. Dysbiosis can then adjust our food choices by altering our food cravings, metabolism, and mood, leading to a cycle where we are stuck perpetually making poor food choices.[15] If you feel like you are in this cycle and are struggling to break it, it may be worth trying a probiotic supplement to help kick-start you onto the right track. Still, always remember to look at your food as it's the most significant change you can make to your life. Foods will help restore imbalance, and you will reap the benefits with more energy, vitality, improvement in bowel movements, and symptom reduction. It will help your body build a balanced, thriving, happy microbiome and immune system. Also, the immune and nervous systems are intricately interwoven; our immune cells regulate the nervous system, and the nervous system influences the immune system. Individuals with endometriosis often have an overstimulated nervous system, impacting their lives in several ways or can manifest with a number of symptoms. Whilst having a healthy microbiome may not resolve these all on its own, it's an integral part of the story that many can benefit from. The degree of central sensitisation will vary from person to person; some may have increased pain perception, whilst others may have cognitive changes such as anxiety. Food is shown to be able to change the gut microbiota, making it a fun and delicious way to provide therapy to your body and help it calm down.[16]

* * *

Low Inflammatory Diet

The typical Western diet is known to be inflammatory due to its abundance of added sugar, processed meats, refined carbohydrates, trans fats, and artificial ingredients.[1,2] This diet is often lacking in fruits, vegetables, legumes, and whole grains, which are known to help manage inflammation.[3,4] While some scientists argue there is no direct link between endometriosis and food, its widely accepted diet can either be the foundation for good health or put you on the road to chronic disease. In fact, a study in 2023 collected data on 3,410 American participants between 1999 and 2006 and found that a pro-inflammatory diet was associated with increased endometriosis risk, suggesting anti-inflammatory dietary interventions may be beneficial in preventing the disease.[5] So, whilst diet alone does not cause endo, it might be a contributing factor. It's important not to overlook the impact of diet on symptom control, inflammation reduction, and disease management. It can be disempowering to believe we have no control over our health or the ability to manage our condition. Many of us turn to food as a means of nourishing and supporting our bodies, choosing ingredients we believe can help us feel better. This study highlights inflammation caused explicitly by diet is vital to acknowledge and an issue we can address. The notion that diet has no relation to endometriosis may stem from a lack of *robust* scientific research rather than because it's untrue.

It's evident that what we consume on a daily basis has the power to bring about changes, whether big or small, noticeable or subtle, that contribute to our overall health and wellbeing. It's easier to recognise the impact of a poor diet because, over time, our body shows us something isn't right through new health issues or disease. For example, enjoying an occasional sugary drink won't cause harm, but habitual or high consumption of sugary drinks can lead to health issues slowly creeping up on a person, such as mood disorders or weight gain.[6] Similarly, the effects of a well-balanced, low-inflammatory diet may be less apparent but equally significant. It's less obvious when what we are doing is working because there's no metric for health; no symptoms flare up to show that your body is happy. Simply, you feel good. If you have pre-existing symptoms coming from an imbalance in the body, maybe over time, these disappear, like noticing your joints don't hurt as much. So, that may be your metric to show what you are doing is working. It's essential to consider food a powerful tool in reducing inflammation and promoting optimal health.

Endometriosis is complex and currently incurable, but modifying diet and other lifestyle factors can be a great way to prevent further issues from developing. One hypothesis for why endometriosis forms in the first place is that inflammation creates a perfect storm for it to grow. By working with this theory and creating a strategy to reduce the inflammation, we can try to prevent creating an environment with our diet where endometriosis thrives. I am not saying a low-inflammatory diet alone will cure or prevent endo, but we should acknowledge the impact of inflammation caused by food, making it a good piece of the puzzle to address. Food can be a valuable part of a broader strategy to support health and manage inflammation. None of this is based on science that says this *absolutely* works, but for many of us, it's logical to try everything we can, using holistic approaches to reduce inflammation and let ourselves feel good. Diet is a powerful tool in this, so by empowering ourselves with knowledge of foods that can either fight or promote inflammation, we can make a real difference in our wellbeing. Remember, this is all about giving you the knowledge to find out what works for you. The key is recognising that there is no 'one-size-fits-all' approach; what works for others might not be suitable for you, and sometimes, there may be foods you don't even want to try for various reasons. In Part 1, we discussed that inflammation is not inherently harmful; it's a crucial part of the immune response that we need to survive. The problems arise when it becomes chronic rather than transient, as seen in response to an infection or injury. We shouldn't view inflammation as bad or the enemy, but rather just that we have too much and want to bring it down to a normal healthy level. How we view things can influence how we feel and heal, so we don't have to have negative connotations around the word inflammation, but it is just something we want to lower. This shift in perspective can positively influence our healing journey. Numerous studies examine the role of certain foods on inflammatory markers or the role of dietary patterns in various diseases. While this book focuses specifically on endometriosis, it's worth mentioning anti-inflammatory diets have been associated with positive outcomes for other conditions as well, so although no specific diet has been conclusively proven to prevent or treat endo, incorporating anti-inflammatory foods into your daily routine can provide numerous benefits.

Anti-Inflammatory Foods

Fruit & Vegetables

Rich in polyphenols, fruits and vegetables are potent antioxidants that can help neutralise free radicals, preventing them from causing harm. This can reduce oxidative stress and inflammation. Key foods include tomatoes, green leafy vegetables, berries, and citrus fruits.

Antioxidant Foods

Foods rich in vitamins A, C, E, and B9 (folic acid) possess antioxidant properties. These help reduce free radicals, which in turn has an anti-inflammatory effect. Key foods include nuts, leafy greens, plus red and orange fruits or vegetables.

Unsaturated Fats

Monounsaturated fats, abundant in olive oil, canola oil, avocado, and nuts, possess antioxidant properties and exhibit anti-inflammatory effects. Polyunsaturated fats, especially omega-3 fatty acids found in fatty fish, play a role in lowering inflammatory cells and even reducing the proliferation of endometriosis tissue in lab tests.[7] If you recall, we should consume more omega-3 than omega-6 to prevent inflammation. Also, omega-3 could affect the pro-inflammatory prostaglandins found in endometriosis and reduce the amount circulating in our blood, possibly reducing inflammatory symptoms.[8]

Herbs and Spices

Herbs and spices are plants used in their natural form or grounded into powders to flavour and season food. They have various healing properties: some are excellent sources of polyphenols, which are potent antioxidants, and others are anti-inflammatory.[9] These can be incorporated into daily meals for a boost of goodness or brewed as teas to drink throughout the day for additional support. Overall, there is evidence that herbs and spices possess antioxidant, anti-inflammatory, antitumour, anticarcinogenic, plus glucose- and cholesterol-lowering properties.[10] So, use your spices and make yummy and nutritious meals full of flavour. Examples include oregano, rosemary, thyme, parsley, cinnamon, cumin, cloves, basil, mint, lemongrass, nutmeg, turmeric, ginger, and marjoram.

Inflammatory Foods

Trans Fats

Trans fats are associated with higher levels of inflammatory messengers and, therefore, increased inflammation.[11] They are commonly found in baked and fried foods and are thought to contribute to 500,000 premature deaths in the world each year.[12] Trans fats are not so much of an issue in the UK due to laws regulating the amount allowed in food. Artificial trans fats are banned in countries like Denmark, Austria, Switzerland, and the United States. If you live in a country without regulations, be careful of your trans-fat consumption.

Sugar

Not only is sugar detrimental to the microbiome, but it's also considered a critical factor in inducing low-grade chronic inflammation and aggravating existing inflammation.[13] Even though maintaining healthy sugar levels can be challenging, it's pertinent to consider when assessing your diet.

Highly Processed Foods

Highly processed foods can cause inflammation in many ways, either directly or indirectly. Processed foods tend to be high in sugar and simple carbohydrates, which can trigger rapid spikes in blood sugar levels, causing insulin and inflammatory molecules to be released into the blood to help break down the glucose. They also disrupt our gut health by changing the balance of bacteria, leading to immune responses and further inflammation.[14]

Advanced Glycation Products (AGEs)

Processed meats contain Advanced Glycation Products (AGEs), which are harmful compounds linked to serious health problems, including chronic diseases. AGEs form in the bloodstream when sugar is combined with protein or fat. When they are made in the body *after* consumption, levels are relatively low, so the body can work to remove them without much issue. However, when meat is processed, AGE compounds are formed *prior* to consumption, especially when cooked at high temperatures. Excessive consumption of AGEs (such as from processed meat) overwhelms the body's natural defences, increasing oxidative stress and inflammation. The primary source of AGEs is diet, so be mindful of your intake.

Refined Carbohydrates

Refined grains are stripped of their bran, fibre, and other nutrients to produce flour. The grain is then used to make white bread, pizza dough, white pasta, pastries, etc. Refined carbohydrates can be inflammatory in a similar way to other processed foods. They are composed of simple sugars or carbohydrates with little or no fibre, creating a higher glycaemic index, which causes blood sugar spikes. They may also promote the growth of inflammatory bacteria in the gut.

Red Meat

Red meat can increase the expression of pro-inflammatory markers in the body, possibly creating an environment that promotes the growth and progression of endometriosis.[15] Although, this likely depends on the quality, type, fat content, and cooking method of the meat consumed.

Fried Food

Fried food includes foods you fry at home, dishes cooked in deep fryers at restaurants, and pre-packaged convenience foods that are fried before you purchase them, like oven chips. Frying foods can form harmful compounds such as AGEs and trans-fat, which directly stimulate and increase inflammation and oxidative stress in the body.[16] Fried foods can also affect the gut microbiome by reducing the diversity of microbial communities and altering the levels of specific microbes.[17] Fried foods tend to have high levels of omega-6 due to the vegetable oils used during cooking. If you consume a lot of fried foods, it's easy for the scales to tip into greater omega-6 than omega-3, perpetuating chronic low-grade inflammation, which naturally you don't want.[18] To avoid this, try air frying, baking, steaming, boiling, or roasting food instead. Although air frying uses oil, it uses a minimal amount of oil to cook your food, so when comparing homemade chips made in the air fryer, they will be less inflammatory than pre-made oven or deep-fried chips.

Our standard diets tend to be pro-inflammatory, containing abundant processed foods, sugar, refined carbohydrates, and insufficient amounts of fruits, vegetables, and healthy fats. By shifting our dietary choices toward an anti-inflammatory approach, we can restore balance in the body. If you know you eat more foods on the inflammatory side, it can be particularly important to look at what you can switch up, as you don't want to fuel your inflammation.

Rather than focusing on what we cannot eat, try to embrace the vast array of foods that can support our wellbeing, making the journey exciting and enjoyable for yourself. Remember, you don't have to cut foods from your diet forever. It's just about changing your everyday food practices to make your body feel good to be in. An anti-inflammatory diet should also include antioxidants to balance the oxidative stress present in chronic inflammatory processes. Foods with anti-inflammatory characteristics may suppress endometriosis-related pain symptoms. If you are curious about dairy, the relationship between dairy consumption and inflammation is a complex and debated topic in the scientific community, with many studies comparing whether it's inflammatory or anti-inflammatory. There are many types of dairy-based foods, so this can impact the answer. If you are considering going dairy-free, be aware the topic is nuanced, and the evidence to date is not strong enough to say either way. If elimination helps you, there's your answer, so continue it.

At the start of your anti-inflammatory journey, take extra time in the supermarket to find your new staples. Find joy in exploring new ingredients and reading food labels to avoid chemicals, preservatives, and words you don't know. Go for the simplest, less processed versions of everything where possible, and organic if you can. For example, if you are able to buy fresh tomatoes to make tomato sauce instead of buying a pre-made sauce, do it. Sometimes, we may be in a position where we need to purchase something processed and ready-made, if so, go for one with the fewest ingredients or words you don't know. If you consume meat, select minimally processed, grass-fed options if possible. Over time, you won't have to spend extra time choosing which foods to buy as you relearn your food shopping habits.

It's crucial to understand that how we perceive our diet is central to our relationship with food. If you believe you are counteracting the inflammation in your body with your food, this can positively affect the outcome, as the way we perceive how we eat is very important. Avoid creating a sense of boredom, restriction, or deprivation around food, as it can undermine long-term adherence. Remember, you are making this choice, no one is forcing you to. Embrace the process and enjoy discovering new flavours and recipes.

While the impact of diet on endometriosis is still an area of ongoing research, it is evident that dietary choices can influence inflammation levels and potentially alleviate symptoms. By incorporating anti-inflammatory foods and reducing your intake of pro-inflammatory foods, you can take a proactive approach to support your wellbeing. Adjustments to your diet can be a process of elimination and experimentation to find what works best for you. Take the time to educate yourself about the potential benefits of various foods and make conscious decisions while grocery shopping. As you embark on this journey, remember that positive changes to your diet can profoundly impact your overall health and wellbeing. Embrace the power of food as a tool to support your body in feeling its best.

* * *

Vegetables & Fruit

Incorporating a variety of vegetables and fruits into your diet is essential for good health, providing fibre, vitamins, minerals, and anti-inflammatory compounds. Even though research is limited, studies have suggested that specific dietary patterns can influence endometriosis disease progression, whilst increasing intake of certain fruits and vegetables may help manage symptoms by supporting hormonal balance and reducing inflammation. Research has yet to establish any definite causal links; but understanding which foods may have a positive impact on disease management can be a valuable tool. Generally, when it comes to fruit and vegetables, you want to 'eat the rainbow', emphasising that you want a variety of colours in your shopping basket. This diversity ensures you consume a broad range of nutrients and phytochemicals, each providing different health benefits. While research is still developing, it can still be fun to know which evidence-based dietary changes can be made to ultimately get you feeling better.

Cruciferous Vegetables

Cruciferous vegetables may exhibit protective effects against oestrogen-dominant conditions. One study found that eating cruciferous vegetables less than once a week was associated with a 13% higher risk of developing endometriosis compared to eating them at least once a day.[1] This protective effect is primarily attributed to the presence of Indole-3-Carbinol (I3C) in cruciferous vegetables. This compound promotes the detoxification of harmful substances in the liver and enhances the conversion of oestrogen into less potent forms.[2] By turning oestrogen into waste products, it promotes its clearance from the body. This is particularly beneficial for those with oestrogen dominance, which is commonly associated with endometriosis.[3] After ingestion, I3C can be converted into 3,3-Diindolylmethane (DIM), which regulates sex hormones and reduces high oestrogen. One of the ways it does this is by inhibiting the enzyme aromatase, which converts testosterone into oestrogen. By reducing this conversion, DIM helps stabilise excess hormone production.[3] The fibre in cruciferous vegetables also helps remove oestrogen via the digestive system. Through both hormone regulation and detoxification, this dual action makes cruciferous vegetables a potentially valuable part of a diet. Research also suggests that regular consumption of these vegetables may reduce the risk of oestrogen-related cancers.[4] To reap the benefits, eating food sources of DIM daily is advised.[5] Thankfully, there are many types of cruciferous vegetables, meaning we don't need to be repetitively eating the same food every day, but can include a variety each week.

Cruciferous Vegetables			
Cauliflower Cabbage Kale Bok Choy	Broccoli Rocket Horseradish Rutabaga	Wasabi Turnips Radishes Garden Cress	Lettuce Brussel Sprouts Collard Greens

Fresh Fruit & Green Vegetables

Research found that women who consume more fresh fruits and green vegetables have a significant reduction in risk of developing endometriosis.[6] Fresh fruits are defined as those that haven't been processed (i.e., canned, preserved, frozen, dried, or pickled). In particular, citrus fruits like oranges and grapefruits have been shown to be protective, reducing the risk of endometriosis by 22% when consumed more than once a day.[7] Strangely, in America, the opposite results were found. A study concluded fruit intake increased disease rates, alongside high intake of β-Carotene found in yellow, orange, and green foods such as spinach, carrots, tomatoes, and mango.[8] These contrasting findings are proposed to be attributed to the high number of pesticides used in American farming, increasing the risk.[9] This highlights the role of toxins in endometriosis, which we will discuss further at the end of Part 3. If you wish to avoid this, prioritise organic produce when possible.

Vitamin C, E and B9 (Folic Acid)

Certain vitamins, such as Vitamin C, E, and B9 (folic acid), may have a protective effect against endometriosis. A large study on ~70,000 women, in which ~1,000 had endometriosis, found consuming foods rich in these vitamins had an inverse risk of developing endometriosis, indicating they may have a protective effect.[10] That being said, the study didn't find the same effect when these nutrients were taken in supplement form, nor were they able to determine if these nutrients could help mitigate endometriosis symptoms. Therefore, it's best to try and consume them through whole foods rather than assuming you can reap the same benefits by relying on supplements. Listed below are foods rich in these nutrients — see if there's any you can incorporate more of into your diet.

Foods Rich in Vitamin C	Foods Rich in Vitamin E	Foods Rich in Folic Acid
Citrus Fruits (oranges, lemon, lime, kiwi, grapefruit)	Plant Oils (wheat germ, sunflower, safflower, soybean, hazelnut oil, rapeseed, olive)	Dark Green Leafy Vegetables (spinach, romaine lettuce, asparagus, kale, cabbage, brussel sprouts, broccoli)
Bell Peppers	Spinach	Beans & Peas
Strawberries	Sunflower Seeds	Sunflower Seeds
Tomatoes	Peanuts and Peanut Butter	Other Fruits (include mango, papaya, grapes, bananas)
Cruciferous Vegetables	Collard Greens	Citrus Fruits (i.e. oranges)
White Potatoes	Spinach	Whole Grains
Guava	Pumpkin	Eggs
Papaya	Avocado	Peanuts
Raw Tomatoes	Wheatgerm	Poultry, Pork, Liver
Brussel Sprouts	Almonds	Lentils

* * *

Organic Food

Organic food comes from farming or food production methods that avoid synthetic chemicals, such as man-made fertilisers, pesticides, growth hormones, and livestock feed additives — instead using only natural substances and processes. Standards are set to define what is considered organic farming, and these may vary worldwide, but generally, they require that at least 95% of ingredients come from organic sources. The aim is to produce high-quality food without exposing consumers or animals to the harmful chemicals sometimes used in other farming techniques, as they are linked to health problems. Considerable care and attention are required to maintain this style of farming without dependence on these chemicals. Instead, organic farmers use natural alternatives to ensure they can still produce ample food without the need for these. Soil health is a critical component in organic farming as maintaining nutrient-dense, healthy soil ensures that crops grow well, plus these nutrients are transferred to the food we eat. Organic food tends to be healthier and more nutrient-rich due to this careful management of soil quality. Certifications like the *Soil Association Organic* label can help consumers identify foods produced to higher standards, ensuring no synthetic chemicals are used.

Regarding animal products, organic farming offers several advantages, particularly in terms of animal welfare and health. It's good to consider the treatment of the meat you consume. Non-organic factory farms often use antibiotics and growth hormones to increase the size of their animals, which can have negative consequences for animal welfare, human health, and the environment. Routine antibiotic use in farming contributes to the global antibiotic resistance crisis, where antibiotics are becoming less effective against infections, posing significant public health risks. Can you imagine a world without effective antibiotics? Scary right. From tonsillitis to surgical procedures, antibiotics are relied on to restore our health when we are not well. We need to take this threat seriously, and this partly stems from the overuse of antibiotics in our food chain. In organic farming, antibiotics and growth hormones are not routinely used. Instead, farmers focus on providing better living conditions, including space, hygiene, and proper diet, to keep animals healthy without dependency on antibiotics. This improves animal welfare and reduces the risk of antibiotic resistance, making organic animal products a more sustainable choice. Organic farming is also better for the environment as it minimises chemical runoff into waterways and protects ecosystems. The absence of synthetic pesticides and fertilisers ensures that harmful substances do not contaminate rivers, oceans, or other natural habitats, promoting better health for the soil, the animals that reside on the farmland, and us.

You may think that all sounds lovely, but organic food is expensive and not everyone can afford to eat only organic, and... how important is it anyway? Well, organic food not only contains fewer harmful chemicals, but one of the key arguments in favour of organic food is that it's often more nutrient-dense than non-organic food, meaning it is healthier for us. Studies suggest that organic produce contains higher levels of essential nutrients like vitamin C, iron, magnesium, and phosphorus.[1] As these are found in a higher quantity, we are fuelling our body with more of what it needs, which can prevent deficiencies. This could be particularly important for those with endometriosis, as various nutrients are crucial in managing inflammation, boosting the immune system, and supporting overall health. We'll explain in more detail in the supplements chapter, but to not have to rely on supplements to consume these nutrients is a step in the right direction. Organic foods also tend to be higher in antioxidant phytochemicals such as flavonoids and carotenoids,[1] which helps protect our bodies from oxidative stress damage and reduces inflammation. Additionally, organic meats, including pasture-fed beef, can have up to 30% less saturated fat and around 23% higher amounts of healthy unsaturated fatty acids, including omega-3.[2,3] We have established the importance of omega-3, and we've also seen that red meat is often villainised for its adverse impact on health. Therefore, if you consume red meat, it may be better to eat less of it, but buy organic when you do, as it provides healthier fats and fewer harmful additives.

So where does this leave us, stuck between choosing the food we know is better...but tends to be more expensive and choosing more affordable food...that has chemicals on it? Don't feel defeated and give up on trying to eat healthy. It's always better to eat five different fruits and vegetables a day (whether organic or not) than to not consume any at all. If budget is a concern, the best option is to buy organic if and when you can, as even occasionally reducing the amount of chemicals in your diet is still helping. Foods with thin skins, such as berries, peaches, and grapes, tend to absorb more chemicals compared to those with thick skins, like avocados and bananas, so if you can buy a couple of items each week, it's good to know where your money is best spent, prioritising organic purchases for produce that absorbs the most chemicals. You can also wash and peel your foods to reduce the exposure to the substances, although this will not eliminate them. To help consumers make informed decisions, organisations like the *Pesticide Action Network UK* release a 'Dirty Dozen' list each year, highlighting the top twelve foods most contaminated with pesticide chemicals known as residues. They focus on multiple residues because of growing evidence that chemicals can become more harmful when combined. The dirtiest foods are named and shamed, helping you decide whether to avoid them or buy them as organic produce to stay away from the chemicals. Similarly, in the U.S., the *Environmental Working Group (EWG)* provides a 'Dirty Dozen' list to match US produce as well as a 'Clean Fifteen' list, showing which foods are safest to buy non-organic.

If you drink plant-based milk alternatives, such as oat or almond milk, it's helpful to know that organic versions are not allowed to have added nutrients, such as calcium and vitamins, a practice typically carried out to match the nutrients of cow milk. This can be an essential source for vegans, so if you rely on these drinks for your calcium intake, consider opting for non-organic fortified versions to ensure you meet your nutritional needs or supplement instead. Organic food also prohibits artificial flavours, colours, or preservatives.

Incorporating organic food into your diet offers several benefits, from higher nutrient content to reduced exposure to harmful chemicals. While organic food can be more expensive, purchasing organic options for certain high-risk foods can still significantly reduce your overall chemical intake. Whether you can afford to go fully organic or just buy a few organic items each week, making informed choices about what to prioritise can help support both your health and the environment.

47

FODMAP Diet

FODMAP is an acronym for
fermentable oligosaccharides, disaccharides, monosaccharides, and polyols

FODMAP foods are short-chain carbohydrates that belong to the acronym above, which are poorly absorbed in the small intestine. When these carbohydrates are not properly digested, it causes them to stagnate, where they can attract water into the gut and become a target for bacterial fermentation,[1] producing gas and symptoms like bloating, discomfort, diarrhoea, or constipation. Foods high in FODMAPs contain certain carbohydrates and sugar alcohols that can cause gastrointestinal distress, while foods low in FODMAPs are generally easier to tolerate. The list was developed to help people struggling with gut symptoms to identify problematic foods in their diet. It's particularly useful for conditions like IBS or SIBO, where sensitivity to FODMAPs is common. This is not to say high-FODMAP foods are inherently bad, but for those with pre-existing bowel issues, they can exacerbate or contribute to the symptoms of these conditions. By eliminating and later reintroducing specific foods, individuals can isolate the problematic ones by detecting whether they provoke symptoms. This then allows them to enjoy meals without discomfort by avoiding specific trigger foods. This is what the FODMAP diet is, where you first eliminate high-FODMAP foods, followed by a gradual reintroduction to determine which ones trigger symptoms. The elimination phase, typically lasting 2-6 weeks, is designed to give the gut time to heal and for symptoms to subside. This allows you to recognise if foods trigger issues when reintroducing them later. During this time, meals are based around low-FODMAP foods. This diet is very restrictive and involves cutting out an extensive list of foods, including numerous fruits, vegetables, legumes, and lactose-containing food, so most dairy products. Therefore, it should only be used in the short term to pinpoint foods. It's important to still try and maintain a balanced diet. If you are struggling to achieve this, consider consulting a dietitian or nutritionist who can work with you to ensure your nutritional needs are met. If you are underweight or have a history of eating disorders, do not try this diet without consulting your doctor.

After the elimination phase, high-FODMAP foods are slowly reintroduced, one at a time, to identify which ones cause symptoms. Keeping a food journal during this phase is crucial for tracking how your body responds to different foods. The reintroduction process typically involves consuming a test food on day one, followed by two days of a low-FODMAP diet again to observe any delayed reactions before trying another new food. This window also allows the body a chance to reset before attempting the next test food. Relying on memory isn't recommended as it can be hard to remember every detail, which is where the journal comes in handy. Once problematic foods are identified, your diet returns to normal, with only those specific foods being avoided. This process can provide peace of mind, allowing you to enjoy your meals without experiencing side effects and regain confidence in your food choices without unnecessary restrictions. If the full elimination phase feels too restrictive, or if you've previously struggled to complete this test, some people may choose to remove one category of high-FODMAP foods at a time, such as eliminating dairy first and then moving on to gluten, et cetera. However, this approach is not part of the standard low-FODMAP protocol.

Day 3
Continue with
Low FODMAP Diet
Record Any Symptoms

Day 1
Try to New Test Food
Continue Low FODMAP Diet

Day 2
Return to Low FODMAP Diet
Record Any Symptoms

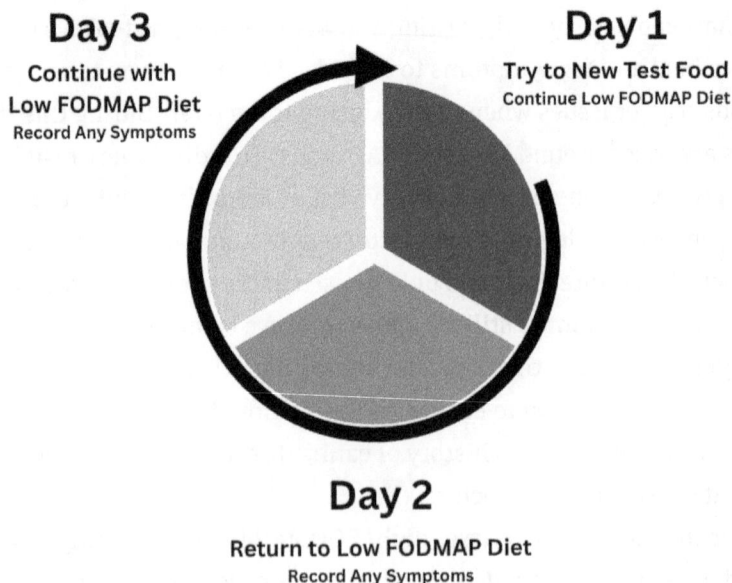

It's important to remember that everyone's digestive system reacts differently to food. What triggers symptoms for one person may not affect another, so following your own experience is essential rather than using recommendations. You cannot replicate anyone else's journey. This is particularly true for people with conditions like endometriosis, which is often linked to gastrointestinal symptoms or issues like IBS or SIBO. A study in New Zealand found that 72% of women with endometriosis experienced significant relief from gut symptoms after following a low-FODMAP diet, with over 50% seeing improvements in bowel symptoms within four weeks.[2] What you eat can sometimes fuel or diminish endo pain, so even if foods aren't inflammatory, they can still cause issues for specific people. Food sensitivities can also cause bloating, a well-known issue for those with endo, so the low-FODMAP diet may relieve stomach distension. Naturally, there is a difference between gastrointestinal and gynaecological bloating; but sometimes it's related to both, so diets like this can be helpful. Dietary modifications, including a low-FODMAP, gluten, or dairy-free diet, can help alleviate various endo symptoms.[3]

For people with both IBS and endometriosis, a stronger case exists for trying the low-FODMAP diet. Up to 86% of IBS patients report improved gastrointestinal symptoms after following a FODMAP approach.[4] If you're considering a low-FODMAP diet, the foods are listed on the next page,[5] but it's crucial to remember this diet is not intended for long-term use. For individuals with bowel endometriosis, this diet may be particularly beneficial as any distortions can make residue in the bowel incredibly painful.

High FODMAP Foods	Low FODMAP Foods
Fruits: Apple, Mango, Nashi, Pear, Canned Fruit, Watermelon, Apricot, Avocado, Blackberry, Lychee, Cherry, Nectarine, Peach, Pear, Plum, Prune, Watermelon, Dried Fruit, Fruit Juice	**Fruits:** Banana, Blueberry, Boysenberry, Cantaloupe, Cranberry, Durian, Grape, Grapefruit, Honeydew Melon, Rockmelon, Kiwi, Lemon, Lime, Mandarin, Orange, Passionfruit, Pawpaw, Raspberry, Rhubarb, Star Anise, Strawberry, Tangelo.
Vegetables: Green Bell Pepper, Mushroom (except oyster), Sweetcorn, Asparagus, Beetroot, Broccoli Stems, Brussel Sprouts, Cabbage, Aubergine, Fennel, Garlic, Leek, Okra, Onion, Shallot	**Vegetables:** Alfalfa, Bamboo Shots, Beat Shoots, Bok Choy, Carrot, Choko, Choy Sum, Endive, Ginger, Green Beans, Lettuces, Olives, Parsnip, Potato, Pumpkin, Red Bell Pepper, Spinach, Squash, Swede, Sweet Potato, Taro, Tomato, Turnip, Yam, Courgette.
Sweeteners: Sorbitol, Mannitol, Isomalt, High Fructose Corn Syrup, Honey	**Sweeteners:** Sucrose, Glucose, Sugar (in small quantities), Golden Syrup, Maple Syrup, Molasses and Treacle (in small quantities)
Dairy: Cow Milk, Goat Milk, Sheep Milk, Custard, Ice Cream, Yoghurt, Cheese (soft cheeses - cottage cheese, mascarpone, ricotta)	**Dairy:** Lactose-Free Milk, Oat Milk, Rice Milk, Cheese (hard cheeses, brie and camembert), Lactose-Free Yoghurt, Gelato, Sorbet.
Legumes: Beans, Baked Beans, Chickpeas, Kidney Beans, Lentil	**Legumes**: Canned Lentils and Chickpeas (both ok in small quantities)
Cereals: Wheat and Rye (e.g. bread, crackers, cookies, couscous, pasta)	**Cereals:** Gluten-Free Bread and Cereal Products, 100% Spelt Bread, Rice, Oats, Polenta, Quinoa, Sorghum, Tapioca

48

Histamine & Allergies

In Part 1, we discussed how individuals with endometriosis often experience allergies, food sensitivities, intolerances, or histamine-related issues. If you find yourself in this category, it's best to avoid all problematic foods, as there is little point in consuming foods that are causing problems for you. Of course, this is especially true with allergies. With food intolerances or sensitivities, removing trigger foods not only enhances your quality of life but also grants your body the respite it needs to heal. Over time, some food sensitivities might dissipate, as they're tied to gut bacteria rather than the immune system. Managing dietary restrictions might seem like a daunting task, especially when it means saying goodbye to beloved foods. Nevertheless, it's paramount for those with endo to manage this area of their lives as it can help reduce symptoms like inflammation and digestive problems. Food-related challenges affect a considerable number of us, and diet is amidst the multifaceted strategy of improving your overall wellbeing. Understanding the significance of diet can be both helpful and transformative.

Among the most gruelling challenges in endometriosis is the struggle with pain. As we've explored, what you eat can either amplify or alleviate this pain, especially if consuming foods that your body reacts negatively to, as this can trigger inflammation. Not only can this make pain management harder by exacerbating pre-existing pain, but it can introduce a new source of pain from gastrointestinal discomfort, including bloating and stomach cramps. Continuing to eat foods that trouble your body is comparable to pouring petrol on a fire; that may sound dramatic, but all it is doing is pairing digestive issues with the pain felt elsewhere, which can be overwhelming and frankly, no one wants to deal with this. Moreover, removing problematic foods can significantly improve other symptoms and your overall comfort. By combining the removal of aggravating foods with adopting a low-inflammatory diet, you may discover a winning formula for feeling better. Properly managing these food-related challenges can significantly improve your digestive health and reduce this added stress on the body. Chronic pain and poor digestive health can also take a toll on a person's energy levels and seep into other areas of their life. Remember, 80% of our immune system lives in our gut. Prioritising proper nutrition and managing intolerances can furnish your body with more energy and wellness, making it easier to cope with the challenges of endometriosis or life in general, as it takes one problem off your plate (excuse the pun). I've personally experienced the impact of allergies and sensitivities. I can attest that unmanaged, they can feel like they're dominating every aspect of your life, from having elevated stress levels to daily concerns about digestive issues and how to cope with them. So, while managing dietary restrictions may appear challenging, the rewards of improved wellbeing and quality of life are well worth the effort. It's not just about what you're giving up; it's about what you're gaining — relief, energy, and a renewed sense of control.

Identifying Food Intolerances and Sensitivities

If you suspect you have a food intolerance or sensitivity, an elimination diet can help identify the culprit. Remove any foods you are suspicious of for at least two weeks, then reintroduce them. If symptoms like gas, pain, nausea, or diarrhoea appear, the food may not be suitable for your body at the moment. Eliminating such foods calms gut inflammation and allows the immune system to repair any damage. Please note that depending on the type of food issue will determine if you can reintroduce the food later. If you're unsure of the specific trigger, a broader elimination diet can be useful to determine the answer. In the FODMAP chapter, we outlined what an elimination diet looks like; it's the same process here, where you remove multiple foods for a duration and then reintroduce them one at a time, keeping a food log to keep track of what you ate and whether it produced any symptoms. You can identify specific sensitivities by removing common problematic foods like gluten, dairy, soy, nuts, and eggs for around a month and reintroducing them one at a time. Don't try to reintroduce multiple foods at once because you won't be able to determine which one is causing you problems. Also, avoid testing foods in a shorter time frame (i.e. every day), as reactions from food intolerances and sensitivities can be delayed for a couple of days, so you need time in between for the body to react. If you are still unable to determine the cause, speak to your doctor. They can refer you to a dietician for professional guidance, or they may run tests to see if they can work out the cause of your symptoms that way.

You may have seen advertisements for at-home intolerance or sensitivity tests using a finger prick blood test to measure IgG results, a type of antibody. These companies then send your results with a list of foods you are reacting to. I am not here to dictate what you should and shouldn't do to improve your health. Dealing with health problems can be exhausting, and the journey to health is frustrating, so it's understandable to be drawn to anything that might offer guidance and relief. However, please know there is no substantial clinical evidence to say these tests (nor any other) are reliable at successfully identifying food intolerances. In fact, the Advertising Agency banned these companies from alluding to or stating they can diagnose food intolerances. The gold standard for identifying food intolerances and sensitivities is the elimination diet. I know many people don't want to hear that, quick fixes are always more desirable, but think of it as a fun way to try out new meals and ultimately get you feeling better.

Histamine Intolerance

A lesser-known issue, histamine intolerance, occurs when there is an excess build-up of histamine in the body, leading to allergy-like symptoms. Although studies in this area relating to endo are lacking, a 2021 study highlighted women with endometriosis were 4x more likely to have intolerances compared to those without endo, with a higher prevalence of histamine intolerance.[1] To be clear, histamine is not bad, is a natural chemical involved in immune responses. Mast cells are the immune cells that release the chemical histamine. When your body perceives an allergen, it activates the immune system, signalling mast cells to release histamine in your eyes, nose, throat, lungs, skin, or gastrointestinal tract, causing allergy symptoms. Therefore, when a person has histamine intolerance, it displays itself in ambiguous allergy-like symptoms. Histamine intolerance is not actually an intolerance, nor is it an allergy; it's simply a state of having excess histamine in the body. It should probably only be called histamine overload, but I guess it's called histamine intolerance because your body cannot tolerate the levels of histamine present without exhibiting symptoms. So how does one get a build-up of histamine in the body? Well, the analogy of a bucket is often used to explain this. Firstly, each and every person has a bucket, symbolising the level of histamine you can tolerate. The size of your bucket is determined by factors such as your genetics and gut health. Each day, your bucket accumulates histamine through foods you consume or chemicals you are exposed to. Different foods and substances contain varying levels of histamine, so your diet might be higher in histamine than someone else's. Environmental factors also contribute to histamine accumulation. For instance, weather changes can affect histamine production. During summer, those with hay fever will experience increased histamine levels and well, all allergies trigger the release of this chemical, adding to your metaphorical bucket as part of the body's response to the allergen. Some medications, gut bacteria, hormones, and even stress levels can further increase your histamine load. As we have histamine receptors throughout our whole body, if the bucket overflows, you can experience a wide range of undesirable symptoms affecting various bodily systems: the respiratory, digestion, nervous, muscular, and reproductive systems. This can complicate the process of pinpointing or understanding why we feel the way we do. Initial symptoms include headaches, itchy eyes, bloating, tummy aches, or other gastrointestinal symptoms such as diarrhoea or vomiting. Existing eczema may worsen, or a person may develop itchy skin, hives, or a rash. It can also cause flushing, particularly on the face and chest, which may be combined with difficulty regulating body temperature, leaving a person feeling extremely hot or sweaty. The heart may sporadically start racing, causing palpitations or low blood pressure. When someone experiences these symptoms, it's easy to understand that they can be quite unpleasant or unsettling. This can be magnified if there's little comprehension of what is happening or why their body is reacting that way. Unfortunately, once the build-up of histamine is overflowing, the body may feel like it's starting to crosswire. Individuals may have allergic-type reactions to foods they are not allergic to or experience symptoms such as flushing or diarrhoea in response to stress or high-histamine foods — which most people wouldn't even know to be aware of. Another possible and horrible side effect is panic attacks. This is attributed to the close relationship between histamine and stress. Stress can stimulate increased histamine production into an overflowing bucket. Subsequently, cortisol, the stress hormone, may be released, triggering the body's fight-or-flight response. If you have ever had an allergic reaction, you will know the panicking feeling they can induce.

DAO, an enzyme covered earlier in the book, is responsible for breaking down histamine. The cause of a histamine build-up might come down to issues with the amount of DAO present in the body. DAO deficiency can be caused by genes, medications, diet, bacterial overload, or IBD. A lack of DAO means histamine is insufficiently broken down, allowing it to accumulate. Other conditions can cause histamine issues; for example, it can be attributed to mast cell dysfunction, possibly through a condition called mastocytosis *characterised by an increase in mast cells*, or also Mast

Cell Activation Syndrome (MCAS), *involving an abnormal rise of activated mast cells.* Eventually, high histamine levels will lower, however, it can take a few months to decrease to a level considered normal. If you are struggling with high histamine levels, consider implementing strategies to accelerate this process. Depending on the cause of elevated histamine will determine whether the strategies can be used for a short time to rebalance your bucket or if they require lifelong adherence.

Bucket Filled By:

Food
Chemicals
Exercise
Hormonal Balance
Environmental Factors
Allergic Reactions
Stress
Medications

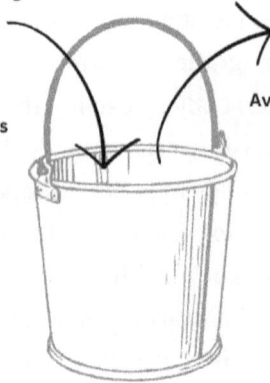

Bucket Emptied By:

Avoid High-Histamine Food
Fresh Foods over Processed
Limit Histamine-Triggering Foods
Avoid Histamine-Releasing Medications
Improve Gut Health
Support Enzyme Function
(DAO supplementation)
Manage Stress
Avoid Allergens
Monitor Hormone Levels
Reduce Environmental Toxins

Size of Your bucket Determine By:

Genetics
Gut Health

Why is Histamine Intolerance a Greater Risk for Those with Endometriosis?

Mast cells have a role in endometriosis, possibly contributing to several features of the disease. Activated mast cells release several proinflammatory substances. When responding to a threat, this is a very good thing, however, endometriosis lesions are reported to have more activated mast cells than in normal tissue,[2] which may have a role in the inflammatory process of the disease. It's believed that oestrogen stimulates the activation of mast cells, causing them to release their proinflammatory chemicals.[3] As there are high levels of oestrogen in endometriosis lesions, it stipulates why there are more activated mast cells than considered normal. If you recall, endometriosis lesions can create their own nerve supply. Due to the close proximity of nerve fibres to mast cells, the various chemicals released can contribute to the formation of a blood and nerve supply to the lesions, triggering inflammation and inducing pain.[4,5] Owing to their enhanced presence, the European Medical Journal proposed that due to considerable evidence, mast cells should be targeted with drug interventions to assist in controlling the pathogenesis or progression of endometriosis and mitigate symptoms.[6] This provides hope there may be future treatments that work at targeting the genesis of the disease. Due to enhanced mast cell activation, there is an increase in the proinflammatory chemicals released, including histamine, causing our buckets to fill up quicker than the body was designed to cope with. For those suffering from histamine intolerance, the bucket is fuller, so in everyday situations where histamine production is triggered, the bucket can 'spill' over causing an inability for the body to tolerate the levels. Studies show it can cause a shift in the allergen-dose response, causing allergy symptoms to be exacerbated.[3] This means consuming food you are mildly allergic to can cause a larger response by the body because the histamine produced in response to the allergen causes the bucket to overflow. This dose-response issue transfers into other areas of people's lives. When the bucket is fuller, tolerance to stress may reduce, or consuming high-histamine foods can cause unpleasant symptoms. The rise in systemic inflammation resulting from histamine intolerance can make it harder to deal with any pre-existing pelvic inflammation, as foods that elevate histamine levels can further elevate inflammation and amplify pain. This presents challenges in creating a balanced and symptom-friendly diet. Furthermore, due to symptom overlap, it may be hard to distinguish from endo symptoms, as existing symptoms like abdominal pain, bloating, diarrhoea, and nausea can be exacerbated. Due to oestrogen's role in activating mast cells, there can be variations in symptoms experienced throughout the menstrual cycle. Histamine levels fluctuate with hormone levels, so at times when oestrogen levels are higher, such as when ovulating, it may be harder to deal with histamine issues. Alternatively, triggers may increase when you're menstruating, possibly due to the increase in inflammation. Dealing with histamine intolerance can cause a lot of emotional distress. If your endo is not well-managed, it can be brutal dealing with the physical and mental stress of the two conditions combined. I want you to know you are not alone, so many people are in the same position as you, dealing with the same fears, issues, and triggers.

How to Manage Histamine Intolerance?

The goal is to keep your bucket empty enough so there is room to deal with the natural fluctuations of life without suffering horrible repercussions. The good news is the bucket can be emptied. Firstly, histamine levels will naturally reduce with time, but how do we speed it up? The best way to manage histamine intolerance is to avoid histamine. Probably the most important factor to look at is your diet. At the end of Chapter 22 we outlined some foods to avoid as they contain high amounts of histamine, foods that cause the body to create histamine, as well as foods that block DAO. If you are struggling and need immediate results, you may need to eat a low-histamine diet to reset, removing all foods high in histamine. I would strongly advise if you are vegetarian or vegan, not to do this unless under the guidance of a dietician. This diet is very restrictive, and you don't want to put yourself at risk of deficiencies as that will only cause more problems, which is not the goal here. Cruciferous vegetables like broccoli contain DIM, which can reduce high oestrogen levels. Consuming foods from this family group may be a proactive step in reducing histamine. While ensuring adequate hydration by drinking lots of water can flush out excess amounts of the chemical. You can also take antihistamine medication to suppress your symptoms. If you don't feel like they are working well enough, your doctor can prescribe stronger antihistamines, although be warned the drowsiness can make you feel like you're on a boat.

There was a time in my life when I was incredibly stressed and experienced a multitude of food issues. I took antihistamines daily to help with the symptoms, including ones I had prescribed by a doctor for when they were particularly bad. It was a struggle, but the good news with histamine intolerance is once it's controlled, the symptoms will diminish. I am now happy to say I am in a place in my life where I don't rely on antihistamines, I don't worry about the symptoms, and my bucket is finally at a reasonable level. I did give up being vegetarian after five years as part of that journey because a lot of my diet prior was heavy in histamine-rich foods, which needed to be replaced. I realised if I started eating meat and fish again, I would maintain a balanced diet. If you are legitimately struggling mentally and physically, I also suggest removing rules. Don't pressure yourself into lifestyle choices that are not working for you at a given moment in time. You don't have to do the same thing as me or anything you do not want to do, and no choice must be long-term. I want to give you hope that if you are dealing with this issue (and you weren't born with it, nor do you have a mast cell condition), it does not mean it's your new normal, and it's not going to be around forever. Your histamine levels will come back down if you take the right steps to help yourself. Reducing stress is an integral part of alleviating symptoms and reaching manageable histamine levels. Not only because stress triggers symptoms but also because it can help balance your hormones, preventing excess oestrogen from activating histamine. Stress can also lower progesterone levels, leading to oestrogen dominance and therefore possibly too much histamine. We will discuss ways to reduce stress later, including mindfulness, meditation, and yoga. I recommend trying some of these to give your body a chance to rebalance and provide your brain a break from worry and anxiety.

Finally, our gut health and microbiome have a role in eliminating excess oestrogen and histamine. Certain types of gut bacteria that produce beta-glucuronidase interfere with oestrogen detoxification. Instead of excess oestrogen being removed in our waste, the bacteria cause greater amounts of oestrogen to leave the bowel, circulating back into the body and increasing your hormone levels. We want to prevent the recirculation of oestrogen, leaving no room for excess mast cell activation. You can treat gut dysbiosis through probiotic supplements, eating probiotic food such as yoghurt, and eating plenty of high-fibre foods to feed the bacteria. If you have tried these options but are still struggling, speak to your doctor, who can refer you to the right specialist. Histamine intolerance is a hard thing to deal with, and you don't have to go through it alone.

49

Diet Summary: Key Takeaways for Endometriosis Management

We have laid out a lot of information on how diet can play a significant role in managing endometriosis symptoms. Here's a recap of the main points to keep in mind:

Avoid Inflammatory Foods: Reduce or eliminate foods that promote inflammation, such as processed foods, trans fats, refined sugars, and excess red meat.

Variety is Essential: Aim to eat a wide, varied diet to ensure you're getting a diverse range of nutrients.

Get Your 5-a-Day: Consume different fruits and vegetables for vitamins, minerals, and fibre.

Omega-3 Fatty Acids: Include sources of omega-3 to help reduce inflammation.

Consume Low-Inflammatory Foods: Focus on incorporating naturally anti-inflammatory foods.

Avoid Trigger Foods: If certain foods aggravate your symptoms, it's best to eliminate them to prevent further inflammation and digestive discomfort.

Gut Health Matters: A healthy gut can improve digestion, support your immune system, and aid in managing inflammation.

Go Organic When Possible: If your budget allows, opt for organic produce to reduce exposure to pesticides and chemicals, as these may contribute to inflammation or hormone disruption.

* * *

Managing inflammation should be a key focus in your dietary approach. Choose nutrient-dense, anti-inflammatory foods, and limit processed foods, refined sugars, or anything that might spike inflammation in your body. This is your journey, so tailor what you are going to implement based on your needs, preferences, and beliefs. You must make choices that excite you and will work best for you. We all have different concerns, so what is working for a friend may be different from what you need to do. Hopefully, you find food choices you enjoy, which, with time, can help manage pain. It's always a good feeling when you know you are giving your body everything it needs to be in its optimal state. Feel free to experiment with different dietary approaches — whether gluten-free, plant-based or another option to see what best suits your body. You can adapt this as you wish, depending on what feels right. You don't have to stick to a particular diet for the rest of your life. There are so many wonderful foods out there; making what you eat feel exciting and fresh is all part of it. Ensure your diet covers the essential nutrients your body needs to help your cells and immune system perform to their best ability. With more research, one day we will hopefully know more about the optimal foods for endometriosis. Until then, we know diet is important and something we can manage. Remember, anyone who says diet cannot help is entitled to their opinion, but if you know it is helping you, that's what you should focus on. In an upcoming chapter, we'll look at supplements you might want to try. However, always remember we don't eat nutrients, we eat food, so supplements should complement your diet, not replace it. Focus on creating good food habits and look at them as a form of self-care, as a healthy diet will protect you from far more than just endo symptoms, it will create a legacy for the rest of your life. Create this change in your life with love and respect for your body.

50

Alcohol

Alcohol comes in all shapes, sizes, flavours and strengths, and everyone has a different relationship to alcohol — some people drink frequently, others rarely or not at all. Each person has their preferences, avoiding certain types whilst gravitating towards others. Some people drink to celebrate and others may drink when feeling low. Alcohol is undeniably embedded into culture, and the health impact of this is not black and white. Studies vary from saying a glass of red wine is protective against heart disease to others stating no amount of alcohol is safe or beneficial. The World Health Organisation (WHO) declared alcohol as a toxic substance, classified in the highest risk category as a 'Group 1 Carcinogen', alongside tobacco, asbestos, and radiation.[1] While I am not here to say you shouldn't drink, it's good to be reminded of this fact and reinstall that alcohol (like everything in this world) is harmful when consumed in excess. Alcohol is inflammatory in a handful of ways. It's metabolised by the liver using enzymes, which lead to the production of free radicals, the unstable molecules that can damage healthy cells, potentially leading to illness and accelerated ageing.[2] Alcohol also reduces the body's antioxidant levels, which are necessary to neutralise these free radicals. By increasing free radicals and inflammation while also impairing the body's ability to regulate them, alcohol contributes to oxidative stress, which can damage healthy tissues.

Alcohol can also affect the Hypothalamic-Pituitary-Adrenal (HPA) axis, which is part of the central nervous and endocrine systems and is involved in stress responses.[3] This axis includes the hypothalamus and pituitary gland in the brain as well as the adrenal glands, which work together to regulate hormones called glucocorticoids in response to stress. When alcohol stimulates this system, glucocorticoid levels, namely cortisol (the stress hormone) increase, which is associated with various health problems. Heightened glucocorticoid levels can allow stored sugar to be dumped into the blood, in effect preparing the body for a fight-or-flight response. This may seem strange as alcohol appears to do the opposite, instead producing a relaxing feeling and calming anxiety — this is because it stimulates GABA, a neurotransmitter in the brain which calms the nervous system. This is why having a glass of wine at the end of the day can make you feel relaxed. However, once the alcohol wears off, you may experience 'hangxiety,' a horrible combination of heightened anxiety and a hangover, as your body works to normalise GABA levels and restore brain activity. Each person's tolerance to alcohol will vary and the impact it has on their body, but generally, with alcohol, less it more.

Though alcohol is metabolised primarily by the liver, it can also alter the gut microbiome, potentially leading to bacterial overgrowth and dysbiosis, which is the reduction in beneficial bacteria and increase in harmful bacteria.[4] This is partly because alcohol promotes inflammation, but dysbiosis itself can cause further gut inflammation. Excessive alcohol consumption can also modify the permeability of the gut lining, a condition known as increased intestinal permeability or 'leaky gut'.[5] This phenomenon allows microbes to enter the bloodstream, potentially reaching organs such as the liver or brain, triggering immune responses and chronic inflammation as the body works to remove these unwanted substances from the blood. A leaky gut can put added pressure on the liver as it works to detoxify and remove these substances. The impact of alcohol on gut permeability varies among individuals, depending on factors such as the amount and frequency of alcohol consumption, genetics, and overall

313

health status.

Alcohol can also significantly impact hormone levels, increasing oestrogen by slowing its breakdown in the liver whilst increasing the conversion of testosterone into oestrogen.[6] For reasons like this, alcohol is considered a risk factor for developing oestrogen-dependent diseases like breast cancer.[7] As you can see, alcohol can affect the body in a variety of ways, which might not be helpful to endometriosis as it's an inflammatory, oestrogen-dependent disease. There is research validating this, showing a strong association between alcohol intake and the risk of developing endometriosis.[8] More research is needed to determine whether this is due to altered oestrogen production and whether different types of alcohol impact the disease differently. It would also be good to understand if alcohol impacts the severity of the disease and whether it exacerbates existing endometriosis. Putting the scientific evidence aside, anecdotally, many people with endo struggle with alcohol as it triggers unwanted symptoms such as fatigue, flushing, pain, bloating, nausea, or leads to an agonising flare. When you are already feeling awful, the added stress that alcohol can cause on the body will feel draining, leaving many choosing to remove alcohol from their life.

Sober-Curious

The term 'sober-curious' refers to a cultural movement where people choose to drink less or abstain from alcohol for personal reasons rather than an issue like alcoholism. Sober-curious individuals may still drink but do so on a mindful and conscious basis rather than being driven by habit or social expectations. If you have felt drawn to reducing your alcohol intake, this approach can be a nice step towards finding the middle ground, as alcohol can cause intolerable side effects in some people with endometriosis. That being said, having endo doesn't mean you must give up alcohol. But, reducing your intake or exploring a sober-curious approach may be a good option for those who are struggling or do not feel in alignment with it at any given time, sometimes due to the health repercussions they experience. Adopting a sober-curious approach might benefit your health and symptoms.

* * *

There was a time when I felt drawn towards sobriety because my body wasn't handling alcohol well. Even small amounts, like a glass of wine, would mean I was unable to function properly the next day due to astonishing fatigue. Hangovers meant being bed-bound, whilst my friends would have the energy to meet for brunch. Not wanting to give up drinking entirely, after some research, I discovered that avoiding high-histamine alcohols like wine and beer helped. I cut out these drinks for over a year and reduced my overall intake. If I were to drink, I would only have tequila with mixers. After giving my body time to recover, I was able to reintroduce white wine without issues.

* * *

Sometimes, our bodies just need a break, but that doesn't mean you have to give up alcohol forever. Listen to what your body needs right now and adjust your habits accordingly. If you're considering cutting back, take it one week at a time. Adjusting your drinking habits will help you discover what works best for you — whether that means abstaining for a while or if you don't feel you have any issues, enjoy that glass of wine when you feel like it.

51

Supplements

Supplements are designed to complement and enhance a person's health when taken alongside a varied and balanced diet by providing additional nutrition. They are not meant to replace food or serve as a substitute for healthy eating. Instead, supplements help to bridge potential nutritional gaps in our diets, ensuring our bodies receive all the vital nutrients necessary for optimal function. Each nutrient has a unique set of roles in the body, working together in tandem to keep us alive and healthy, from sending nerve signals, healing wounds, maintaining the immune system, and regulating our hormones. The term 'essential' signifies the human body cannot produce these nutrients, necessitating their intake through diet. Supplements are derived from plants or animal sources and are available in various forms, including capsules, tablets, or liquids. These products are concentrated sources of vitamins, minerals, amino acids, essential fatty acids, enzymes, fibre, or various plant or herbal extracts. Although only required in small amounts, these nutrients are crucial for maintaining health. It's wise to approach supplementation with caution, as excessive intake of certain nutrients can lead to adverse side effects and, in some cases, toxicity. This chapter outlines supplements you may want to consider as part of your endo treatment. The evidence on some of these nutrients may be weak (meaning a small number of studies have been conducted) or inconclusive. I don't want this to be a breeding ground for misinformation, so the science behind each supplement will be untangled so you can make appropriate selections for what feels right for your body. Always consult with a healthcare professional before incorporating new supplements into your regimen.

Do You Need Supplements?

No, for most individuals, you can get everything you need from food, but sometimes it can be a struggle to obtain them *all* solely through diet. We might not always be able to factor in everything we need each day, and that's where supplements can be helpful. Failing to provide the body with sufficient nutrients can cause disease, as some health conditions are rooted in lacking specific nutrients. For example, iron deficiency anaemia stems from a lack of iron absorption, and an underactive thyroid (hypothyroidism) can be caused by an iodine deficiency. It's usually safer and better to eat food over taking supplements as nutrients obtained from whole foods are generally more potent and efficiently utilised by the body than those contained in supplements. Foods not only contain the desired nutrients but also a host of other beneficial substances that often interact synergistically, enhancing their effectiveness. The main exception to this rule is folate (Vitamin B9), which is better absorbed as a supplement.[1]

Supplement Ingredients

Many supplements contain added ingredients or nasty additives we want to avoid excessive amounts of. Choosing high-quality supplements with minimal additives and steering clear of products containing excessive artificial ingredients is advised. Common additives include:

Fillers: As nutrients are only needed in small amounts, fillers boost the product to achieve the desired pill size.

Bulking and Binding Agents: These are used to hold the supplement together to make a digestible tablet form, ensuring they don't crumble.

Coating Agents: Improve texture, appearance, taste, or odour and make pills easier to swallow.

Flow Agents: Ensure smooth processing during manufacturing, preventing ingredients from clumping together in the machinery.

Colouring & Flavour Agents: These can be natural or synthetic, added to enhance taste and appearance.

Doses

National health bodies establish the recommended daily intake of vitamins and minerals. In the UK, the Scientific Advisory Committee on Nutrition (SACN) provides Dietary Reference Values (DRVs), which outline the recommended amount of nutrients required for maintaining health based on age and sex. While supplements can help individuals meet these recommendations, taking high doses excessively can result in nutrient imbalances and undesirable health outcomes. SACN also sets safe upper limits, representing the maximum daily intake of a nutrient that is unlikely to pose health risks with long-term use. It's essential to adhere to these guidelines and avoid consistently taking supplements at 'maximum strength' unless directed by a healthcare professional. Overloading the body with nutrients from both supplements and food sources won't make you healthier. Supplement labels often include the '% NRV' (Nutrient Reference Value), indicating the percentage of the daily nutritional intake provided by the supplement. This information can help guide safe supplementation. For instance, a supplement providing 100% NRV supplies the entire daily recommended amount for the average person. Please consider the nutrient intake you also receive from your diet when determining the appropriate dosage.

Bioavailability

Bioavailability refers to the extent to which a nutrient or substance is absorbed and utilised by the body. This is not as straightforward as what goes into the body the body uses. The body is complex, and various chemicals are needed for each process to be optimally carried out. Several factors are involved to explain why deviations in bioavailability occur. Firstly, some nutrients are naturally easier for the body to absorb than others, and then interactions with other substances can further enhance or impair bioavailability. Some nutrients require the presence of other nutrients for absorption, so the body gets the most nutrition when combining them with these. On the other hand, foods can hinder the absorption of certain nutrients. For example, oxalates in tea inhibit iron absorption. Some supplement manufacturers incorporate ongoing research on bioavailability when designing their products, aiming to optimise their effectiveness by including critical components. For instance, turmeric supplements often contain black pepper to help absorption. This is not always the case, so be aware of these considerations when selecting your supplements.

Contraindications

Supplements are not always suitable for everyone. Please be vigilant if you have a medical condition or are taking medication. Contraindications refer to situations where a supplement could cause harm to a person due to factors like their medical history or age or interact negatively with other treatments, so it should be avoided. It's critical to be aware of potential contraindications before taking any supplement. For example, high-dose vitamin E supplements can interfere with blood-thinning medications.

Pregnancy

If you are pregnant, you may require a higher amount of nutrients, such as folic acid or calcium. On the other hand, there may be supplements to avoid, such as Vitamin A (retinol), as it can harm your baby's development. If you are pregnant or breastfeeding, please speak to your doctor before using supplements.

* * *

Iron

As discussed earlier, iron has a significant role in the body, and there may be a heightened risk of deficiency among people with endometriosis. While food serves as a primary source of iron, the increased blood loss during menstruation can elevate our iron requirements. Depending on your dietary habits, it may be challenging to obtain a sufficient amount of iron solely from food. Iron deficiency is the most encountered nutrition deficiency in humans,[2] making it a prime candidate for supplementation, particularly for individuals with a history of iron deficiency, are vegan or vegetarian, experience heavy prolonged periods, or exhibit symptoms suggestive of low iron levels. Individuals with endo often contend with heavy or frequent bleeding, which can deplete the body's iron stores, necessitating greater requirements of this vital nutrient. Therefore, it's crucial to replenish iron either through food or where required, supplements. Given the widespread occurrence of iron deficiency, if you experience any of the symptoms listed below, ask your doctor to assess your iron levels with a blood test to determine if you need to increase your intake. Some people may decide to take iron supplements on their period, extending a few days before and after to mitigate the risk of deficiency symptoms. Others may find an occasional supplement sufficient to maintain their iron stores.

Dose

UK RNI is 14.8 mg for females (aged 19-50 years)
   The maximum recommended daily intake for long-term use is 17 mg.

Symptoms of Deficiency

Extreme fatigue, weakness, pale skin, cold hands and feet, brittle nails, chest pain, fast heartbeat, or shortness of breath.

Bioavailability

Vitamin C is required for adequate absorption of non-haem iron, the type that comes from plants. This is particularly important for vegans or vegetarians. Some supplements may contain this, but you could take them with orange juice if they do not. Phytate fibre (found in whole grains, seeds, and legumes) and tannin-containing drinks (tea, coffee, and wine) can reduce iron absorption. Depending on your routine, taking iron first thing in the morning on an empty stomach with orange juice is preferable. Then, if possible, wait an hour or two before eating or drinking tea or coffee. If you have your first coffee or eat breakfast at work, this might be easier for you to achieve.

Contraindication

Iron supplementation may cause other drugs to work less effectively. Talk to your doctor if you are taking tetracycline, penicillin, ciprofloxacin, or medications used for Parkinson's disease or seizures.

Pregnancy

During pregnancy, your body has higher iron requirements because the mother's body transfers iron to the foetus through the placenta for the infant's development. *However*, as your periods also cease, your iron requirements tend to balance out. You should not need an iron supplement during pregnancy, but on a case-by-case basis, your midwife or doctor may recommend one, which is safe to take. In the second and third trimesters, the iron requirements of the foetus outweigh the amount the mother's body can absorb each day, so this balance is met by using the mother's iron stores.[2] Therefore, if you have low iron stores at the beginning of the pregnancy, your doctor may advise supplementation.

Food Sources of Iron	
Haem Iron	Red Meat, Beef, Liver, Oysters, Fish, Turkey, Mussels.
Non-Haem Iron	Spinach, Tofu, Dark Chocolate, Pumpkin Seeds, Lentils, Cashews, Chickpeas, Beans, Dark Green Leafy Vegetables, Raisins, Quinoa, Sesame Seeds, Chia Seeds, Fortified Foods

Zinc

Zinc is a cofactor for over 200 metabolic enzymes, meaning it's required for many bodily processes. It has a major role in immune function, growth, DNA synthesis, and hormone release. Due to its role in the immune system, particularly in inflammation and tissue repair, it has been investigated to understand whether there is a relationship to endometriosis. Several research papers state an association between low zinc intake and lower zinc levels in the blood of women with endometriosis compared to women without the disease.[3,4] Unfortunately, the mechanisms of why or how this could relate to endo are not understood; more research is needed to understand the relationship better. Zinc deficiency is associated with increased inflammation and impaired immunity, which may trigger an inflammatory response capable of aiding endometriosis.[5] Supplementation of zinc might, therefore, assist in reducing inflammation and oxidative stress as it inhibits free radical production.[6] Zinc might also help alleviate period pain,[7] premenstrual symptoms, and irregular periods, all of which commonly present as issues, making supplementation potentially useful if you suffer from these. This can be a case of trial and error to see if they help. One very small study suggested that zinc deficiency contributes to endometriosis cyst development, with supplementation potentially suppressing cyst development.[8] Zinc can also be beneficial in the treatment of PCOS.[9]

Dose

UK RNI is 7 mg a day for females (aged 19-50 years)
The maximum recommended daily intake for long-term use is 25 mg.

Bioavailability

Studies show women taking the oral contraceptive pill have lower levels of zinc in their blood, meaning the pill might reduce the absorption of zinc.[10]

Symptoms of Deficiency

Hair loss, rashes or skin roughening, white spots on fingernails, lethargy, frequent infections, or poor wound healing.

Strangely, I cannot take zinc supplements as they trigger severe nausea. I tried several brands to find one that would work for me and found that if I take it in a combined supplement with magnesium and calcium, I do not experience any side effects. If you have experienced this, consider taking a combined supplement. Nausea is also common if people take a high dose of zinc, as it can irritate the stomach, so avoid buying maximum-strength capsules.

Food Sources of Zinc	
Red meat Seafood (particularly oysters) Eggs	Cheese Whole Grains and Pulses (in lower quantity)

Magnesium

Magnesium is the fourth most abundant mineral in the human body and plays a role in more than 600 enzyme reactions.[11] Over half of the body's magnesium is stored in bones and teeth, while the rest supports essential functions such as energy production, nerve signalling, and maintaining healthy tissues, including the brain, muscles, and blood vessels. Magnesium ensures the heart beats properly, facilitates communication within the nervous system, and supports dopamine production, a neurotransmitter associated with happiness. Only a handful of enzymes can work without magnesium, so it's imperative we get the right amount into our bodies. Magnesium deficiency has been linked to several health concerns, including increased susceptibility to stress, anxiety,[12] and depression.[13] In turn, sufficient magnesium levels can have a soothing, calming effect on the body. Unfortunately, a vicious cycle occurs whereby stress depletes magnesium levels, but low magnesium also contributes to higher stress levels. Usually, less than 1% of our magnesium is found in our blood; however, during times of stress, whether that's physical, psychological, or even stress caused by a lack of sleep, increased magnesium can be found in blood and urine, meaning the body is expelling magnesium from its stores during stressful periods.[12] Given that endometriosis can cause multiple forms of stress, individuals may be at a higher risk of magnesium deficiency. Magnesium is also essential for cellular energy production, meaning we depend on magnesium to produce energy for the body. Low magnesium levels can lead to cellular dysfunction and, in severe cases, premature cell death, potentially explaining why a deficiency is associated with chronic fatigue. Since energy production heavily depends on magnesium, supplementation could improve fatigue and low energy levels if it's a contributing factor. In addition, magnesium may have a role in alleviating gynaecological symptoms, with research suggesting supplementation can effectively reduce Premenstrual Syndrome (PMS), painful periods, and menstrual migraines in some individuals.[14] Magnesium deficiency is common; the UK National Diet Survey found substantial gaps in the number of people failing to meet their magnesium intake targets.[15] The good news is you can get magnesium from many food sources. It can be found in chocolate, which may be why many of us crave it during our periods — to help PMS symptoms and energy production (as we utilise more calories during menstruation). You can also use magnesium creams, topical sprays, or soak in magnesium bath salts for the skin to absorb magnesium.

If you consider that magnesium intake is often insufficient, making deficiency common and that stress further depletes magnesium levels — when you couple this with research suggesting deficiency significantly contributes to chronic low-grade inflammation and increases the risk of various diseases,[16] there may be a potential relationship between endo and magnesium deficiency — but is this true? Some women with endometriosis have fallopian tubes that do not contract at regular intervals; instead, they have spasms or seizures due to dysfunction in the nervous system.[17] Theoretically, this might contribute to retrograde menstruation.

Magnesium relaxes smooth muscles, which could reduce this occurrence, suggesting a plausible connection to endo through influencing retrograde menstruation. We know the disease is not solely attributed to this, however, studies consistently demonstrate a relationship between magnesium intake and endometriosis: higher dietary magnesium intake correlates with a lower risk of endometriosis.[18] This could be attributed to several factors, like the potential to lower inflammatory markers or maybe its the ability to influence the proper functioning of the fallopian tubes.

Another facet of endometriosis development involves angiogenesis, the growth of new blood vessels to supply oxygen and nutrients to diseased tissue. A study on rats sought to evaluate the potential benefits of supplementation in endo due to magnesium's established role in managing various gynaecological conditions. The findings revealed that magnesium reduced Vascular Endothelial Growth Factor (VEGF), the most important regulator of angiogenesis, and reduced oxidative stress — both significant components of endometriosis.[17] This suggests a potential protective effect of magnesium in conditions characterised by these processes, such as endo. However, human studies are necessary to determine whether magnesium can yield the same results.

If you are dealing with PMS, anxiety, high stress, pain, low mood, menstrual migraines, or bloating — supplementing magnesium may be helpful.

Dose

UK RNI 270 mg
The maximum recommended daily intake for long-term use is 400 mg. Taking more than 400 mg over a short-period can cause diarrhoea.

Bioavailability

While taking a magnesium supplement, ensure a sufficient intake of calcium because they work closely together and can compete for absorption if one is present in higher quantities in the body. Similarly, high intakes of zinc or vitamin D through supplementation may interfere with magnesium absorption. This is why it's always good not to exceed the recommended amounts set by governing health bodies by taking high-dose supplements. High doses do not mean better results and should only be taken if a registered health professional recommends them.

Symptoms of Deficiency

Loss of appetite, nausea, fatigue, weakness, cramps, palpitations, low blood sugar, and diarrhoea.

Food Sources of Magnesium	
Whole Grains (i.e., wholemeal bread) Leafy Vegetables (i.e., spinach) Soy	Avocado Chocolate Seeds

Selenium

Selenium is a trace element needed in our diet in very small quantities. The name selenium comes from Selene, the Greek Goddess of the moon. This mineral is required for normal cell growth and immunity as it stimulates the production of antibodies and cells that fight infections. Selenium also repairs DNA and enhances a liver enzyme called P450 that detoxifies cancer-causing chemicals. It's a powerful antioxidant that might help prevent cancer as it's involved in triggering programmed cell death (apoptosis) of abnormal cells. It's important for both male and female fertility, and excessive levels of deficiency have been linked to miscarriage, preeclampsia, and preterm birth.[19] While there is no strong evidence that selenium directly plays a role in endometriosis, its antioxidant and anti-inflammatory properties suggest potential benefits. Selenium's ability to regulate the immune system is also important, as both acute and chronic inflammation have been associated with selenium deficiency. Food sources acquire their selenium content through the soil they are grown in, but this requires the soil to be rich in selenium for food to be also. Therefore, dietary sources are not always the most reliable. Some countries, such as China, may need supplementation to ensure adequate intake if their soil is selenium-poor. Brazil nuts are a rich source of selenium, so eating one or two of these nuts a day is sufficient to meet requirements.

Dose

UK RNI is 60 micrograms.

The maximum recommended daily intake for long-term use is 350 micrograms.

Toxic levels can cause garlic odour on the breath or metallic taste in the mouth, fragile or black fingernails, dizziness, nausea, and hair loss.

Symptoms of Deficiency

Infertility, fatigue, hair loss, increased infections, and mental fog.

Contraindication

Do not take selenium supplements without consulting your doctor if you have an underactive thyroid (hypothyroidism) or skin cancer.

Food Sources of Selenium		
Liver Kidney Brazil nuts Crab	Mushrooms Onion Garlic	Broccoli Cabbage Cereals

Vitamin B

There are several B vitamins as follows:

- B1 - Thiamine
- B2 - Riboflavin
- B3 - Niacin
- B5 - Pantothenic Acid
- B6 - Pyridoxine
- B7 - Biotin
- B9 - Folate and Folic Acid
- B12 - Cobalamin

Each B vitamin has a distinct role in the body, is derived from different food sources, and exhibits unique deficiency symptoms. They are all water-soluble, meaning the body cannot store them, so any surplus is flushed out in our urine. Consequently, consistent daily intake of B vitamin-rich foods is necessary. This is not always achievable, supporting the case for supplementation to maintain optimal levels in the body. You can purchase vitamin B complexes containing some or all types. Vitamin B6 is the most studied in relation to endometriosis.

Vitamin B6

Vitamin B6 is a group of compounds converted into pyridoxine in the body. Pyridoxine is a cofactor for over 60 enzymes. It's involved in protein metabolism and the creation of amino acids. It has a role in controlling or regulating the function of sex hormones and gene expression. Animal studies show a deficiency in B6 increases the uptake and retention of sex hormones in tissues and enhances organ responsiveness to low doses of oestrogen.[20] It's easy to see how this may be detrimental to endometriosis. Additionally, B6 works with the immune system, increasing the production of antibodies and other immune cells. Vitamin B6 may also improve PMS and depressive symptoms.[21] More research is needed, but it may be worth trying as an affordable, non-invasive, and safe way to support your body. There is also some evidence that low dietary intake is associated with a risk of endo.[22]

Dose

UK RNI is 1.2mg

The maximum recommended daily intake for long-term use is 10 mg.

Please note: toxicity levels can occur at low doses of Vitamin B6, so do not exceed 10 mg.

Deficiency Symptoms

Recurring mouth ulcers in the corner of the mouth, split lips, swollen tongue, headache, anxiety, irritability, and bloating.

Food Sources of B6		
Nuts Seeds Oily fish Meat	Seeds Green Vegetables Whole Grains Avocado	Garlic Egg Yolk Legumes (pulses, beans, groundnuts)

Vitamin C

Vitamin C, also called ascorbic acid, is perhaps best known for preventing scurvy in sailors in the 1400s. Like vitamin B, it's water-soluble, so the body cannot store it and must be consumed regularly. It's needed for over 300 metabolic reactions, assisting in the production of collagen growth and tissue repair, including your skin, bones, and teeth. As a potent antioxidant, it protects against oxidation and genetic mutations, which may have a role in cancer protection. It also has antiviral and antibacterial characteristics, although its ability to protect against the common cold is heavily debated. Vitamin C may balance and indirectly reduce the amount of cortisol in our body (the stress hormone). However, this relationship is complex and not fully understood, so it's not considered a form of treatment.[23] Vitamin C plays various roles in reproductive health. As an antioxidant, it can reduce free radical damage, potentially improving the health of the reproductive system and protecting eggs from oxidative stress-related damage. Studies suggest vitamin C may have a role in preventing preeclampsia, particularly in high-risk individuals, although further research is needed to confirm this.[24] Furthermore, it may positively impact fertility in individuals with luteal phase defect, which occurs when the ovaries don't release enough progesterone or the uterus lining does not adequately respond to progesterone, leading to difficulties in conception.[25] Vitamin C's role in supporting hormone synthesis and reproductive tissue health may contribute to its ability to address some underlying factors associated with luteal phase defect. Several animal studies have been conducted to determine whether vitamin C treatment may affect endometriosis. The results indicate it may prevent endometriosis implantation or have a role in the regression of lesion size,[26] including ovarian endometriosis.[27] It is suggested the anti-inflammatory and anti-angiogenic effects of the vitamin facilitate this.[26] Furthermore, vitamin C and E supplements have been found to effectively reduce painful periods, painful intercourse, and severity of pelvic pain experienced by women with endo.[28] Biochemical evidence supports this with a study demonstrating a reduction of inflammatory markers in peritoneal fluid after supplementation.[29] A single serving of blackcurrants or guava provides 5x the daily reference intake, making them excellent sources of vitamin C.

Dose

UK RNI is 40mg

The maximum recommended daily intake for long-term use is 1000 mg.

If you smoke cigarettes, cigars, or vapes, consider your sources of Vitamin C, as nicotine may induce a higher intake requirement.

Deficiency Symptoms

Pre-scurvy syndrome includes frequent colds, infections, lack of energy, weakness, and muscle and joint pain. Scurvy will develop if there is chronic inadequate vitamin C intake, but this is rarely seen.

Contraindication

If you have blood disorders, including thalassemia, sickle cell disease, G6PD deficiency or haemochromatosis, you should only take Vitamin C supplements under the advisement of your doctor.

Food Sources of Vitamin C		
Fruit (especially citrus and guava)	Berries Capsicum Peppers	Green Vegetables Tomatoes

Vitamin D

Vitamin D is a fat-soluble vitamin occurring in five forms. Vitamin D2 is found in plant sources and vitamin D3 is derived from animals, including humans, and is produced in our skin when exposed to UV light. During the UK winter months, from October to March, we often do not produce enough vitamin D, so supplementation is recommended at 10 micrograms daily. The research into the effects of vitamin D on endometriosis is varied; some show no relationship whilst other findings pose the suggestion for further studies. For example, animal studies have found supplementation can reduce inflammation, the spread of endometriosis cells, and angiogenesis, which can prevent or limit the growth of endometriosis.[30,31] On the contrary, other studies showed no improvement in symptoms with vitamin D supplementation. Despite a lack of hard and reliable data, this vitamin was included in this book as a reminder that supplementation in winter is recommended for everyone to ensure good health. If there is a chance that this can help prevent the implantation and cause regression of endometriosis tissue, then that's a win-win. The body can receive vitamin D through exposure to the sun from UV light or by consuming vitamin D-rich foods. Supplementation is particularly important for individuals who spend a lot of time indoors (as many of us do) or cover up their skin when outside.

Dose

UK RNI is 10 micrograms

The maximum recommended daily intake for long-term use is 25 micrograms.

Supplements containing vitamin D3 are generally more effective in maintaining blood levels than vitamin D2.

Deficiency Symptoms

Fatigue, poor sleep, bone pain or aches, depression, hair loss, muscle weakness, and loss of appetite.

Bioavailability

Vitamin D is a fat-soluble vitamin requiring dietary fat for enhanced absorption.

Contraindication

Do not take vitamin D supplements unless advised by a doctor if you have hypercalcemia, hypervitaminosis D, or any other malabsorption conditions.

Food Sources of Vitamin D	
Oily Fish Fish Liver Oil	Mushroom Egg Yolk Cheese

Vitamin E

Vitamin E, a fat-soluble vitamin, acts as an antioxidant protecting cell membranes and nerve cell sheaths while strengthening and repairing muscle fibres — which can help relieve muscle cramps. Its antioxidant properties have linked high levels of vitamin E with enhanced brain health and a potential delay in cognitive decline.[32] Additionally, it can promote immunity by working with selenium to bolster antibody production. It has a mild anti-inflammatory role, which, combined with its immune-enhancing activity and antioxidant role, can be effective in the prevention and reversal of various diseases.[33] Studies indicate vitamin E levels tend to be lower in patients with endometriosis compared to those without the condition.[34] Lower levels of vitamin E have also been detected in the blood of infertile women with moderate to severe endometriosis when compared to those with minimal to mild stages.[35] This highlights the need for further research to elucidate the potential impact of systemic oxidative stress from endometriosis on infertility and to evaluate whether vitamin E supplementation provides improvements. As highlighted earlier, vitamin E and C supplements were able to effectively treat endometriosis symptoms in some individuals, including painful periods, painful sex, and severity of pelvic pain.[28] Inflammation causes pain, so reducing inflammation alongside oxidative stress may reduce clinical symptoms.

Dose

UK RNI is 3 mg

The maximum recommended daily intake for long-term use is 540 mg.

The recommended dose of Vitamin E widely varies as it largely depends on your diet, specifically how much Polyunsaturated Fatty Acids (PUFA) you consume. The higher your PUFA intake, the more vitamin E you need. PUFA is found in salmon, vegetable oils, and nuts and seeds. It's best to take vitamin E with other antioxidants, such as vitamin C or selenium.

Bioavailability

Vitamin E is a fat-soluble vitamin, so dietary fat is required to be absorbed. Taking a supplement with a meal or snack containing a portion of fat increases absorption.

Deficiency Symptoms

Vitamin E deficiency is rare and only seen in those with severe fat mal-absorption or rare genetic disorders. Lack of vitamin E can lead to issues with the nervous system, including muscle weakness, poor coordination, lethargy, and poor concentration. It can also depress the immune system and reduce antibody production.

Food Sources of Vitamin E		
Plant-Derived Oils Nuts Spinach Carrots	Avocado Apricot Freshwater Fish Wheatgerm Oil	Butter Wholegrain Cereals Seeds

Omega-3

There are three primary sources of omega-3: ALA (*short chain*), DHA (*long chain*) and EPA (*another long chain*). The body can use short-chain fatty acids to produce long-chain fatty acids, although not very efficiently, so it's advised to consume sources of both long and short-chain fatty acids, as health issues can arise with insufficient omega-3. Long-chain fatty acids, particularly DHA, have well-documented health benefits, so ensure you eat the foods listed. Plant-based sources are harder to come by. It's primarily found in algae, which is useful for vegans and vegetarians. Still, not everyone will enjoy the taste of these foods or know how to incorporate them into their diet regularly. This is where omega-3 microalgae supplements can be of use. This is the original source of omega-3 that fish feed on, storing it in their bodies. The main source of DHA in the Western diet is oily fish. Please note, tuna, whether fresh or tinned, is not considered an oily fish. Omega-3 can be found in other fish and shellfish but not as much as oily fish contains. Omega-3 is frequently consumed via cod liver oil supplements, derived from the liver of cod fish, which has the added benefit of also containing vitamin A and D. UK citizens are recommended to consume two portions of fish a week, one serving should be oily fish. Short-chain ALA food sources come from plants, which is good news for those who do not eat fish.

Omega-3 is beneficial as it forms part of our cell membranes throughout the body, affecting the functioning of these cells. They provide the starting point for hormone production that supports heart and lung health by regulating abnormal heart rhythms, maintaining healthy arteries, lowering high blood pressure, and reducing the risk of blood clots. They can also provide benefits to the brain, eyes, and immune system. Omega-3 has a role in reducing inflammation, whilst insufficient amounts may detrimentally lead to inflammation, which is linked to various diseases' progression.

Omega-3 is valuable for those with endometriosis as it has been scientifically proven to have anti-inflammatory, anti-apoptotic, anti-proliferative, and anti-angiogenic effects.[36] These characteristics postulate a role of omega-3 in suppressing endometriosis or, on the other hand, lead to the disease in a deficient state. Several studies researched this possible relationship. One study found women with the highest intake of omega-3 were less likely to have endometriosis than those with the lowest intake, suggesting a protective role of omega-3.[37] Furthermore, high intake of the long-chain fatty acid called EPA was associated with a considerable reduction in endometriosis rates validating the need to ensure adequate sources of this type.[38] A lab study supported the notion of high omega intake being beneficial, as the survival of endometriosis cells in vitro significantly reduced in the presence of a high omega-3: omega-6 ratio.[39] Animal studies have similar results, with omega-3 preventing the implantation and growth of peritoneal endometriosis.[40,41] Another literature review on fat intake and endometriosis found fish oil reduced period pain.[42] As you can see, there is considerable evidence suggesting omega-3 has a use for endo, helping manage the disease and symptoms. Whilst these studies are not conducive to denote it will heal endo, they are still a step in the right direction, and supplementing can benefit overall health.

Deficiency Symptoms

Dry, scaly, or irritated skin, fatigue, insomnia, brain fog, mood swings, sleep issues, joint pain, and stiffness.

Contraindication

Consult your doctor before taking omega-3 supplements if you have bipolar disorder, liver disease, diabetes or if you are on anticoagulant medicines or warfarin (Coumadin®).

Pregnancy

Fish liver oil contains vitamin A, so it should not be consumed when pregnant as it can harm the foetus. Consult your doctor before taking omega-3 supplements.

Short Chain Omega-3 (ALA) are found in:	
Whole Grains	Chia Seeds
Legumes	Soy/ Edamame
Flaxseed	Avocados
Pumpkin Seeds	Walnuts
Long Chain Omega-3 (DHA/ EPA) can come from oily fish such as:	
Salmon	
Cod	Sardines
Herring	Mackerel
Long Chain Omega-3 (DHA/ EPA) plant sources include can:	
Seaweed	Nori
Spirulina	Chlorella

Diindolylmethane (DIM)

Diindolylmethane (DIM) is a bioactive compound formed in the body during the digestion of cruciferous vegetables. Research suggests that DIM can affect oestrogen metabolism, leading to interest in its potential for managing hormone-related conditions such as breast cancer, endometriosis, menopause, and acne. Specifically, DIM affects the balance between different forms of oestrogen by promoting the conversion of oestradiol (a potent oestrogen) into less active forms. This mechanism has led to investigations into whether DIM could play a role in controlling oestrogen-driven disorders.

Dienogest is a prescribed progestin medication we described earlier, which can be used in birth control pills as a treatment for endometriosis. A 2018 study analysed the effects of DIM in conjunction with dienogest in eight women with endo.[43] The researchers found that DIM not only reduced oestradiol secretion from endometriosis tissue, but when combined with dienogest there was an enhanced effect, leading to a significant reduction in endometriosis-associated pelvic pain and bleeding. However, given the small sample size of this study, the results must be interpreted with caution. Larger, well-designed clinical trials are needed to confirm these findings and determine the safety of DIM supplementation. While abnormal oestrogen levels or oestrogen dominance is sometimes observed in endometriosis, it's important to note this is not universal. DIM supplementation may only be beneficial for those who demonstrate oestrogen imbalances. Individuals interested in using DIM for hormonal regulation should consult a healthcare provider, especially since the compound can influence hormone levels and interact with medications like hormone therapy. At present, no standardised dosage recommendations for DIM supplements exist due to the limited scope of research. Clinical guidelines based on more extensive studies will be essential to determine the optimal dosage and effects. As it is being used in practice by some clinicians, I have included it in case you wish to discuss this with a doctor, naturopath, or dietitian. Alternatively, dietary sources of DIM, such as cruciferous vegetables, offer a safe way to increase intake of the compound without the potential risks associated with supplementation.

Probiotics

Probiotics have gained significant attention in recent years due to their versatile role in supporting various aspects of health, particularly gut and immune function. Emerging research suggests that gut bacteria may influence the development and progression of several conditions, including endometriosis. This research endorses that we should all pay more attention to our gut and strive for a healthier microbiome. Whilst maintaining a balanced diet is often sufficient for promoting gut health, supplements can provide targeted support by delivering specific strains of beneficial bacteria. Furthermore, probiotic-rich foods like yoghurt and kimchi might be great food sources of bacteria, but not everyone can tolerate them. For instance, having lactose intolerance means you will struggle with dairy-based sources, while fermented foods can aggravate histamine sensitivities. In such cases, probiotic supplements can be a viable alternative to help restore gut balance, especially when signs of imbalance arise, manifesting as bloating, diarrhoea, gas, or stomach pain. Probiotics may also support mental wellbeing; approximately 95% of serotonin, a hormone linked to mood regulation, is produced in the gut. Nicknamed the 'feel good' chemical, serotonin affects not only mood but also influences pain perception, general wellbeing, and even sexual desire. Maintaining a healthy gut could, therefore, positively impact these aspects of health.

Antibiotics, designed to eliminate harmful bacteria, can also reduce populations of beneficial bacteria in the gut. In addition, stress, a common factor in endometriosis, can negatively impact the microbiome's diversity, making a case for supplementation during periods of high stress or after a course of antibiotics. Note that you are given antibiotics after surgery through a drip to prevent the risk of infection, so supplementing with probiotics post-treatment can help restore gut health. The term antibiotic somewhat stands for *anti-life*, designed to kill bacteria and viruses, ensuring they don't pose a risk to the host, meaning you and your body. However, this also means antibiotics can inadvertently diminish populations of beneficial bacteria, which is far from ideal. Probiotics, on the contrary, mean *pro-life*, assisting in replenishing and diversifying the gut microbiota, fostering a healthier balance, so they can help restore any imbalance once treatment is completed. Probiotic supplements are formulated with specific microorganisms intended to reload the gut microbiota, nurturing diversity which can help eliminate harmful bacteria. This supports your immune system and can mitigate inflammation, leading to a spectrum of health benefits. While probiotics are associated with numerous health claims, let's focus specifically on their potential impact on endometriosis. One valuable strain of bacteria, *Lactobacillus,* is renowned for its health-promoting benefits. Unfortunately, research consistently shows that women with endometriosis tend to have reduced levels of *Lactobacillus* in their microbiota.[44] To investigate whether restoring *Lactobacillus* levels could provide benefits, clinical studies found supplementing for 8-12 weeks significantly improved endo-related chronic pelvic pain and menstrual discomfort without any adverse side effects.[45,46] Furthermore, in an animal study, mice with endometriosis were supplemented with two probiotics, either *Lactobacillus Acidophilus* combined with *Saccharomyces Boulardii,* or *Saccharomyces Boulardii* alone.[47] Both groups presented with reduced size and volume of the endometriosis lesions. Interestingly, *Saccharomyces boulardii* alone was more effective at reducing pain.

Many people with endo also experience IBS or symptoms similar to the condition on occasion. Probiotics have been researched for their role in relieving IBS symptoms such as abdominal pain, bloating, gas, and urgent bowel movements. A review of several studies concluded various strains could be effective in reducing all these symptoms whilst reducing the number of bowel movements needed in a day.[48] This suggests probiotics could be beneficial if you are struggling with IBS.

Choosing the right probiotic supplement can be overwhelming due to the wide variety of strains, doses, and brands available. What many companies don't want to tell you is that there is a substantial reduction in the bacteria you take compared to the amount that reaches the bowel alive (where you need them to be). Bacteria need to survive the mouth, stomach, small intestine, large intestine, and colon — all of which have unique anatomical mechanisms that can influence the survival rates. To provide the desired health benefits, they must survive each part of the digestive system. For instance, the stomach is full of acid, vital to help break down food, however, it can also break down probiotics with its low pH level, so bacteria must survive long enough in these conditions to make it through the stomach. After that, they enter the small intestine, where the acidity is neutralised; however, they must now survive the abundant pancreatic juice, bile, and digestive enzymes. The probiotics can survive this if coated with a protective shell, ensuring enough bacteria reach the large intestine. You see, not all probiotics are equal — many bacteria do not survive. Before making any purchases, research brands, look into how they are designed, and what mechanisms will increase their survival through the digestive process. This will ensure you invest in high-quality probiotics and spend your money wisely. With their potential to support your immune system, alleviate inflammation, and promote overall wellbeing, probiotics may play a valuable role in your self-care regime and management of endo. If you struggle with bowel issues, probiotics could help ease symptoms, *but* still evaluate your diet to ensure you're not consuming foods that are aggravating your bowel. If you choose to supplement, it's advised to take them consistently for at least three months to allow time for them to take effect. If symptoms persist, you may consider trying a different strain or brand.

Antioxidants

Antioxidants perform a crucial role in combating oxidative stress, which may contribute to the development and progression of endometriosis.[49] Researchers have explored the potential of several antioxidants in managing this condition and alleviating symptoms. While the benefits of vitamins C and E have been previously discussed, there is exciting research surrounding other antioxidants which may offer additional therapeutic advantages.

Alpha Lipoic Acid (α-LA)

Alpha-lipoic acid (α-LA) is a powerful antioxidant that the body produces naturally. It's present in every cell, where it plays a critical part in converting glucose into energy. Beyond its metabolic functions, α-LA recognition for its antioxidant properties means it's often used to manage conditions linked to oxidative stress, such as diabetic neuropathy. While many health claims are associated with α-LA, not all are strongly supported by research. Scientists have also begun exploring the antioxidant and anti-inflammatory effects of α-LA in the context of endometriosis. One animal study found α-LA reduced oxidative stress and decreased the size of endometriosis lesions.[50] In humans, α-LA has been tested in combination with Palmitoylethanolamide (PEA), a compound naturally found in foods like egg yolk and peanuts; two separate studies showed that this combination significantly reduced symptoms like painful periods, painful sex, and chronic pelvic pain.[51,52] A further animal study investigated the combined effects of α-LA and PEA with bromelain, an enzyme found in pineapples. This resulted in a reduction in the size and number of endometriosis cysts.[53] Although more research is needed to fully understand the therapeutic potential of α-LA as a treatment for endometriosis, early evidence suggests that its antioxidant and anti-inflammatory properties may help inhibit the progression of the disease.[54] Given its track record in managing oxidative stress, α-LA is worth considering as a part of a comprehensive treatment plan as it could relieve pain and improve quality of life. However, as with any supplement, please consult a healthcare provider before incorporating α-LA into your routine, especially since research is still in its early stages.

Bioavailability

When taking alpha-lipoic acid as a supplement, it's not recommended to consume it with food, as this reduces bioavailability. It should be taken on an empty stomach or 30 minutes before eating.

Contraindication

Consult your doctor before taking alpha-lipoic acid if you have diabetes, malnutrition, thyroid conditions, or are having chemotherapy.

Food Sources of Alpha Lipoic Acid (α-LA)	
Spinach Broccoli Tomatoes	Carrots Red Meat

N-Acetylcysteine (NAC)

An exciting supplement you may want to try is N-acetylcysteine (NAC). After ingestion, NAC is converted into the amino acid L-cysteine, which the body uses to produce glutathione — a powerful antioxidant. NAC offers both antioxidant and anti-inflammatory effects as it helps reduce levels of proinflammatory cytokines and oxidative stress. It also has the ability to replenish other antioxidants after the body has used and depleted them. NAC has been approved in clinical settings for the treatment of cystic fibrosis, chronic obstructive lung disease, and paracetamol overdose. Additionally, emerging evidence suggests NAC may have potential benefits for conditions such as PCOS, fertility, immune function, and liver health, though more research is needed to validate their efficacy. NAC has also been studied for its potential to manage endometriosis. In both in vitro and in vivo models, NAC has successfully reduced the proliferation of endometriosis cells.[55-57] A 2010 animal study further demonstrated that NAC treatment significantly decreased the size of implanted endometriomas.[58]

It was suggested that this was achieved by switching the endometriosis cell behaviour to a less invasive and proliferative phenotype while decreasing tissue inflammation. Other studies indicate NAC could improve pain symptoms caused by inflammation and provide a safe and effective way to improve fertility without side effects. This hypothesis was later tested on humans, producing encouraging results. Not only were the results for symptom improvement better than reported from using standardised hormonal treatments, but 24 patients treated with NAC cancelled their scheduled laparoscopy due to their endometriomas either shrinking or disappearing, alongside significant pain reduction.[59] Due to evidence of NAC's effectiveness in managing endo, a study in 2023 concluded oral supplementation reduced endometriosis-related pain symptoms, endometrioma size, and also blood levels of CA125.[60] Furthermore, combining NAC with alpha-lipoic acid and bromelain was also shown to improve pain symptoms in patients considerably.[61] Naturally, these results would make anyone want to run out and buy this to see if it works. Whilst the evidence is insufficient to confirm its effectiveness on a wider scale, the demonstrated benefits in smaller trials make it a potentially valuable addition to your treatment regimen as a low-cost, low-risk, and possible high-reward supplement.

While NAC can only be taken as a supplement, cysteine, the amino acid it produces, can be found in protein-rich foods such as meat, fish, seafood, and eggs, as well as plant-based sources like legumes, onions, and broccoli in smaller amounts.

Resveratrol

Resveratrol is a polyphenol, a group of compounds known for their powerful antioxidant properties. It's primarily found in the skin of red grapes, so products created with grapes, such as juice and red wine, may contain it. This may partially explain why red wine is said to be good for you. Resveratrol is also classified as a phytoalexin, a compound synthesised in plants as a defence mechanism in response to stress or parasites (such as a fungal attack), helping them to prevent or recover from threatening circumstances and promote disease resistance. These phytoalexin properties may transfer to humans when they are ingested, promoting human health in a similar way. Certain phytoalexins, including resveratrol, have shown to possess various bioactive properties, including antioxidant, anticarcinogenic, antidiabetic, antiparasitic, cardioprotective, neuroprotective, and hypoestrogenic effects[62] — all sounds great right? Research on resveratrol's potential to help manage endometriosis also looks promising. Lab studies have shown it can ameliorate endometriosis progression, perhaps through its ability to lower the levels of two inflammatory enzymes, MMP-2 and MMP-9, which are known to play a role in endometriosis disease progression and invasion.[63] Animal studies further support these findings, showing that resveratrol supplementation decreased the number and size of endometriosis lesions and suppressed vasculature, inflammation, and cell survival by increasing apoptosis.[64] These findings suggest resveratrol could be a natural treatment option for endometriosis, with its ability to target inflammation and reduce lesion size. Of course, further testing of its impact on humans is required before the compound can be considered an official treatment option. That being said, one study concluded that "the role of resveratrol in reducing the volume of endometriotic lesions and chronic abdominal pain is a proven fact", highlighting its potential as a complementary treatment for the disease.[65] Resveratrol supplements are available, typically derived from an Asian plant called *Polygonum Cuspidatum*, red wine, or red grape extracts. If you choose to supplement, ensure the product is high quality and contains at least 98% pure trans-resveratrol — the active form of the compound most beneficial to health.

Food Sources of Resveratrol	
Wine Peanuts Pistachios	Blueberries Cranberries

Epigallocatechin-3-Gallate (EGCG)

Epigallocatechin-3-Gallate (EGCG) is a potent plant compound found in green tea, extensively studied for its potential impact on a wide range of diseases. Over 1,000 studies have explored the influence of green tea on cancer alone. Its benefits are believed to stem from green tea's high polyphenol content, particularly catechins, with EGCG being one of the most prominent.[66] Research shows that EGCG acts as a powerful antioxidant, protecting healthy cells from free radical damage. In addition, its antiangiogenic effects (meaning it can prevent the growth of new blood vessels), are essential in the context of endometriosis, where lesions thrive by developing their own blood supply. EGCG has also exhibited abilities in suppressing pro-inflammatory chemicals, making it a potential ally in reducing chronic inflammation associated with many diseases, including endometriosis. You can obtain the benefits of EGCG by drinking green tea or matcha, but if you are not a fan of the taste, EGCG supplements offer an alternative. Excitingly, the potential role of EGCG in treating endometriosis has garnered significant research interest, with encouraging results from animal studies. In 2008, a study demonstrated that EGCG treatment led to the regression of endometriosis lesions by inhibiting both angiogenesis and blood flow to the lesions without affecting ovarian function.[67] It's not entirely clear how this mechanism works, although it's thought that EGCG inhibits Vascular Endothelial Growth Factor (VEGF) expression, similar to how it may exert anti-cancer effects. In 2013, another animal study found that after just two weeks of treatment, EGCG significantly reduced the growth of endometriosis lesions.[68] Not only did it inhibit the development of lesions, but there was also a decrease in the lesion size, as it enhanced apoptosis (cell death within the lesions). A year later, further research suggested that EGCG prevented the progression of fibrosis in endometriosis, which is the dense tissue that can lead to scarring, pain, and altered organ function.[69] Based on these findings, EGCG was proposed as a potential drug candidate for the treatment and prevention of endometriosis. More recently, a 2021 study showed that EGCG can also block oestrogen receptors in endometriosis tissue by binding to them instead, effectively suppressing the further development of the disease.[70] The researchers concluded that EGCG affects multiple stages of endometriosis development, making it a strong candidate for managing the disease. ECGC could also benefit other gynaecological conditions such as PCOS[71] and adenomyosis.[72] While these animal studies are positive, human clinical trials are necessary to determine whether the same could be achieved. Ensuring there are no side effects and determining the proper dosage is also critical. Until more research is available, consuming green tea or low-dose EGCG supplements may provide some of these potential benefits. If you struggle with nausea when drinking green tea, try consuming it with food instead.

Contraindication

Talk to your doctor before consuming green tea or supplements if you have high blood pressure, kidney problems, liver problems, stomach ulcers, or psychological disorders.

Do not take EGCG supplements without medical approval if you have renal failure, liver disease, or a heart condition or if you take medications to control cholesterol or blood pressure.

Quercetin

Quercetin is a plant pigment and part of a group called flavonoids, which give many fruits and vegetables their vibrant colours. Flavonoids are known to have many medicinal benefits, mainly due to their ability to function as antioxidants. Quercetin, in particular, also possesses anti-inflammatory and antiangiogenic properties, making it a beneficial compound in endometriosis. In animal studies, quercetin supplements have shown promise. Daily supplementation inhibited the growth of lesions, promoted apoptosis (cell death) in endometriosis tissue, and reduced inflammation.[73] Additionally, quercetin exhibits both anti-oestrogenic and progestogenic effects,[74] which may offer benefits in hormone-dependent conditions like breast, ovarian, and cervical cancers.[75-77] This quality suggests further possible use in treating endometriosis, which is oestrogen-dependent. Moreover, quercetin can help stabilise mast cells, regulating the release of histamine. This could offer a mild antihistamine effect, reducing the release of chemicals that trigger allergic reactions.[78] While further research is required to confirm these benefits in humans and establish its role in endometriosis therapy, quercetin remains an important compound for overall health. You can boost your intake of quercetin through a diet rich in fruits, vegetables, and green tea. However, some people may still wish to take it as a supplement occasionally to enhance the effects. It's important to note that quercetin is not water-soluble, and the body absorbs it poorly. To improve bioavailability, supplements often include vitamin C or bromelain to aid absorption. Be sure to keep an eye out for this and buy high-quality supplements to get the maximum benefit.

Food Sources of Quercetin		
Red Wine	Red Grapes	Broccoli
Green Tea	Kale	Raw Red Onion
Apples	Tomatoes	Olive Oil
Berries	Cherries	Ginkgo Biloba

* * *

Supplements may have a helpful role in managing endometriosis. Whilst it's unclear if they can be impactful in preventing disease escalation, they may still have a pivotal role in reducing your symptoms or improving your quality of life. Though supplements alone may not make substantial changes in your disease status, they are a form of complementary treatment, so they can be a valuable addition to a comprehensive approach to health, complementing a healthy diet, medical treatments, or lifestyle changes. You may want to trial different supplements at different points and see if you find any improvements in how you feel. With time, research will catch up, and advancements in the data will show what supplements are effective in endometriosis and what the best dose is to receive the benefits without any side effects. Supplements can be easily incorporated as part of your toolkit, though it's best not to look at them as a strategy you do for one month, then never again, expecting to reap the benefits. Also, don't rely simply on supplements without working on a healthy diet, as supplements will struggle to elicit any benefits if there's poor consideration of what else you put into your body. Furthermore, taking a long list of supplements each day is not ideal, especially if you remember the list of all the additives supplements can have. Ensure you buy non-GMO and organic options where possible. The Food Standards Agency in Europe has strict regulations on what can be included in food supplements, regulations in the US tend to be less rigorous. Capsules, liquids, or bulk powders tend to have fewer unwanted ingredients or additives in them compared to tablets. Liposomal supplements are coated in a layer of fat, which might increase absorption and bioavailability. The moral of the story is, you can still enjoy supplements and the benefits they bring, but always buy the highest quality you can afford, don't overconsume them, and still eat good food.

52

The Four Pillars of Health - Movement

Movement is one of the four pillars of health, as it's essential to living a healthy life. Moving your body and engaging in exercise contributes to the wellbeing of your mind, body, and soul through various mechanisms. The four key types of exercise are aerobics, strengthening, balance, and stretching. Maximising the benefits of movements involves incorporating a blend of these four types. Let's explain them in more detail:

Aerobics

Aerobic exercise, often called cardiovascular exercise or cardio, increases your heart rate and changes your breathing. Examples include a brisk walk, swimming, jogging, cycling, or dancing. Engaging in aerobic exercise improves cardiovascular health by strengthening your heart and blood vessels, helping your heart pump blood more efficiently throughout the body; in turn, this can lower blood pressure and improve brain health. Simultaneously, it can aid in weight management and improve sleep. Even if you're in too much pain to go jogging or cycling, a low-impact activity around the house can provide similar benefits for that day, like cleaning or gardening. The most accessible form of aerobics is walking, as it's low-impact and free to do. The goal of 10,000 steps a day is a recommendation often floated around as it's associated with numerous health benefits. Although, several factors can influence how achievable this goal feels. Your lifestyle, your job, where you live, and whether you need to drive everywhere will determine whether this goal is easily reached or seems daunting. If you live a very sedentary life, particularly if you work from home, 10,000 steps might feel unachievable. In this case, consider breaking it down into manageable segments. For example, getting up 30 minutes earlier to go for a brisk walk can add around 3,000 steps — nearly a third of the way there. Don't forget, all the steps you take count, so this includes the ones you do around the house too. A morning walk may not be practical or suitable for you, so it's about arranging your goals to be attainable for your life. Summer can be a great time to go for an evening walk, or if you take a bus to work, getting off a stop earlier to walk from there can build up your step count. So, whilst 10,000 is a great goal to work towards, the key is making it fit your life. If accountability is a more pronounced obstacle, you could consider joining a running club or sports team and enjoy the more social aspect.

Strengthening

Strong muscles allow us to feel healthier and fit in our bodies and capable of doing everyday tasks with ease, like carrying groceries or getting up from the floor. It's crucial for long-term health as our muscle mass naturally decreases when we age, leading to a greater risk of frailty, weakness, or falling. No one wants to be in that position. Strength training also has the benefit of building bone mass, which is vital for preventing osteoporosis. This is generally important for women, but also on account of some of the hormone treatments used for endo. As we all know from yoghurt and milk adverts, we want strong, healthy bones. It may seem odd to some that our bones are living, growing tissue. We might assume that once we stop growing, so do our bones, but this isn't the case. Our bones are responsible for many tasks throughout our lifespan, including storing minerals and creating blood.

There are various ways to incorporate strength training. You can lift weights, use gym machines, or workout using just your body weight, like push-ups or squats. Resistance bands are an excellent option for at-home workouts, adding resistance to your movements to build strength. Even simple activities like taking the stairs instead of the lift are strengthening exercises. You could wear a weighted vest when going for a walk or even around the house for an extra kick of strengthening without majorly changing your lifestyle. Whatever method you choose, strength training will help you feel fitter and healthier in your body.

Balance

Balance exercises improve muscular strength and coordination, which are essential for stability. Even if improving your balance doesn't seem important now, ageing affects our vision, inner ear function, and muscles, making falls more likely. Balance exercises can slow or prevent this decline, so working on movements contributing to our lifelong health is an act of self-love. That being said, balance exercises aren't just for your future-you; they can improve your core, coordination, reaction times, and body awareness. They are particularly helpful for those struggling with joint pain or arthritis, as muscles around the joints are strengthened, improving joint function and alleviating discomfort. Strengthening your core can also improve back pain by reducing the pressure off your spine.

Simple balance exercises include standing on one leg with open or closed eyes, doing step-ups on a platform, or walking heel-to-toe. If you feel your body wobbling and moving a lot, this is signalling that your body is learning to maintain balance, so continue on, and you will see improvements as you build these muscles. Yoga is another excellent way to improve stability while strengthening and stretching the muscles, contributing to balance.

Stretching

Finally, there's stretching, which involves lengthening your muscles to improve flexibility and range of motion. Not only can stretching feel delicious, but it also keeps your muscles healthy, reduces the risk of injury during exercise, and enhances mobility. Be sure to stretch gently and avoid pushing yourself too hard or to a point that's painful. It's good to warm up the muscles first by moving around to increase the blood and oxygen flow, as this will make stretching easier and more effective.

Benefits of Movement

All types of exercise release chemicals like dopamine and endorphins, which can help reduce our perception of pain and make us feel good, happier, and relaxed. The ability for exercise to bring down our stress levels may also be a welcoming thought. At first, the idea of incorporating four types of exercise may seem overwhelming, however, it also shows us that exercise doesn't have to be complicated or expensive. Simple activities like going up and down your stairs a handful of times then doing gentle stretching can be beneficial. Exercise is not restricted to spending money on a gym membership, nor does it require you to work out at the gym every day. Movement is not exclusive or unachievable — it's accessible to everyone. Regular physical activity is one of the most important things you can do for your health. The endorphins and health benefits reaped can make it extremely rewarding, but it will also keep you in the best shape as you age, allowing you to lower your risk of disease whilst prolonging your independence.

Movement and Endometriosis

The symptoms of endometriosis, like fatigue or pain, can sometimes make exercise feel like a challenge or dreaded activity. But engaging in movement activities is still valuable and encouraged. It can positively impact your quality of life, improve your cardiovascular health, and make you feel good in your own body, both physically and mentally. Depending on where you are in your endometriosis and fitness journeys will dictate how you approach incorporating movement into your toolkit. You may need to start gradually, allowing yourself to build trust in yourself that you can and will carry out these activities. Giving yourself too big a goal can mean you don't end up doing it, or you might find it negatively impacts your body, causing you to give up while creating a self-belief that you cannot stick to your goals. Fear avoidance can become a big issue with endo, where we avoid activities due to the fear it will increase pain. If you make exercise too strenuous or arduous, you may increase your inflammation or trigger a flare. This has the potential to form a negative mental feedback loop that exercise is bad for you. Creating bite-sized goals means you're more likely to adhere to them while working on self-trust. You may want to start gradually with low-impact movement exercises, so you are not putting a lot of strain on your body. This is particularly helpful if you experience a lot of pain. Naturally, the goal isn't to increase your pain but to reduce it. If you feel with time, like trying out some higher intensity exercises, go for it, but if your body cannot handle them, listen to your body and adjust accordingly.

Exercise can help reduce inflammation. Studies show you attain an increase in anti-inflammatory chemicals and a decrease in the production of proinflammatory substances.[1] Even a twenty-minute walk can reduce the body's inflammatory response.[2] Conversely, a sedentary lifestyle can lead to the accumulation of excess body fat. Whilst body fat is incredibly important and needed to maintain health, when we have excess fat, increased inflammation can come from the fat tissue. So, by neglecting movement it can increase our pain later down the line. You see, exercise can fight inflammation, whilst being sedentary can intensify it, so we really are doing ourselves a huge favour by engaging in movement. It may take a few weeks or months to notice the difference in your body. But every step we take towards reducing our inflammation is a step closer to feeling better.

Another benefit of exercise is the ability to reduce your overall stress levels. Living with a chronic condition like endo can raise stress, which directly suppresses how our immune function functions through mechanisms like decreasing the number of immune cells in our body. In a growing field of study called psychoneuroimmunology, scientists explore how our mind, the nervous system, and our immune system interact with each other. There is a complex relationship between these facets of the body. This realm of research suggests that both physical and psychological stress can weaken the immune system, but also how we handle or perceive stress is a large indicator of how much immunity is suppressed.[3] We need our immune systems to be on their 'A game' to help remove harmful pathogens and substances from our body, to protect, heal and repair our tissues, and to correct the imbalances endo can provoke. Even though stress is unavoidable, how we manage it is connected to our health. Whilst some endo-related stress is related to the physical aspects of the disease, making it harder to change, how you look at or handle it can still be critical. Moreover, exercise can be a fantastic tool for alleviating physical and psychological stress, which can then benefit our nervous and immune system health. Even the simple act of having some time to pause your day and clear your head, knowing you can use exercise as an outlet, is lovely. When you pair that with the endorphin release and sense of pride we have in ourselves for showing up, it can be a winning combination. Studies on psychoneuroimmunology also show that a positive psychological wellbeing, where you feel happy or grateful, can improve the human body's responses, creating a more spiritually and physically prosperous life.[4] This is where 'Hot Girl Walks' may be productive, defined as going for a walk where you think about what you are grateful for, your goals, and how you will achieve them — so doing this might accelerate benefits on multiple levels. Generally, your mind will be calmer and sharper from exercise, so numerous benefits can unfold. Whichever way you incorporate exercise into your daily routine, make it something you enjoy, ensuring you feel optimistic about it and what you are doing for your body. Start with low-impact, and if your body is reacting well, with time, you can increase intensity if you desire. Similarly, if something is not working, switch it up and try something else. There are many types of exercise to enjoy. Pilates and yoga are often suggested for endo as they promote stretching and strengthening, which can relieve muscle pain and improve any muscular imbalances that have occurred. These options also encourage relaxation and stress-reduction, which psychoneuroimmunology suggests supports our immune system. We'll explain these in more detail to provide a better understanding of how they can help, but the key is to listen to your body and stay consistent.

Yoga

Yoga incorporates all four types of exercise. Whilst there are many different types of yoga, they universally comprise a set of specific poses or 'asanas' designed to connect the body, breath, and mind. The word 'yoga' is often interpreted in translation as 'union', reflecting the connection of these three things. You may know some anglicised terms for common poses, such as *downward dog* or *child's pose.* During yoga practice, you move through physical positions that improve strength, flexibility, balance, and endurance. Focusing on your breath or engaging in the breathing exercises integrated into the class can reduce stress and promote mindfulness. Encouraging stress reduction positively impacts both mental and physical wellbeing. Yoga helps take your mind off everything else except what you are doing with your body, bringing your attention to the present moment — this creates a meditative state that can improve concentration, mental clarity, and emotional balance. Additionally, yoga can alleviate physical pain, making it a valuable complementary therapy.

The movements increase blood flow, so may aid detoxification and enhance digestion. Finally, and very importantly, the practice has a calming effect on the nervous system, helping regulate emotions and reduce any anxiety. As a practice that benefits both physical and mental health, yoga is highly recommended for endometriosis to help manage symptoms, relieve tension, reduce pain, and encourage relaxation. Pelvic pain and adhesions caused by the disease can lead to stiffness as your muscles tense in response. Yoga can be an excellent method to counteract this act and improve the mobility of your muscles and nerves, supporting their optimal function. We know nerves have a crucial role in driving both the progression of the disease and in generating pain. There is some understanding of the sensory and sympathetic nerves involved in endo, but the vagus nerve's role is less documented. The vagus nerve, the longest and most complex nerve in the autonomic nervous system is considered the communication superhighway as it carries messages between the brain and body's organs. A study found decreased vagal tone in people with endometriomas, showing evidence of vagal nerve dysfunction.[1] This decrease may also be true of superficial and deep endometriosis, however, the study did not test for these forms. Reduced vagal tone manifests as hypersensitivity to stress and a slower recovery from stressful situations, meaning it takes longer to relax after experiencing stress. It can also provoke anxiety, poor emotional regulation, changes in heart rate, and digestive issues like abdominal pain and bloating. Improving your vagal tone activates the parasympathetic nervous system, which promotes faster relaxation and better emotional regulation. Yoga is an effective way to enhance vagal tone through the use of specific poses and a breathing technique called *ujjayi breathing*. This technique involves constricting the back of the throat and taking deep breaths, creating a soft sound with each inhale and exhale. By combining *ujjayi breathing* with yoga poses, the practice stimulates the vagus nerve, improving vagal tone and, in turn, enhancing mood, heart rate regulation, and stress perception.[2]

In yoga philosophy, a person's mental state, specifically stress, is considered the root of all physical illness, making mental healing a key component to the overall healing process. Do you remember earlier we mentioned the field of study called psychoneuroimmunology which studies the relationship between psychological stress, the nervous system, and immune function? Well, this philosophy aligns with this modern scientific field, so it appears the ancient yogis of India understood, as far back as 5000 BCE, what science is only now beginning to confirm. Yoga promotes relaxation, improves vagal tone, and reduces pain; collectively, this cultivates a lower stress response. Additionally, the practice was shown to reduce the amount of circulating cortisol, the body's primary stress hormone, and decrease inflammatory markers,[3] both of which are valuable for limiting the progression of endometriosis and managing its symptoms. Incorporating yoga into your routine, even just one class per week or every couple of months, can be highly beneficial. It offers a chance to stretch, relax, and strengthen your vagal tone whilst building physical strength and improving balance. Evidence supports the benefits of yoga for people with endometriosis, showing a reduction in pelvic pain and improved quality of life.[4]

About eight months after my second surgery, I was still struggling with anxiety, so I sought advice from my GP, who encouraged me to try yoga to calm my nervous system. I had always been drawn to yoga, but it was the push I needed to incorporate the practice into my life. I started with a class on YouTube, and I was surprised when, during the practice, I found myself bursting into tears for no apparent reason. I was confused, but since I was at home and alone in my bedroom, I went with it, allowing myself to feel the emotions. About a week later, I did another class, and the same thing happened — I began crying again without being aware of any clear trigger as to why it was happening. After researching online, I learnt that stress is stored in the body according to the ancient Ayurvedic medicine system. In yoga, the hips are considered the seat of emotions, where energy from past and present experiences can accumulate, leading to imbalances. Yoga can help release these emotions, particularly hip-opening poses, which allow deeply rooted emotions and energy to be released. After realising that I had been doing many hip-opening asanas and experienced an intense release of emotion — twice! I felt even more encouraged to continue practising yoga. It felt like a worthwhile thing for me to do for my healing. If you ever have a rush of emotions in yoga, you're not alone, and it's a good sign. As yoga helps release deeply held emotions, it allows physical and emotional healing to occur.

Pilates

Pilates is another excellent form of exercise that focuses on balance, posture, strength, and flexibility. It was developed in England in the 20th century by a German man named Joseph Pilates. Joseph believed that mental and physical health were interconnected, so during World War I, he designed a method of exercise to ameliorate ill health. In its early days, the practice was used to rehabilitate seriously injured veterans, and Joseph designed specialised equipment to accelerate the benefits of the process — one of which, *the reformer*, is widely used today in reformer Pilates classes. Understanding the origins of Pilates helps dispel the misconception that it's just a trendy exercise for influencers and yummy mummies. In reality, it's a low-impact exercise designed to realign the body, strengthen the core, engage the mind-body connection, build muscle, increase flexibility, and improve posture and balance. Central to the practice is breathwork, which helps engage and activate the right muscles during movement. When we experience pain, our muscles tend to contract, and when we are in chronic pain, our muscles can become stiff and rigid. This lack of motility affects how we walk, stand, and move. Pilates can positively impact the entire body by relieving tension to promote mobility and reactivating neglected muscles to allow for proper realignment.

The pelvic floor is one of the areas that can be affected by endometriosis. Inflammation and scar tissue can weaken the pelvic floor, leading to pain and muscle spasms, particularly after intercourse. Engaging in Pilates positions with proper breathwork can aid these muscles in releasing and lengthening, whilst strengthening them can improve various aspects of life, including sexual health and incontinence. Alternatively, chronic pain can cause pelvic muscles to remain overly tense, persistently contracting without proper relaxation. Over time, these muscles can become too strong, so they are unable to relax, which can create a host of issues. If this occurs, a trip to a physiotherapist is required instead.

Pilates can form part of your pain management plan as it improves flexibility and core strength. The gentle stretching involved can alleviate muscle tension associated with endometriosis pain. It also builds the core muscles in the trunk of the body, including the abdominals, lower back, pelvic, and hip muscles. A strong core ensures proper load distribution across the pelvis and spine, allowing these muscles to work together harmoniously. This provides additional support to the pelvis can reduce discomfort and pain. It may also help alleviate bloating and swelling in the abdomen. In essence, Pilates is an exercise that benefits various aspects of health. It promotes a strong mind-body connection, teaching you to identify and manage your pain triggers while adjusting your movements to avoid exacerbating discomfort. The breathing techniques used in Pilates can reduce stress, tension, and anxiety, making it an effective practice for both physical and emotional wellbeing.

Lymphatic Movement

Your lymphatic system is a network of lymph nodes, vessels, organs, and tissues. It's essential this system remains healthy to ensure that destroyed bacteria, abnormal cells, toxins, and other waste matter flow in a one-way system towards the heart so that it can be filtered and then expelled from the body by the liver or kidneys. This process is essential for overall good health, not just endo. Diseases such as lymphedema, certain cancers, fibromyalgia, or rheumatoid arthritis can provoke a decrease in lymphatic drainage. Although you don't need to have these conditions to benefit from supporting your lymphatic system. If you've recently had surgery or suffer from aching joints, abdominal swelling (think endo-belly), or swelling in the legs or arms, promoting lymphatic movement can be especially helpful.

If you recall from Part 1, we discussed the possible involvement of the lymph nodes in the pathogenesis and spread of endometriosis. The lymphatic system plays a vital role in immune cell function and surveillance. In endo, immune cell function is disturbed, and studies suggest that the lymph nodes draining the pelvic region may be impaired. This reduced drainage might contribute to the persistence and spread of endometriosis, as the body is less effective in clearing diseased cells.[1]

The lymph system is also involved in regulating hormones circulating in the body, particularly the female sex hormones, oestrogen, and progesterone, which, as we know, have a role in endometriosis.[2] A healthy lymphatic system supports the flow of progesterone, helping to balance oestrogen levels. Yet when disrupted, progesterone may not flow as efficiently, causing oestrogen to build up. Stimulating lymphatic flow can help eliminate excess hormones and maintain balanced oestrogen levels, which could positively impact endo management. Even though the connection between the lymphatic system and endometriosis isn't fully understood, we do know there is an association between the two. The lymphatic system also has a crucial role in regulating the immune and inflammatory responses in the body. Promoting lymphatic drainage can therefore, help reduce inflammation, eliminate toxins, and improve immune system function — key factors in managing endometriosis. Movement is one of the best ways to stimulate the lymphatic system. Physical activity increases heart rate, helping lymph fluid circulate and eliminate any build-up of toxins and inflammatory chemicals. This can reduce fluid retention, swelling, and even improve pain levels. Dry brushing can also stimulate lymphatic flow, ideally done before showering, but remember to brush towards the heart. Deep breathing exercises promote lymphatic circulation by increasing oxygen flow and encouraging drainage. Furthermore, drinking plenty of water is vital for flushing out toxins and keeping the system functioning efficiently. You may want to try a lymphatic drainage massage from a qualified practitioner as a relaxing, non-invasive way to stimulate the system. Lastly, Pilates and yoga can provide benefits, although indirectly. They can stimulate muscle contractions near the lymph nodes, which may help propel lymph fluid through the vessels. They also improve blood circulation through muscle engagement and breathing techniques, which enhance the removal of waste products.

Physiotherapy

Physiotherapy is a science-based treatment in which professionals train to a degree level, specialising in restoring physical health. Their core mission is to promote recovery, enabling individuals to regain movement and reduce pain or stiffness. Physiotherapy can play a crucial role when someone has been affected by an injury, illness, or disability by restoring any impaired movement and function. The scope of physiotherapy is broad, covering a wide range of treatments. A physiotherapist can design a customised treatment plan to meet your needs, incorporating exercise, massage, or other techniques like heat therapy and electrotherapy. Physiotherapy can be beneficial in managing endometriosis, depending on the specific ways it has impacted the body — factoring in the location and extent of damage to healthy tissue. Chronic localised inflammation sometimes leads to scar tissue formation and adhesions within the pelvic or abdominal cavity, encouraging organs to be displace from their original positions. This displacement can impede organ mobility and disrupt normal function, thereby restricting the body's natural movement. For example, scar tissue on the bowels may cause pain or digestive issues such as difficulty emptying your bowel properly. Adhesions can tether organs to the abdominal lining, giving rise to issues with posture or the way we hold ourselves. In some cases, this damage leads to muscular imbalances, where certain muscles overcompensate for dysfunction, altering how we sit, stand, or move. During surgery, a doctor can confirm whether adhesions or distortions are present. If they are, physiotherapy may be beneficial to restore alignment. It's important to note that surgery is the only definitive way to remove adhesions. However, surgery is typically only recommended if part of another procedure to treat endometriosis or the patient has an advanced case necessitating it due to the increased risk of exacerbating adhesion growth. Physiotherapy can help address adhesions or scar tissue through techniques that stretch and loosen them. While physiotherapy doesn't directly remove them, it can reduce their impact on surrounding tissues by easing tension and relaxing tight muscles, improving mobility and pain. This treatment may also help restore the proper functioning of any affected nerves.

It's not uncommon to find dysfunctional pelvic floor structures with endometriosis. This is sometimes attributed to elevated stress levels, including fear or anxiety, stimulating muscle tightness. While everyone's response to stress varies and not everyone experiences the same manifestations, during fight-or-flight, the tailbone can tuck under. As the pelvic floor muscles are attached to the tailbone, chronic stress can cause the muscles to tighten and shorten over time. Combined with pain and inflammation in the pelvic region, this can lead to a *hypertonic pelvic floor*. In this condition, the pelvic floor muscles remain overly tight and fail to relax. Symptoms may include pelvic pain, constipation, urinary incontinence, painful urination, and painful intercourse. If these symptoms resonate and you have concerns, seek a specialised physiotherapist with advanced training in gynaecological conditions who can help. The cause of a hypertonic pelvic floor differs in each person, so it's crucial your physiotherapist identifies the root cause of what is driving the dysfunction to provide effective treatment. For those who feel they might have a hypertonic pelvic floor but think they can resolve it on their own, please don't read the term 'pelvic floor dysfunction' and assume Kegels will fix it. Kegels strengthen your pelvic floor, and since the muscles in the hypertonic pelvic floor are already too tight, it's not recommended to do Kegels as it can worsen the problem by further increasing tension.

Sex can be a painful experience for many with endometriosis, sometimes leading to the inability to have intercourse altogether. Some people may also find that inserting a tampon triggers pain and discomfort. Ideally, sex should be enjoyable and not something associated with pain or fear. If you're finding sex painful, you could benefit from seeking out a specialised physiotherapist. Painful intercourse can create anxiety or fear, which only amplifies the problem, making it challenging to enjoy intimacy. This can be important to address early on as if you continue to have sex whilst simultaneously creating strong fear connotations, realistically, it's only creating further issues to resolve. For those looking to get pregnant, painful sex can provide its own form of contraceptive. Knowing you must go through a profoundly painful experience to try and create a baby can naturally diminish the sense of excitement. Resolving issues with pain before attempting pregnancy can be incredibly important for mental and physical health. While there are several causes of pain during intercourse, it can be caused by musculoskeletal problems, pelvic floor dysfunction, or connective tissue issues. A physiotherapist can assess the cause and create a personalised treatment plan to suit you. If pelvic floor dysfunction is identified as the issue, they can help either strengthen or relax the muscles as needed. Manual therapy techniques such as *myofascial release* can ease tension by applying pressure to areas that feel tight or rigid instead of elastic and moveable. Additionally, physiotherapists can provide education and pain management strategies, as well as address the emotional or psychological aspects of painful sex. They can also help treat conditions such as vaginismus or vulvodynia.

Endometriosis can affect the bladder in various ways. Sometimes, adhesions on the organ prevent it from expanding and contracting fully, resulting in pain and difficulty emptying. Alternatively, pelvic floor dysfunction can prevent the muscles supporting the bladder from working effectively, leading to urinary incontinence or difficulty initiating and stopping urination. Physiotherapists can offer specific exercises and techniques to strengthen the pelvic floor, improve bladder control, and reduce urgency or leakage. They can also provide guidance on proper bladder-emptying techniques and use manual or heat therapy to alleviate discomfort.

Physiotherapy is a valuable treatment at any stage of endometriosis, helping to manage a range of complications and improve quality of life. It can complement surgical treatment by restoring optimal body function and mobility. This may be what you need to feel you've put your disease in remission with the lasting impact of the disease being put to rest. The restoration of mobility in the body can allow for any disrupted flow of blood, fluid, and lymph move freely again, supporting overall recovery and wellbeing. This restoration of multiple facets of the body can help down-regulate the nervous system, moving it from fight-or-flight to the rest and digest mode. If you suspect a physiotherapist could benefit you, it's essential you consult a certified and highly specialised women's health practitioner. Some pelvic pain clinics within the NHS have physiotherapists who work alongside gynaecologists, so speak to your doctor to see if this is available for you. Keep in mind that physiotherapy isn't a quick fix; improvements may take a few months to truly notice a difference, and ultimately, not every approach works for every person. It's essential to have realistic expectations of what a physio can provide, as persistent pain can be challenging to treat, so complete pain resolution may not be possible. However, physiotherapy can still offer valuable tools to help you self-manage this long-term condition. It may be precisely what you need to thrive.

53

The Four Pillars of Health – Sleep

"O Sleep, O Sleep, Nature's Soft Nurse"
– William Shakespeare

Sleep is often undervalued in society or overlooked in our pursuit of health, with many of us focusing solely on food or exercise. Sleep is the time when our body rests, recovers, rebuilds, and regrows. Without sufficient sleep, it can lead to a wide range of adverse and detrimental effects on the body, ranging from simply lacking energy to more serious consequences and the increased risk of various diseases. It's crucial to never relegate the priority of a good night's sleep, even when tempted by the allure of the next Netflix episode. Achieving a proper sleep routine considers multiple factors. It's not just about the duration of your sleep, although getting enough hours each night is an important component. It also consists of:

Depth of Sleep – Ensuring you get enough *deep* sleep.

Sleep Continuity – Limiting the number of times sleep is interrupted.

Regularity of Sleep – A routine and bedtime you stick to helps to regulate your circadian rhythm. Try to aim for a consistent sleep schedule, going to bed and waking up at the same time every day, even on weekends.

Naturally, some of these aspects may be out of our control; night shifts or having young children who wake you up in the night can make creating a better sleep routine more challenging. Regardless of your personal situation, it's still important to consider all these aspects when assessing your sleep routine. Are you getting the most out of your sleep and getting high-quality rest?

When we sleep, a small pea-sized gland in the brain called the pituitary gland secretes hormones into the blood, aiding the healing process in our bodies, repairing our muscles, and creating new tissues. This maintenance and repair work is a vital aspect of keeping us healthy and flourishing. While we slumber, our immune system springs into action, replenishing immune cells to help the body fight off infections, disease, or recover from any illnesses. When sleep is limited, our immune activity decreases, including a drop in the number of Natural Killer (NK) cells detectable in the body, which are responsible for destroying infected and diseased cells.[1] We want our NK cells performing at their optimal best, as reduced functioning is associated with a 1.6 times higher risk of dying with any cancer,[2] and endometriosis often already shows impaired NK cell function so we don't want any further issues.[3] Sleep deprivation or a disturbed sleeping pattern can lead to other alterations in the immune system, promoting higher inflammation, which can progress to increased levels of stress hormones.[4] You can probably tell from that last sentence how sleep is vital to incorporate into your toolkit. Prioritising quality sleep is a potent weapon in maintaining health and preventing disease. During sleep, our brain undergoes a cleansing process whereby harmful toxins and waste products accumulated throughout the day are filtered and flushed out, restoring the brain. Cerebrospinal Fluid (CSF) is a clear fluid that surrounds the brain and spinal cord, bathing the central nervous system and delivering the required nutrients. When we sleep our CSF pulses, cleaning away the harmful waste products. Scientists believe this may be why diseases like Alzheimer's are associated with a lack of sleep, as this process is protective of your brain and health. This cleansing process occurs primarily during deep sleep, supporting the need to look at multiple aspects of how we sleep. This is a crucial task for the body to carry out at the end of the day. Sleep benefits are not just limited to brain or immune health; rest is involved in all the body's major physiological systems, including cardiovascular and endocrine health. Essentially, sleep is your superpower to prioritise, especially as there is a higher prevalence of insomnia and poor sleep quality in endometriosis.[5,6] A plausible explanation for this is the symptoms, namely pain, which can directly cause sleep disturbances. However, the high prevalence may also be caused by hormonal fluctuations and mood disorders. The female sex hormones oestrogen and progesterone are involved in a variety of processes that regulate sleep, whilst oestrogen dominance or an imbalance in these hormones is capable of causing sleep struggles. Most people won't know if their hormones are out of balance, leaving them unsure why they are bad sleepers. This partly explains why endometriosis is associated with fatigue — a lack of sleep impairs how you function in the daytime, causing you to feel tired and unable to carry out your tasks effectively. It can be pretty gruelling when poor sleep is combined with the other factors contributing to endo fatigue. The world is not exactly built to accommodate people who cannot get enough sleep at night by allowing them the grace to work less or have rest periods. Instead, everyone is expected to continue waking up at the same time and carry out their roles and duties accordingly. This seems like a practical and proper way to carry out society until you're personally hit with these sorts of issues. The structure of our lives can lead to a horrible cycle where we are unable to catch up on needed sleep due to our commitments like work, yet when we are back in bed and trying to sleep, there is a frustrating continuation of sleep disturbances. Over time, this can feel like your quality of life just isn't the same, always one step behind with fatigue clouding every activity you try to do. This can be depressing or mentally draining in of itself. Unfortunately, this ability to impact your waking hours and escalate with time, isn't simply because you didn't sleep enough. An abundance of complex processes in the body designed to optimise our health will not occur if there is a lack of sleep. Yet the shortage of sleep simultaneously causes adverse processes to occur, making you feel worse. Very annoying right? During deep sleep, our immune system produces certain anti-inflammatory cytokines activating parts of the immune system to protect the body, promote healing, and fight excess inflammation.[7] When we curtail our sleep schedule, there is an increase in inflammatory cytokines, triggering chronic low-grade inflammation and immunodeficiency.[8] So, getting enough sleep decreases inflammation, whilst, on the other hand, insomnia does the opposite — possibly resulting in disease progression.[6] We are aware by now that inflammation can stimulate or cause pain, exacerbating many endo symptoms. Pain also has an established relationship with insomnia or disturbed sleeping patterns, with research showing women with insomnia are more susceptible to pain symptoms.[6] Furthermore, sleep deprivation can elevate anxiety and depress mood, possibly due to increased cortisol (the primary stress hormone). Even if you do not suffer from anxiety or depression, a lack of sleep can increase your stress response due to the hormones released, causing lowered tolerance to symptoms like pain.

So how do you improve your sleeping habits, or as it's otherwise termed, sleep hygiene? First, look at your sleep duration. Do you have a lot of disruptions, or do you sleep well and deeply? Plus, do you have a consistent sleep schedule that works for you? You need to assess what you are doing well and what could do with some improvement. Think about why some aspects of sleep are easy and why you struggle with others. For example, if you sleep a good number of hours each night but wake up a lot, causing disturbed sleep, is it because you get too hot, need to pee, or maybe because you wake up thirsty. Understanding the cause can help determine what you need to do to try and improve on these. In relation to the examples above, proactive steps to improve sleep could involve buying a duvet with a lower tog so your body can breathe better, or if it's related to your bladder, you may need to stop consuming fluids a couple of hours before bed, on the other hand, you may require to drink a glass of water before bed. Furthermore, create a sleep schedule that suits the time you need to be up, then allow for eight hours of sleep to calculate the time you need to be asleep by. You may want to add some extra time to determine your ideal bedtime, allowing for sleep routine practices and the act of falling asleep to occur (unless you are someone who falls asleep the moment your head hits the pillow). Next on the list is creating a relaxing bedtime routine. We have all heard it, but this means limiting your screen time to 30-60 minutes before going to bed. You may want to use lavender spray on your pillow, so you associate the smell with sleeping. You could also meditate, read, do breathwork, or gentle stretches to slow down the mind and create space between your day and the transition into rest and sleep. If you struggle with a racing mind before bed, part of your routine could be journaling to get your thoughts out or plan your day tomorrow so that you don't start thinking about everything you need to do while trying to sleep. Decipher if changes need to be made to your sleep space to encourage better sleep, such as buying a new pillow or blackout blinds. Consider a traditional alarm clock so you can leave your phone outside your bedroom. Also, examine your daily habits and how you prepare for good sleep later in the evening. You could limit caffeine to two cups a day, both of which must be consumed before 12 pm. Or do you need to move your body and exercise, so you are tired later? Exercise has been shown to improve sleep quality and mood and calm the nervous system, all of which can complement your desire for good sleep. When creating your new sleeping plan, create a routine that makes you excited for bed and do things that will make you feel cosy and happy to be winding down. Adjusting your sleep schedule can be valuable to reduce pain, balance hormones, reduce stress levels, control inflammation, and improve quality of life. Feeling good in your body on a day-to-day basis is soup for the soul, and if a good night's sleep can help, then it's worth considering.

If you have overburdening fatigue not caused by a lack of sleep but the status of the disease, sleep hygiene can still help. Endo fatigue can feel all-encompassing and as though all the sleep in the world could not resolve it. No matter how hard you try to shake it, sometimes you need to just rest, because staring at your computer screen forcing yourself to get a task done, but really, are unable to think through the fatigue, is not helping.

That incredible urge to lay down may sometimes be the most productive thing you can do. Getting additional sleep is what your body is asking you to do for a reason. It's looking for the downtime to heal and fight off the inflammation and stress hormones in your body. The four pillars of health are all tied together. If you do not consider sleep in addition to your other goals, it can cause the other pillars to suffer. When you are tired, you don't make healthy food choices, nor do you have the energy to exercise. Yet, when we are well-rested, the opposite is true. Plus, our nervous system calms down, so we perform better. It's all intertwined. Sleep is essential to health, not a luxury. If you are feeling unusually tired, please remember to have your iron levels checked by your doctor in case iron deficiency anaemia is contributing to your fatigue; this is important to determine and can be easily treated.

There was a time in my life when sleep was my priority every night, particularly on weekdays, when I had to be up for work and then try and make it through the day, struggling to stay awake. If I were invited to do something after work, which would mean going to sleep at a later time or drinking alcohol... then I wouldn't go. I knew how horrible that would make me feel the next day so it would be the worst choice for myself. At the time, my body was incredibly sensitive. I could not handle any additional energy use. Sometimes, self-love is making an effort to see friends and family, but sometimes, the act is not going out and instead doing what your body needs. With time taking care of my health, I am happy to say I am not in that state anymore. My body is better equipped to handle busier days because my body doesn't react the same way it once did. Give yourself the same grace if it needs it and know bad periods may not last forever.

54

The Four Pillars of Health – Wellbeing

The fourth pillar, wellbeing, represents a dynamic state characterised as being comfortable, healthy, and happy. It reflects how we perceive and respond to our internal and external environments and encompasses how we feel in our bodies and about ourselves. Cultivating wellbeing involves finding strategies to navigate daily life, manage day-to-day stress, and overcome any obstacles that are impeding our wellbeing. It also means doing things that bring us joy. This pillar entails developing a positive outlook on life and creating a sustainable lifestyle that nurtures the mind, body, and soul. Core facets of wellbeing include connection, social and emotional health, and finding time for relaxation. As mood disorders are prevalent in endometriosis, this chapter primarily concentrates on how to navigate through these. However, you do not need to be struggling to still work on this pillar.

Connection and Social Health

Connection is a sense of belonging — feeling part of something larger than ourselves that enriches our emotional lives. This includes social connection to our friends and family but also to nature, the world, our bodies, and spiritual connection. Activities like going outside for a walk in a park or meeting a friend for a coffee are both ways to enhance connection.

The benefits of feeling in this state are numerous: it can lower rates of anxiety or depression, boost self-esteem, strengthen our immune system, and enable us to enrich our relationships.

Self-connection is equally as important as our social connectedness, as when we feel connected to ourselves, with time, we cultivate self-awareness and compassion. This allows us to manage our emotions better, create healthy boundaries, and make conscious choices about what we want out of life. A scientific framework proposed for developing self-connection includes three aspects: awareness, acceptance, and alignment.[1] To achieve awareness, we need to start listening to our bodies and recognise what we are craving and why. A common example I hear Endo Warriors talking about is feeling compelled to stop drinking alcohol, yet many don't do it because of work or societal pressures, or they feel like they'll be missing out. Ignoring what our body is asking us to do keeps us away from the next stage of acceptance.

Another aspect of awareness is paying attention to our thoughts and emotions, which so often flow in and out of our heads without us ever sitting with them, leaving us unaware of what we tell ourselves repeatedly. Most of us have negative self-talk patterns which don't do any favours for our wellbeing. Although these can be a challenge to rectify, if we start to notice them, it can enhance our emotional intelligence and help us identify patterns in how we look at the world. As the first step is awareness, this process can be enlightening. From there, we can work on reformulating the way we *allow* ourselves to think. Done correctly, this act should encourage positive self-talk whilst diminishing negative speech. As self-connection grows, so does acceptance of who we are, our strengths, and our aspirations. This allows us to start addressing our needs, which can benefit us in a multitude of ways. Alignment, the third stage of self-connection emerges as we evolve with a greater appreciation of ourselves and what *we* want to do. Ultimately, leading us to a more meaningful and fulfilling life.

Furthermore, engaging in self-compassion creates a positive feedback loop, increasing our happiness and facilitating better relationships with others.[2] Understanding our feelings improves how we articulate them, which is important in our endometriosis journey because there can be many hurdles, fears, and grievances along the way to deal with and process. Knowing how to communicate these and work through them is needed to achieve wellbeing. Humans are social creatures, and building connections with the people in our lives is an essential form of medicine. Social ties bring us laughter, joy, entertainment, love, and a sense of belonging. All wonderful things we want more of. Research links strong social bonds to improved physical and mental health, even influencing factors such as BMI, cancer survival, and overall wellbeing.[3] Belongingness is also one of Maslow's hierarchy of needs, important for psychological growth and development — a widely used and respected theory for understanding human behaviour. Maintaining relationships enhances your belongingness and can uplift your mood and wellbeing. Even if you're very busy or are struggling with a flare, making an effort to call someone for a catch-up on your commute to work can still make a difference. It's paramount to find ways that suit your lifestyle. Endo can be a little isolating at times. Cancelling or declining invitations when your endo flares can make you feel like your social life is falling by the wayside. Even if you think you don't have the energy or the time to work on your social relationships, would it help if I said it will truly make you feel better?

A final component of connectedness is to nature. The World Health Organisation describes nature as "our greatest source of health and well-being". Our relationship with nature and how much we notice, appreciate, and connect to our natural surroundings is critical in supporting good mental health. How often do you touch the earth, smell the flowers, or listen to the birdsong? This won't be frequent enough for many of us, and certainly not a daily experience as it's meant to be. Nature can help clear the mind, generating calmness and creativity whilst reducing anxiety and depression. For those who live in cities and urban jungles where green and blue are lacking in our day-to-day lives and our ability to be exposed to nature and animals is rare, this act of connecting to nature is particularly important. Green prescriptions exist whereby doctors encourage their patients to engage with nature as treatment. They started in New Zealand at the tail end of the 20th Century, although in Japan, forest bathing has been recommended since 1982 due to the positive physiological effects on human health. By 2020, the UK launched a two-year green-prescription pilot to test the benefits. If you are wondering why health professionals prescribe nature as this seems outside their usual scope? Well, the health benefits have been long recognised, and with the current mental health and chronic disease epidemic, doctors are looking at factors in our lives that have changed generationally and deciphering what is pertinent to reincorporate. Most people should connect with nature more often, whether going for a walk in the park, gardening, hiking, or swimming in a lake. Do something that appeals to you and try to make it a habit you stick to. This also relates to two pillars, movement and wellbeing, highlighting their interconnectedness.

Vagal Tone and Social Anxiety

Earlier, we discussed how people with endo sometimes have decreased vagal tone, so the vagus nerve is less active and responsive than it should be. This manifests in several ways, impacting both our physical and mental health. It can lead to digestive issues, cause a less flexible or adaptive cardiovascular system, heighten the inflammatory response, reduce the ability to manage stress (which can lead to anxiety or depression), and diminish immune system efficiency. Vagal tone is often fundamental in managing our disease, and lifestyle changes can improve this. We've discussed yoga and breathing exercises, and later, we will explain how meditation can help improve vagal tone, but connection to a friend or family member can also help. When we see someone we know, we give them a hug, a kiss, or even a handshake. This touch stimulates the vagus nerve, allowing the nervous system to relax by activating our parasympathetic nervous system, slowing down our heart rate, and inducing calmness. Even our hormones can change when we experience intimate or affectionate touch, as it encourages the brain to release oxytocin (nicknamed the love hormone). So, right off the bat, being with loved ones can help improve our vagal tone. Connecting with people and engaging in supportive, nurturing, or meaningful conversations also allows us to feel emotionally supported, enhancing our emotional regulation. Whilst receiving guidance or offering support can build healthy, trusting relationships. The old saying "a problem shared is a problem halved" is true, and many of us feel better and brighter after relieving the thoughts plaguing us or getting us down. Even a productive conversation with a co-worker or pleasant interaction with a stranger provides benefits. All aspects of positive social interactions can activate the vagus nerve, improving our physical health and stimulating favourable emotions.[4] Furthermore, when we engage with others, we affirm positive associations towards social situations, something particularly important for those dealing with social anxiety.

If your vagal tone is poor, the heightened response to stress or anxiety can often lead to over-anticipating threats. These aren't the kind that would typically be described as 'threats', i.e., when something could jeopardise your safety. Anxiety threats or social threats describe the way someone will be biased in their thinking habits towards negativity, perceiving things which aren't threats, *as threats*. Therefore, their fight-or-flight response will be easily triggered. When we perceive stress in a social situation, whether the threat emerges or not, it's harder to adapt, rest and recover after the moment has passed. Meaning a person has built up emotions and chemicals in their body that are difficult to come down from. It's hard to connect to others when in fight-or-flight, so it's understandable if you have reached a place in life where you are struggling with this aspect of life, as negative thought patterns start to occur around socialising. As social anxiety is found in those with decreased vagal tone, fears or anticipated threats are common. This can spread like wildfire in your brain, escalating normal things so we instead perceive them with a sense of stress. For example, having social anxiety about going out with your friends may filter into fearing bumping into someone you know on the street. If you give into the controllable fear by not seeing friends you have arranged to see (due to the symptoms of decreased vagal tone), then it can mean you're allowing your brain to fester on the uncontrollable and unpredictable issues that may arise in life. However, if you choose to put your energy into connection and building your vagal tone, it establishes trust in yourself that you can engage socially with others and that you enjoy it. In turn, this increases your vagal tone, reducing stress whilst promoting relaxation. Over time, the more you stimulate your vagus nerve, the quicker your body can return to normal after a stressful moment, easing your heart rate and breathing and reducing any fight-or-flight response. Once you start building confidence in your body that you can recoup quicker after a moment of anxiety, it improves your mental and physical health. If this all sounds good, but you don't have people in your life who can offer you this right now, you can still make improvements by looking at every social interaction as a chance to leave with a smile on your face. Smile at people on the street if you feel safe doing so, or talk to people in your gym class. There are many ways we can fabricate a world where we receive lots of small but positive daily interactions that can increase our vagal tone. This may seem daunting or weird for some, but it gets easier the more you do it. You will notice the changes in how it makes you feel, and you will start to enjoy it.

Loneliness can be contagious, but following these small steps is a good way to kick back at it whilst improving your health at the same time. You could consider joining a club or community in something you find interesting. When my brother moved to London, he found it considerably lonely, so he joined a gym where you are encouraged to work in pairs or groups and found himself with a new group of friends and a great social life. Taking action to achieve what you want is a valuable lesson to learn, and loneliness is not an exception to the rule. Some of you reading this may not relate, whilst it's an overwhelming concern for others, so take what's relevant to you.

Incorporating Relaxation

Managing stress and incorporating relaxation into our lives is another vital aspect of wellbeing. If you are Italian or have seen the movie *Eat, Pray, Love*, you may recognise the saying "dolce far niente", which translates in English as "the sweetness of doing nothing". In our fast-paced, modern, Westernised world, we never do *'nothing'*. Our brains have even been so degraded by social media that it's changing our brain structure and function. Have you ever found yourself watching a movie but also scrolling on your phone...? The act of relaxation through watching television has even been turned on its head as our brains are looking for more stimulation, so we must do two things at once. There are many examples of this, such as listening to music to walk somewhere or being on your phone whilst on the toilet or in the bath. Acts that were once a moment for mental restfulness have become a time for more multitasking. So, how does this relate to stress? Well, our attention spans have never been shorter, and research determined that individuals who get distracted easily are more prone to suffer psychological distress and mental health issues, with social media usage being highlighted for its problematic mental health consequences.[5] Social media also exposes us to more stressors than previous generations would be, and the rise in mental health problems speaks for itself. We have access to a world of bad news at our fingertips. We have information overload, comparison fears, fear of missing out, or some people may even suffer from cyberbullying. This is not to say social media is inherently bad or something that cannot be used effectively. Still, it's an important part of the story of how our brains are currently functioning, which, in turn, limits the ability to relax. Naturally, there are far bigger stressors than social media that people deal with on a daily basis; they are also part of the story of achieving wellbeing. If you feel you struggle to relax or you are addicted to your phone, then it might be time to look into your social media usage and whether any adjustments should be made. Allocating time for your brain and nervous system to unwind is part of building a healthy lifestyle and achieving wellness. We cannot avoid stress; it's how we are programmed and sometimes it can be extraordinarily helpful. Stress is an essential and inevitable component of life, and too little of it can lead to boredom and depression. It can give us the drive and energy to face challenges, motivate us to reach goals, excite us, and show us what matters to us. Where we don't want to end up is in a state of chronic stress, as this is related to a wide range of illnesses, as prolonged periods of elevated stress hormones and high blood pressure are detrimental to the body. Additionally, chronic stress can make it harder to sleep, create bowel and bladder urgency, suppress our immune system, cause reproductive problems, and increase inflammation. These can be existing problems for people with endo, so it's important to look at how you deal with stress to avoid aggravating these symptoms. Decipher any causes of stress in your life and whether you could benefit from adjusting your daily habits.

Having endometriosis can be stressful at times. Pain is taxing, as are many of the other symptoms, but stress also comes from work, family, fertility issues, or fears. Whatever the reason may be for each person, clinical studies indicate endometriosis is associated with high levels of chronic stress.[6] The main stress hormones cortisol, noradrenaline, and adrenaline all play a significant role in the body's fight-or-flight response. These hormones are crucial to our health and essential for survival, but as we've mentioned, chronic or prolonged exposure can have complex effects on the immune system. For example, cortisol can suppress immune function, increasing susceptibility to infections or impairing the ability of the body to mount effective immune responses. Stress can also contribute to further pro-inflammatory responses by releasing inflammatory cytokines. Whilst stress hormones like cortisol can suppress the production of anti-inflammatory cytokines. The sustained activation of these chemicals can cause chronic inflammation, leading to tissue damage and dysfunction.

Stress can even disrupt the balance of gut microbiota, as our microbiome is closely linked to immune function. If we don't find ways to manage stress, it can impair vagal tone, cause central nervous system sensitisation and functional changes to our brain, as well as induce epigenetic modifications. This might sound depressing, but it's another clue to how we can help our health and protect our bodies. If you are stressed, you may detect signs such as headaches, muscle tension, changes in appetite, a rapid heartbeat, hair loss, and skin problems, or you may feel irritable or overwhelmed. Stress can manifest in different ways for different people, but if you recognise your body is stressed, it might be time to step back and look at what you can change or improve. That said, how you view stress is a significant factor in how it affects the body. If you believe it to be helpful, manageable, or beneficial to you, it better equips you to handle the stress rather than seeing it as harmful and bad. If you experience any of those symptoms, it's a sign of imbalance, and part of the needed change is starting to tell yourself that stress is good, helping you achieve what you need to do.

Overall, finding ways to relax, calm down your CNS, and give your body and mind a break is essential for wellbeing. The ultimate way to relax and quieten the mind is with meditation. Spending as little as five minutes a day closing your eyes and focusing on your breathing will help restore an inner calm. If that doesn't tickle your fancy, you can try guided meditations where you listen to a narration encouraging you to enter a world of your imagination, designed to get you relaxed and free of daily thoughts. Other forms of relaxation include having a bath or shower that isn't rushed, taking the time to enjoy it, washing your body, and maybe listening to gentle music to help you unwind. Another idea is having a massage, whether you pay for a service, get one off your partner, or do it to yourself — it can be a wonderful way to connect to your body, providing it with love, time, and care. Your relaxation method could even be sitting on the grass and watching the clouds. Whichever method you choose, acknowledge the feeling that nothing is more important than what you are doing at that moment. You are calming down your body, easing pressure, allowing hormones to rebalance, and blood pressure to go down — that is all important. Improving wellbeing, seeking positivity, and giving your mind space to relax, slow down, and see the beauty in life can improve pain levels. Whilst emotions like stress, depression or anxiety all increase pain levels experienced, which, with a condition like endo, is likely the opposite of what you need. Interestingly, individuals who feel supported through illness or a stressful period in life report less pain, validating the importance of working on your wellbeing through your community to ensure you feel better.

* * *

The four pillars all work synergistically, so if you can work on each in a small way, you'll be closer to healing your nutrition, stress response, identity, and body. You will feel better about your life and your place in it, and most importantly, you will feel good being in your body again. If you don't know where to start, get a piece of paper, create headings with the four pillars, and write out some actions you would most like to try, then start working towards those. It's a wonderful recipe for creating long-term health and promoting vibrancy in your life. Even if you don't personally struggle with any mental health concerns, high stress levels, or nervous system issues, wellbeing remains a cornerstone of living a vibrant, healthy life.

55

Alternative Medicine

Alternative Medicine, or complementary medicine, comprises a broad variety of healing practices used across the world. Many of these are ancient practices where the knowledge has survived to this day. They fall outside the realm of conventional Western medicine, offering alternative approaches to healing. Often focusing on holistic wellbeing, they recognise the interconnectedness of the mind, body, and spirit as elements of health, so emphasise the importance of treating the whole person. Alternative medicine encompasses a range of therapies, treatments, and philosophies, each with its own principles and methods. They often prioritise non-invasive techniques, focusing on natural healing and remedies. This might include herbal remedies or mind-body practices that stimulate the body's ability to heal itself. Whilst alternative medicine is not without its controversy and criticisms, there is still much to be gained from this approach to health, providing support alongside Western medicine practices. If you wish to try any of these, please always source an accredited and highly trained professional to ensure you get the safest and best experience. You may consider visiting a naturopath who incorporates many of these or seeking a practitioner who specialises in one. If you are considering skipping this chapter because you think it's a bunch of woo-woo, the NHS has previously provided me with a leaflet for endometriosis recommending complementary therapies such as acupuncture or homoeopathy as people have found great relief in their symptoms using them. There is a place for all practices of healing, and knowing how these practices work can support you on your healing journey.

56

Herbal Medicine

Herbal Medicine, also known as phytotherapy or botanical medicine, is a traditional approach to healthcare, utilising active ingredients from plants such as leaves, stems, roots, seeds, or flowers to restore and support the body's health. These plant materials can be used in their whole form, dried, powdered, or as extracts. Herbal medicine aims to heal the body or support its natural processes to regulate itself thereby preventing conditions. By focusing on the root cause of health issues rather than merely treating symptoms, herbal medicine offers support to our physical, mental, and emotional health problems. It can assist a wide range of ailments, from respiratory conditions to digestive issues. Herbal remedies can be prepared in various forms, such as teas, tinctures, capsules, salves, and essential oils. The method of preparation, *meaning how you use the product*, depends on the specific herb and its intended use. Herbal medicine has been an integral part of human history, used across cultures for centuries. Many ancient cultures had a deep-rooted belief in the healing power of nature and maintained a spiritual connection to plants. Communities had to rely on plants readily available in their environment to help them treat ailments, which led to cultures having individual traditions within herbal medicine. It was observational learning, using trial and error to observe the effects of plants on health and then passing down this wisdom to the next generation. Many traditions still thrive today, including Traditional

Chinese Medicine (TCM) and Ayurveda from India. Each culture has a distinct approach and variety in plants used, as they were developed from the plants indigenous to their differing geographical areas. This chapter covers a handful of accessible herbs which may be beneficial for managing endometriosis. These are generally considered safe for most people and are easy to incorporate into your life. However, it's always advised to consult a specialist in herbal medicine for personalised advice. If this chapter inspires you to learn more about herbal medicine, many books and resources are available to deepen your understanding. Also, while many herbal remedies are considered safe, it's essential to understand they can have side effects or interact with medications. It's crucial to read the leaflet that comes with any medicines you take, as some specify herbal remedies not to take alongside them. For example, oral contraceptive pills often state not to take St. John's Wort whilst taking them. If you are ever in doubt as to whether something is safe, consult a qualified herbalist before using it, especially for treating chronic or serious medical conditions. It's also important to note that although herbal medicine has a long history of use and well-documented benefits, it should not be considered a replacement for conventional medical treatments in serious or life-threatening conditions. Certain herbs and plant compounds have been studied extensively in scientific research to determine their safety and effectiveness, leading to the development of herbal supplements and standardised extracts. Nevertheless, not all products are created equal; select organic options where possible and purchase from a reputable brand you trust to make optimal products. It's always good to be an educated consumer. Research any new herbs before trying them to understand potential side effects and the proper dose to take (especially if you are on other medications). Starting with a low dose is a good way to test your sensitivity to new herbs. Without further ado, here are a few options you may want to consider incorporating into your endo toolkit.

Turmeric and Curcumin

Turmeric is the root of a flowering plant called *Curcuma Longa*. It has a similar look to ginger, except when cut into, it has a distinct bright orange colour. It's commonly used in cooking, particularly in Indian cuisine, but also for its potent medicinal properties. It has been used for hundreds of years in Ayurvedic and Chinese Medicine. Turmeric contains an active substance called curcumin, famed for its antioxidant and anti-inflammatory properties. Both turmeric and curcumin have been subject to thousands of scientific studies and tested against a variety of diseases. Turmeric is rich in phytonutrients known for their ability to protect the body by neutralising free radicals, shielding cells from damage. It's particularly valued for its effectiveness in reducing inflammation, swelling, and muscle soreness.[1] This single factor may appeal to those with endometriosis to utilise it, yet turmeric possesses several other relevant benefits, such as reducing anxiety, bloating, indigestion, and boosting liver function.[2] Several studies have shown turmeric's effectiveness in improving IBD symptoms, particularly pain and quality-of-life[3] and has shown promise as a treatment for Ulcerative Colitis (UC), a type of IBD. In one study, whereby 50 patients with UC were given either a curcumin supplement or placebo, showed that over half of the participants who took curcumin supplements alongside their medication achieved remission within four weeks — an impressive result, especially as no one taking a placebo achieved this.[4] In fact, a systematic review accredited curcumin as a possible safe and effective therapy for maintaining remission of UC when administered alongside standard treatments.[5] Turmeric's potential anti-cancer effects are also being explored. Chemoprotective agents are generally divided into groups based on which stage of cancer development they help fight. Curcumin may act as both a carcinogen blocker, *preventing the initial DNA mutations*, and an antiproliferative agent, *inhibiting tumour growth and spread*.[6] Due to some similarities between cancer and endometriosis, curcumin's ability to inhibit cellular proliferation makes it a potential candidate for managing endometriosis

389

as well. Research supports this, demonstrating curcumin has an anti-inflammatory, antiproliferative, anti-angiogenic, and pro-apoptotic effect on endometriosis.[7] This means there may be a viable role for turmeric in the prevention and treatment of endo. This is not to say it's a cure-all; there are certainly not enough studies to state that. However, the possible benefits suggest it can be a valuable addition to your toolkit in a multifaceted approach to healing. Turmeric works by blocking the action of inflammatory molecules in the body, neutralising free radicals, and interfering with various inflammatory signalling pathways. This helps calm down existing inflammation, which in turn reduces angiogenesis — *the formation of new blood vessels*, a vital part of endometriosis' survival and progression. While decreased inflammation can reduce this process, turmeric also has a direct ability to inhibit angiogenesis through the suppression of Vascular Endothelial Growth Factor (VEGF) and Fibroblast Growth Factor (FGF). These potent growth factors have a role in driving the vascularisation of endometriosis lesions.[8] Reducing the amount of these minimises their ability to vascularise lesions needed for survival. Inflammation is a source of pain for many, so decreasing inflammation can reduce this, not just in the pelvis but also in other parts of the body, such as the joints and muscles. There is also a growing body of evidence that curcumin exerts anti-oestrogen and anti-androgen effects,[9] which in vitro was able to directly reduce endometriosis cells and slow growth.[10] Several animal studies further support curcumin's capacity to reduce the development, size, and spread of endometriosis lesions.[11,12] It was also shown to diminish the appearance of cysts in the ovaries of mice, resulting in a healthy follicle appearance, which can improve ovarian function in diseases like endometriosis and PCOS while reversing the amount of oxidative stress.[13,7]

Due to endo's ability to strike any moment with a flare or cause terrible periods, we may sometimes go through sedentary periods, where we don't move very much or are unable to reach our desired exercise goals. While trying to maintain physical activity is fundamental, for moments where you want to crawl up in a ball, turmeric can help. Curcumin can impact endothelial function, which is the ability of blood to keep moving through the body smoothly. A dysfunctional endothelial function is associated with stroke and heart attacks, so we want to keep this operating healthily. Eating nutritious food and exercising is the best way to achieve healthy endothelial function, but consumption of turmeric can provide assistance. One study on postmenopausal women found it had a similar effect on endothelial function as one hour of aerobic exercise.[14] Naturally, this should not replace exercise, but it can offer support when needed when we are bed-bound or unable to exercise. Another time we spend a lot of time lying down is during surgery recovery — turmeric may be able to help you here too. Due to its anti-inflammatory, antioxidant, and analgesic properties, it might accelerate recovery after an operation. Research has found caesarean wounds healed at a faster rate[15] and incision-induced inflammation and pain also reduced.[16]

Overall turmeric may be beneficial in supporting various aspects of our health, so it's worth incorporating into your life if it hasn't been already. Turmeric has an earthy, peppery taste, added to cooking to give flavour, colour, and nutrition. It's commonly found in curries or scrambled tofu to improve the colour and taste. A small amount can be added to smoothies, and depending on the flavour of the smoothie, it may go unnoticed. You can make or purchase turmeric shots or turmeric lattes. Watch out though, turmeric has a potent pigment; if you cook with fresh turmeric, it can stain kitchen surfaces and utensils. If you don't want to take that risk, you can buy powdered versions, which can be spooned straight onto your food. If the taste is not for you, or if you can't find enough ways to incorporate turmeric, supplementation can be helpful. Supplementation can be found in both turmeric and curcumin varieties. As we mentioned earlier, curcumin is the active ingredient found in turmeric and has been the focus of numerous medical studies, so you may be compelled to use curcumin supplements. However, turmeric has also demonstrated remarkable results, and it remains uncertain whether curcumin is the sole component in turmeric capable of achieving health benefits. Nature has provided a divine product with therapeutic effects, so rather than select one of these compounds, it's often best to consume the whole product the way nature intended. At the end of the day, you will still get curcumin in a turmeric supplement, whilst with curcumin-only varieties, you diminish the possible benefits turmeric can offer as they have been extracted away. When you consume turmeric, add black pepper to your serving or ensure your supplement has this added, as an active ingredient called pepperine can increase the absorption of turmeric by 2000%.[1] Always follow the dose on the bottle, and be aware that high doses of curcumin, as often found in supplements, can interact with certain medications, including reducing the effects of aspirin or ibuprofen. Supplementation may also not be suitable for those having chemotherapy or are on immunosuppressive drugs, blood thinners, or those with a family history of kidney stones.

Ginger

Ginger root, derived from a flowering plant, has been used for thousands of years as a spice in food and a remedy in herbal medicine due to its flavour and numerous health benefits. It contains bioactive compounds like gingerol that possess anti-inflammatory properties, making it helpful for combating inflammation. This can be valuable in conditions characterised by chronic inflammation when heightened pain sensitivity or tissue damage is experienced. Incorporating ginger into your routine can be a flavourful and natural way to address these concerns, tapping into its remarkable anti-inflammatory benefits for pain management, including muscle soreness, joint pain, and menstrual cramps. Ginger is *so* good at relieving pain that one scientific paper suggested it may be as effective as mefenamic acid and ibuprofen in relieving period pains.[17] With endo, sometimes traditional painkillers don't work, so why not try getting ginger into your diet to see if it can provide an additional layer of pain relief, especially during times of PMS or period pain. Ginger is safe to take alongside ibuprofen and paracetamol, so it doesn't have to be one of the other, but a powerful combination. Beyond its pain-relieving effects, ginger is widely used to alleviate digestive issues. It can help manage indigestion, motion sickness, and nausea (including morning sickness). For those who experience endo-nausea, try sipping ginger tea or sucking on capsules. Whilst ginger may not appeal to all taste preferences, the benefits of a natural and effective way to minimise nausea can outweigh the taste... and like anything else, you will soon get used to it. Ginger can also strengthen the immune system, aiding the body's defence against infections and illnesses. This benefit is partly attributed to ginger's anti-microbial properties, which have the potential to help combat various pathogens.[18] Immune regulation can be impaired in the presence of many inflammatory and oxidative processes occurring. Getting these under control using foods like ginger can further improve immune function. Due to these properties, ginger can be used to soothe sore throats and coughs and may help reduce symptoms of respiratory conditions. If you already enjoy honey and lemon water when you have a cold, add fresh ginger slices into the mix for an extra boost. Ginger is rich in a vast number of antioxidants, nearly 40 types, helping to protect cells from free radical damage and perhaps treat the symptoms of various inflammatory conditions like endo.[19] The science even suggests these antioxidant and anti-inflammatory properties make ginger a candidate for being protective against life-threatening diseases such as cancer.[20] In Ayurveda, ginger is recommended for combatting anxiety as this emotion is an expression of excess vata. In layman's terms, anxiety is a cold energy, so the individual has an imbalance that requires bringing warmth into the body to rebalance their constitution and restore harmony. Ginger has a hot or warm energy, so sipping ginger tea or having a bath with ginger powder can rebalance anxiety symptoms. Ginger's spicy and zesty flavour gives it versatility, allowing it to be incorporated into various dishes, from vegetable soup to curries and sweet treats like ginger biscuits. In cooking, the taste usually mellows and dissipates depending on the amount of ginger used. It can be employed in various forms: fresh, dried, powdered or oil. Make sure to use it in moderation, as excessive consumption can lead to gastrointestinal issues. Additionally, ginger can interact with certain medications, so be sure to check with a healthcare professional. Other ways to consume more ginger in your diet include ginger shots, ginger ale, or adding fresh ginger to hot water in the morning, which is a great digestive aid.

Ashwagandha

Ashwagandha is a shrub found in Asia and Africa and has been a staple in traditional herbal practices for centuries. Often referred to as a superfood or adaptogen, it possesses a range of health-promoting properties. Adaptogens help the body adapt to stress, either physical, environmental, or psychological. They assist in many facets of bodily regulation: improving mood, balancing hormones, fighting fatigue, and boosting the immune system. To qualify as an adaptogen, a food must be nonspecific, meaning it relieves a wide range of stressors, helping the body maintain homeostasis without harming its normal functions. Simply, adaptogens *adapt* to your body's needs, so you see how they got their name. As an adaptogen, ashwagandha is already off to a great start and may be find exciting to try. Like the other herbs selected for this book, it also possesses antioxidants and anti-inflammatory properties, making it useful in conditions characterised by chronic inflammation. Ashwagandha has been tied to improving energy, vitality, stress levels, cognitive function, mental health, hormonal balance, and sleep improvements. Regrettably, there are no studies examining ashwagandha's impact on endometriosis. Despite that, just because research does not exist doesn't mean it can't help.

Let's explore some of the reasons you may want to incorporate ashwagandha. A 2016 systematic review highlighted it could support reproductive system function in many ways.[21] Due to ashwagandha's ability to improve hormonal balance, it enhanced LH and FSH hormone levels, both of which are vital in a delicate balance to achieve follicle maturation, ovulation, and pregnancy. Fertility challenges can be caused by various factors, including iron accumulation in the reproductive organs; this is common in conditions like haemochromatosis, characterised by excessive absorption of dietary iron. This is worth mentioning as iron overload is also a concern in endometriosis, primarily due to the accumulation of iron from chronic bleeding in lesions. Iron overload can be found in the ovarian follicular fluid of individuals with endo, which is associated with oocyte maturation disorder.[22] Although this will not affect everyone. Iron overload can lead to oxidative stress, potentially impacting ovarian function. A study found the active ingredients in ashwagandha appear to restore iron-overload infertility by acting on iron chelation and capturing iron free radicals.[23] This makes ashwagandha a cheap and enjoyable natural medicine that can be utilised if you are experiencing infertility due to iron overload and want to try everything you can. If you're unsure if this relates to you but are struggling with unexplained infertility, speak to your gynaecologist to see if they can assess the likelihood.

As we know, to achieve pregnancy, it takes having sex, which can be a struggle for those who experience pain or fear avoidance. Ashwagandha is known for its aphrodisiac properties, potentially boosting libido by reducing stress and improving overall sexual wellbeing. Stress, whether physical or psychological, can negatively affect sexual desire, and as an adaptogen, ashwagandha helps mitigate these effects. Its ability to support hormonal balance, increase energy, mood, and blood circulation are also all important in sexual health. A study found daily consumption may translate into improved sexual health in several ways: desire, arousal, lubrication, orgasms, sexual satisfaction, and pain.[24] That all sounds wonderful doesn't it, but naturally, we need to question if this can do the same for those with endo. While no studies specifically address its impact on individuals with endometriosis, it may be worthwhile trialling and experimenting to determine whether ashwagandha can have the same effect on you.

Ashwagandha is one of the best nervine tonics of Ayurveda, meaning it could have neuroprotective effects. Studies have shown it might be helpful in various central nervous system-related disorders such as Parkinson's and Alzheimer's.[25] The mechanisms behind ashwagandha's influence on the CNS are not fully understood. However, it's shown to promote the formation of neurons and potentially inhibit the production of amyloid-beta plaques, a hallmark of Alzheimer's disease.[26] The ability to improve nervous system health whilst fighting off stress can induce calmness and limit anxiety — a welcoming thought for many. Academic studies support this, highlighting a reduction in anxiety and depression levels and improvements in sleep when taking ashwagandha.[27] Blood work also confirmed this with reduced morning cortisol levels, validating it wasn't just a placebo effect.[28] An animal study also noted comparable reductions in anxiety and depression levels when ashwagandha was trialled against leading drugs, benzodiazepine lorazepam and the anti-depressant imipramine.[29] Although animal studies don't guarantee identical results in humans, the potential side effects of those conventional medications make ashwagandha a compelling alternative. Its analgesic effects help soothe the nervous system's pain response, as shown by its efficacy in managing chronic pain, including joint discomfort,[30] which can be particularly beneficial for Endo Warriors. If you are interested in taking ashwagandha, it's typically purchased in powdered form or as a supplement. It can be added to smoothies and desserts or made similarly to instant coffee with hot water and milk. Ashwagandha has an earthy taste, so you may want to sweeten your drink with buttermilk, honey, or cardamom.

Cinnamon

Cinnamon, derived from the inner bark of several tree species, has been traded over the world for over 3000 years and was once more valuable than gold. Known for its warm, sweet flavour and fragrant aroma, it's commonly used in cooking and baking, boasting an array of health benefits. Cinnamon is rich in vitamins and minerals such as magnesium, zinc, manganese, and beta-carotene. There are different types of cinnamon and not all are made equal. The most common variety is cassia, which has a stronger flavour than its biggest counterpart, Ceylon cinnamon, native to Sri Lanka. All cinnamon contains a compound called coumarin, which can be harmful to the liver when consumed in large amounts. Ceylon cinnamon is believed to be superior as it has much less coumarin than cassia cinnamon, making it the safer option to pick, especially when planning to use it regularly. Cinnamon's anti-inflammatory properties, derived from compounds like cinnamaldehyde, make it a valuable tool in managing chronic inflammation. Additionally, its antioxidant content contributes to overall health and wellbeing. Cinnamon may also help regulate menstrual cycles. A study on women with PCOS, a condition that causes irregular periods, found supplementation improved menstrual cyclicity, compared to no improvement seen in the placebo group.[31] Further research showed cinnamon reduced the amount of menstrual bleeding, pain levels, as well as nausea and vomiting experienced during menstruation.[32] Given that painful, heavy, irregular periods are common issues in endometriosis, if implementing more cinnamon in the diet can partially improve some of these, it may be worth the try, especially as cinnamon has a delicious taste many can get on board with. Cinnamon, however, may take more time than drugs such as ibuprofen to act as an effective pain reliever. Therefore, if you want to test cinnamon as a natural pain relief alternative, increase your intake several days leading up to your period to ensure your body can reap the benefits.[33] Cinnamon is easy to incorporate into your diet, but if you are not keen on the taste you may want to try supplements, but please use these in moderation (particularly in cassia form). Cinnamon can be added to your breakfast, sprinkled into porridge, yoghurt, or over granola. You can also dust cinnamon on top of coffee, add it to smoothies or try cinnamon tea or chai drinks. It also pairs well with savoury dishes, adding depth to curries, stews, and rice dishes, as commonly used in Middle Eastern and Indian cuisines. For those with a sweet tooth, cinnamon is widely used in baking, from cinnamon swirls to apple crumbles, or healthier options include cinnamon dusted on apples.

Cacao

Cacao is the seed or bean from which cocoa and chocolate are made. Despite chocolate being associated with sugary foods, you may have heard that dark chocolate is good for you. This is because the cacao bean from which chocolate is made can provide numerous health benefits. As an antioxidant, it reduces inflammation and can lower the number of antibodies released during an allergic reaction.[34] Cacao has more polyphenols with a higher antioxidant ability than green tea, black tea, or red wine.[35] Polyphenols can delay or inhibit damage to our cells, snuff out free radicals, and regulate inflammation in the intestines, leading to a reduction in proinflammatory enzymes.[36] Cacao is also thought to be the food with the highest source of magnesium found in nature. This can be amazing for those with endo to relax tense muscles and help with cramps. It's also one of the highest plant-based sources of non-haem iron known. This is particularly useful for vegetarians or vegans who don't get iron from meat. You can reap these benefits from eating chocolate, but know darker varieties are better than milk or white chocolate. The higher the percentage of cacao, the greater the benefits. You can also drink cacao, which has been popularised in recent years. Raw cacao is made by cold pressing unroasted cacao beans, which retain the living enzymes while simultaneously removing the fat content, called cacao butter. You can use raw cacao powder to make a drink with hot water and/or milk. It can be a healthy alternative to hot chocolate or provide a low-caffeine substitute for one of your cups of coffee a day.

57

Traditional Chinese Medicine (TCM)

Traditional Chinese Medicine (TCM) is an alternative holistic system boasting a rich history. It has been practised in China for over 2,500 years and is still widely used all over the world. TCM is based on a unique understanding of the body; it's a complex system with its own distinct philosophy and diagnostic methods. The concepts of disease are based on ancient schools of thought, so differ greatly from the Western medicine approach. The basic concept of the practice is to rebalance Qi (pronounced "chee"), the vital force of life coursing through the body along invisible energy highways called meridians. While these meridians aren't tangible physical structures, and there is no conclusive evidence to say they exist, TCM ensures uninterrupted flow along them. The harmonious balance of opposing forces that make up Qi, known as Yin and Yang, are the keys to maintaining health. If there is a blockage in Qi or an alteration in the Yin and Yang, such as too little or too much energy, then disease and illness can occur. To regain equilibrium, you must balance the internal body organs and the elements of earth, fire, water, wood, and metal. This intricate balance allows Qi to flow through your body freely so that you feel relaxed and energised. TCM is a broad range of medicine, offering various traditional techniques and products to address problems. These include:

Acupuncture
The insertion of fine needles into specific meridian points to stimulate and balance the flow of Qi.

Moxibustion
The burning of herbal leaves near or on the body to stimulate healing.

Cupping
Placing glass or plastic cups on the skin whilst creating a vacuum to suck on the skin to stimulate blood flow.

Tui Na
A specialised massage involving hand and arm techniques to realign the body.

Herbal Remedies
Herbs are prescribed in a combination or mixture to address patient concerns. They may be taken as daily tea, pills, tinctures, syrups, topical applications, or herbal baths.

Tai Chi
A mind-body practice combining slow and intentional movements, practised for self-defence and to promote health.

Qigong
Another mind-body practice, using coordinated movements, deep breathing, and meditation to promote mental and physical health.

Gua Sha
Gua Sha has been popularised in the 21st Century for beauty purposes, but its true benefits go beyond aesthetics. Gua Sha translates to scraping or rubbing. When used with the correct technique, it produces petechiae on the skin to release stagnant blood and toxins.

Nutrition

Guidance on foods categorised as hot or cold may be provided to align a person's constitution and correct imbalances.

A practitioner may employ a combination of these to provide individualised care to their patients, although you can also seek out treatment for certain practices individually. TCM is described as pseudoscience because the majority of the treatments have no logical mechanisms of action, at least if you look at it from a Western medical perspective. As there is no evidence the concepts in Chinese medicine are true, many feel there is no basis or validity to the treatments. Although its practices and theories do not align with conventional Western medicine, its efficacy is subject to ongoing debate and research. In recent years, efforts have been made to integrate some aspects of TCM into Western healthcare systems while ensuring rigorous scientific evaluation. This is because many people are drawn to alternative or complementary approaches to managing their health. Its holistic and natural methods can be an attractive option over taking pharmaceutical medicines to resolve health concerns. Despite this stigma, some practices, like acupuncture, have been shown to provide patients with notable benefits in certain health conditions, particularly pain management. Additionally, herbal remedies or medicines can be very effective but may also have side effects.

In Chinese medicine, endometriosis is not one distinct disorder but rather a complex condition manifesting differently in individuals. As TCM has its own diagnostic framework and views disease in a unique way, endo is often diagnosed and treated based on patterns of disharmony in the body. People with endo have varying problems and scales to these issues, so the pattern of disharmony and symptoms will determine how a practitioner approaches treating the patient. With multiple potential patterns, treatment varies from person to person. For example, a TCM diagnosis might identify a pattern of blood stagnation or Qi stagnation in the pelvic area, often accompanied by heat or dampness in the lower part of the body. The treatment strategy would then be tailored to resolve these patterns. As most endo patients suffer from symptoms of pelvic inflammation, the accumulation of heat and blood stasis are the main pathologic changes alongside dampness.[1] TCM can be employed to reduce pain and inflammation or improve fertility or mental health. It can even be sought out to improve the appearance of periods. Whilst what defines a normal and healthy appearance for a period will vary between people, periods that are consistently dark or contain large clots are not typically considered normal and can be a sign of underlying factors such as fibroids or endometriosis. In TCM, blood clots are viewed as blood stasis, where blood is slowed or obstructed in the body. This indicates Qi stagnation or cold stagnation, causing symptoms such as severe pain relieved by warmth. In this instance, you may be offered acupuncture to dispel the cold and warming herbs to promote blood flow and circulation.

There are a handful of medical papers on the herbs used in TCM and their ability to treat endometriosis. One study treated 76 women with a pill containing rhubarb as the main ingredient to remove blood stasis.[2] It was effective in 80% of patients, covering symptoms such as dysmenorrhoea, pelvic pain, intercourse pain, and even diminishing size of a mass. These results are consistent with other papers testing various herbs or techniques to remove blood stasis with substantial improvements in symptoms.[3,4]

Quyu Jiedu is an approach to clearing out dampness, heat, and toxins; it can incorporate herbs, acupuncture or other TCM modalities to resolve these qualities. This approach was tested among patients with and without endometriosis alongside a pharmaceutical drug used for endo called gestrinone.[5] To measure the effectiveness of Quyu Jiedu, they monitored the endometrium levels of Vascular Endothelial Growth Factor (VEGF) and cell proliferative nucleoprotein antigen (Ki-67) before and after treatment. Both these compounds have been found to be higher in women with endometriosis, so they can give insight into the activity of endo within the body.[6,7] Upon initiating the study, these were tested, and the expression of these markers was higher in the endo patients than the healthy women, confirming it was a useful marker to understand the clinical significance of the herbs. After three months of treatment, these markers were tested again in the same phase of their menstrual cycle as they were first tested. Both the Quyu Jiedu and the gestrinone drug groups showed positive results, with the VEGF and Ki-67 markers significantly lower than before treatment commenced. Although there were no significant differences in the results between Quyu Jiedu and gestrinone, making neither one of them more effective than the other, this was a win for TCM as gestrinone has heavy side effects and induces a menopause state, so it's not appropriate for those wanting to get pregnant in the near future. Gestrinone is not even available in the UK, making Quyu Jiedu the alternative option. This study also put forward a theory on how TCM techniques work to improve symptoms — it may be related to lowering VEGF expression.

Another paper review on 158 women affirmed that 100% saw some improvement in symptoms from using TCM.[8] That is an exciting statistic, offering plausibility for using TCM — even if it can't cure you or make you feel perfect, it may still provide improvement, which for many will be enough of a draw.

Going beyond symptom control, a clinical trial was also able to show promise from using Chinese medicine to prevent recurrence after surgical removal in those with stage 3 or 4 endometriosis.[9] The patients were divided into two groups: the test group were given a formulation of five Chinese medicinal plants, whilst the control group were given goserelin acetate injections, a type of hormone therapy, over a duration of three months. The blood levels of CA-125 and IL-18 were measured at a six and twelve-month check-up. IL-18 is a cytokine involved in various immune diseases and is suggested to play a pathogenic role in endometriosis, making it a useful marker.[10] Both groups displayed a significant reduction in each blood marker, showing that both treatments were effective. While there were no significant differences between the IL-18 markers, the group that received Chinese medicine had a lower amount of CA-125. This study validates how the use of TCM alongside conservative surgery can work harmoniously and effectively with lasting effects. Again, the side effects of the drug goserelin, also known as Zodelex®, may not appeal to some as it prevents the ovaries from producing oestrogen, instigating a temporary menopause.

Animal studies on rats with endo showed TCM reduced the volume of lesions, induced cell death, and inhibited cell proliferation of endometriosis.[11] This was after only 28 days of treatment, which tested both high and low doses of fourteen plant herbs called Gui Xiong Xiaoyi Wan, commonly used to address conditions related to gynaecological health. This rat-model study demonstrated this combination of Chinese herbs was effective in suppressing the growth of endometriosis. However, what happens in rats does not mean the same will happen in humans, so it's important not to assume so. Further studies would need to validate if the same results could be achieved in humans.

Overall, these studies, and many others, show herbal remedies in TCM may help individuals at different stages of their journey. More clinical tests are required to understand these practices better, their potential application in endometriosis, and how they can work as therapeutic alternatives for different stages of the disease. What's certain is there are people out there benefiting from TCM in the management of endo. If you plan on trying TCM, find a certified practitioner to ensure authentic and safe treatment. When you attend the appointment, your practitioner will do a physical exam of your body, examining your tongue, skin, hair, eyes, nails, and voice. They will ask questions about your health, such as your medical history and why you are there. From their assessment, they will decipher which organ networks are affected and need rebalancing. They will then correct these by providing a combination of therapies. For all serious health conditions, please always consult your regular GP, but Chinese medicine can be useful alongside your regular treatment and for other conditions that don't require medical attention. Chinese medicine can help with nausea, back pain, IBS, recurring cystitis, arthritis, stress, and sleep problems, among many others. If you become pregnant during a course of herbs, always consult your practitioner to ensure they are safe to continue. Although TCM may not be able to replace conventional medical approaches, it may be useful alongside them.

58

Acupuncture

Acupuncture is a fundamental component of Traditional Chinese Medicine (TCM). It is one of the most well-known and widely used therapies, often sought out as a standalone method of healing, so it warrants its own section to understand the principles and therapeutic potential. Acupuncture involves the insertion of small, thin needles into specific points scattered across the body's skin surface. These strategic acupuncture points are believed to be located along intricate energy pathways known as meridians. Although meridians do not represent physical entities like our nervous system would, they are energetic channels. There are twelve standard meridians, which are divided into Yin and Yang groups, as well as a handful of other energetic pathways. Each meridian is associated with different types of energy, depending on the direction energy flows, temperature characteristics (ranging from cooling to warming), and their interconnectedness with various organs and emotional states. They are mapped throughout the body and are believed to function as a network connecting various organs and tissues to other parts of the body. The whole body is considered to be interconnected, so imbalances in one area cause symptoms in another, manifesting in both physical or emotional levels, depending on which meridian an issue is arising. This implies a problem with your gallbladder may cause you to have a neckache. The practice aims to rebalance the flow of vital energy, or Qi, through these meridians to resolve symptoms. The rationale behind this is that meridians can become blocked or stagnant due to stress, illness, or poor lifestyle habits. When there is dysregulation in the meridian flow, it gives rise to systemic issues in the whole body, leading to illness, pain, or emotional issues. Acupuncture endeavours to rectify these imbalances and restore harmony in the body, enabling health promotion. You can visit an acupuncturist for an array of issues, from pain management, migraines, fertility, osteoarthritis, nausea, respiratory disorders, some skin disorders, anxiety, and even general wellness, as it can boost immune system function. Your treatment can tend to a single symptom or multiple at once.

Acupuncture is incredibly helpful in treating pain. By stimulating nerves, muscles, and connective tissues, it can release tension and stress, alleviating pain. Although the mechanism of how it works is not entirely understood, studies show acupuncture can also enhance endorphin release, the hormones that help reduce pain and stress, and improve the sense of wellbeing.[1] Serotonin and dopamine can increase, which are, respectively, the happy and pleasure hormones, helping to regulate your mood and reduce pain sensitisation.[1]

Acupuncture has been historically used to treat inflammatory conditions, including allergic rhinitis. It's believed to have anti-inflammatory effects by regulating the HPA axis, which is critical in the body's stress response. By regulating this axis, acupuncture can modulate both the sympathetic and parasympathetic nervous systems, leading to stress reduction and potential improvements in anxiety symptoms.[2] When the nervous system works effectively, improvements can also be seen in the digestive system and bladder function. Acupuncture might even exhibit small antihistamine effects and downregulation of proinflammatory cytokines.[2]

Studies on acupuncture for endometriosis management show it helps alleviate symptoms and may be particularly effective in relieving painful periods and pain duration while improving wellbeing and quality of life. In one study, women received a thirty-minute session three times a week, and by twelve weeks, all the women had significantly improved test scores.

However, the improvements faded after treatment was discontinued.[3] Medical literature also suggests acupuncture can reduce CA-125 levels in the blood.[4] Therefore, if you want to try acupuncture for pain management, it's nice to know there's evidence it can help in many ways. Having the right expectations from treatment is always beneficial, so whilst acupuncture may not offer long-term protection, many find a significant reduction in pain intensity during their course of treatment. It's also a safe form of therapy that can complement surgery without the side effects of hormonal treatments.

In studies focused on individuals seeking IVF, electro-acupuncture was able to improve menstrual health by improving blood flow to the uterus and ovaries, helping regulate the menstrual cycle whilst also reducing stress.[5,6] Electro-acupuncture is a modern technique whereby electricity passes through the needles to enhance the treatment. Interestingly, acupuncture is often used as a fertility treatment, providing positive results in both men and women. In some instances, it's been able to restore fertility by improving ovarian function, balancing the endocrine system, and regulating fertility hormones.[7] For those using IVF, having acupuncture alongside may help with implantation rates, pregnancy rates, as well as live birth rates.[8] If you have had several rounds of failed IVF, it may be worth considering acupuncture alongside your fertility treatment, as studies show combining the treatments significantly improves the number of mature oocytes regardless of age.[9] Naturally, with any form of treatment, what works for some and not others is complicated and often unclear. Whilst there is no guarantee acupuncture will promote pregnancy, there is plenty of anecdotal and medical research to say there is a possibility it can help.

When choosing a practitioner, check their training and credentials, including a three-year degree-level course. In the UK, acupuncture is accessible for chronic pain through the NHS. If you are in the U.S., some medical insurance will cover the treatment. During your first appointment, the practitioner will run through some questions to understand more about you, why you are there and your health status. They will ask to look at your tongue and measure your pulse on your wrist. You will then be asked to lie on the bed, face up or down. Remember to wear loose clothing or a vest so the practitioner can insert needles across the body. The needles are inserted into your skin at varying depths and in differing amounts each session. You may not feel them being inserted, but they can cause a mild sensation in some locations. Once the needles are in, you will be left to relax. Enjoy this moment; it's a time when you cannot do anything but accept the rest. Appointments can be up to 60 minutes. When the session ends, the acupuncturist will let you know how often you should return for treatment. It may be weekly, but your practitioner will work with you and your budget. After your session, you should avoid strenuous exercise, caffeine, alcohol, and stress for the rest of the day and drink plenty of water. When using acupuncture, understand that results may not occur immediately; sometimes, it can take up to three months to notice a difference, depending on your concern. Multiple factors contribute to the variability in acupuncture's therapeutic effects, including number of needles used, the duration of the session, the technique, the accuracy of the acupuncture points, and the number of treatments you have had, among others. Talk to your practitioner if you have any issues or feel your treatment is not working. They may be able to make changes in your sessions, although sometimes acupuncture may not be right for you or what you need to resolve your particular concern.

59

Homeopathy

Homeopathy, also known as homeopathic medicine, is a system of alternative medicine developed in Germany over 200 years ago, using remedies derived from various natural sources, such as plants, minerals, and animal products. These remedies are often prepared into small sugar pellets to be placed under the tongue, a more palatable option compared to some other herbal treatments such as Chinese teas, which can have strong or unusual flavours. Other homeopathic products include ointments, gels, drops, creams, and tablets. Homeopathy is based on some unconventional principles that diverge from mainstream medical science. The two key concepts include:

1. The Law of Similars: At the heart of homeopathy is the idea that 'like cures like'. This principle proposes that illness can be cured by giving a patient a substance that, if used on healthy people, would produce the same symptoms as the condition.

2. Minimum Dose: Homeopathic remedies are highly diluted substances, as it's believed that the more diluted a substance, the more potent its therapeutic effect becomes. This is intended to enhance the remedy's effectiveness while minimising potential toxicity. Consequently, homeopathic treatments provide the smallest possible dose.

Homeopathy shares some similarities with Chinese Medicine as it operates on the premise that the body possesses vital life energy, and when imbalances occur or energy is disrupted, it can lead to illness. Homeopathic remedies are believed to stimulate the body's vital force to restore balance and promote healing. Another key aspect is the emphasis on providing individualised treatment. Homeopaths take into account not only a person's physical symptoms but also their emotional and mental state before prescribing remedies. As a result, two people with the same condition may receive different treatments based on their unique symptom profiles. This contrasts with conventional Western medicine, which often applies a more standardised approach to diagnosis and treatment. It also differs from mainstream medicine in recognising different clinical patterns.

Homeopathy can treat many symptoms or conditions, including stress, high blood pressure, allergies, dermatitis, and asthma. However, its effectiveness remains a topic of debate. In 2017, the UK's NHS stopped funding homeopathy and advised that doctors should not recommend it due to a lack of strong scientific evidence supporting its effectiveness in treating various conditions, with results often comparable to placebos. Despite this, homeopathy's popularity continues, especially as a complementary therapy. For example, Cancer Research UK notes homeopathy is one of the most common complementary therapies used by people with cancer alongside their treatment. Many patients report feeling better, *despite* the absence of scientific evidence supporting its efficacy.[1] I was also recommended homeopathy on the information leaflet the hospital provided me when they diagnosed me with endometriosis. *Even if these effects are attributed to the placebo effect, the placebo response can be powerful and have a meaningful impact on health, so it shouldn't be underestimated. Studies have shown that sham surgeries, whereby patients are told they had surgery to treat their condition *but did not have anything more than incisions in their skin*, lead to desired improvements in up to 75% of patients, particularly in pain-related conditions.[2,3] This demonstrates the significant influence and power that belief can have on health outcomes. While the scientific basis for homeopathy is weak, it may still offer value to some individuals, particularly those who find comfort in its treatments. It helps many people, so even if the science is not there to validate it, I thought it was worth sharing. If you're interested in trying homeopathy, seek a registered practitioner. Homeopathic remedies are also widely available over the counter in pharmacies or health food shops.

60

Meditation

Meditation has gained remarkable popularity in the 21st century, becoming an essential aspect of conversation around improving mental health. This comes as no surprise, given the alarming rise in anxiety levels worldwide. For instance, in England, 1 in 6 people experience a mental health issue like anxiety or depression in a given week,[1] whilst in the United States, 19% of adults have an anxiety disorder.[2] Anxiety is more frequently reported among women and younger individuals, with around 28% of those aged 16 to 29 experiencing some form of anxiety.[3] Whether you have a diagnosed mental health disorder or are simply looking to reduce stress and stay present, meditation offers an effective tool for managing these challenges. It can serve various purposes, from improving sleep quality to facilitating spiritual growth. Meditation does not have to be considered a boring or unattainable practice but rather an exciting and enriching journey.

Meditation involves sitting in silence with closed eyes, with the intention of resting the mind, clearing thoughts, and connecting with oneself. It grants the mind a precious moment to relax, focusing on your breath and entering a state of tranquillity. It serves as a tool to refocus when feeling overwhelmed, allowing you to set aside responsibilities and worries. Through regular practice, meditation helps achieve a state of equilibrium, generating calmness that allows you to recentre. Meditation can be a soothing experience for the mind and body, reducing stress levels and providing rejuvenation. It enables reconnection back to your inner self, offering a space for reflection on your thoughts and experiences. It promotes a deeper understanding of your feelings, beliefs, and desires by eliminating distractions, allowing you to concentrate on yourself in a non-judgmental attitude. Deep breathing techniques during meditation can have a highly therapeutic effect on chronic pain. By focusing on your breath, tense muscles can relax, alleviating tension and, therefore, any related pain.

Start your meditation with deep diaphragmatic breathing, consciously breathing deep into the stomach, allowing it to swell and expand, filling your lungs with as much oxygen as you can, then exhale slowly, letting your stomach contract inwards and deflate. Deep breathing lowers your blood pressure and can relieve stress. This method can also help shift your body out of fight-or-flight mode, where the breath can become short and rapid, helping you reach a relaxed state. Starting your practice this way can be a helpful tool to get yourself ready for meditation before gradually bringing your breathing back to normal.

There are many types of meditation, incorporating various techniques that go beyond focused breathwork. Choosing a mantra to chant is popular and involves choosing a word or phrase you will repeat during meditation. There are traditional options, such as the Sanskrit chant of 'Om', believed to be the primal sound vibration of the universe. Alternatively, you may choose something that relates to you and holds personal significance, like an affirmation. For example, you might say or repeat in your head, "I am healthy" or "I am loved". Repeating mantras during meditation, when your mind is clear and you are in a deep state of relaxation, can be a powerful method to reinforce positive thoughts. It serves as a point of focus during your time of relaxation and may also be able to bypass the critical, analytical mind and instead communicate directly with the subconscious. You can try guided meditations; these are readily available on YouTube or meditation apps, providing sound to listen to during meditation. Some are designed to help you enter a deeper sense of relaxation, whilst others are targeted towards a specific goal, containing affirmations within them.

This may be a more fun way for beginners to learn to relax the mind.

When dealing with health conditions, meditation can provide solace from a multitude of problems you are facing. Some moments are harder than others, and meditation can be a place to enter during challenging times. Not only can it provide a reduction in pain,[4] it can also help calm down the central nervous system and promote healthy emotional wellbeing. It can recalibrate your thoughts about who you are and what you want. It's even better to adopt daily meditation into your schedule as those who meditate regularly are more likely to yield significant results. One scientific study stated meditating for thirteen minutes a day for eight weeks decreased negative mood and anxiety whilst enhancing attention and memory.[5] Meditation is a form of mind-body therapy, as shown through studies affirming it can significantly improve all types of endometriosis-related pain, which in turn can have a positive impact on mental health.[6] This is important as the interconnectedness of physical and mental health is well-established, with one strongly influencing the other. Feeling good in your body can help make you happy in your mind, but positive mental health is also critical to living a long and healthy life.[7] Helping one aspect of your health helps the other, and vice versa, highlighting the importance of nurturing both aspects for overall wellbeing. Meditation stands as a powerful tool for enhancing mental health, offering respite from the fast-paced world we live in, and providing an avenue for reflection, relaxation, and self-connection. By incorporating meditation into your daily routine, you can experience profound benefits for your mental and physical health, ultimately contributing to a more enjoyable, healthier life.

61

Other Treatments

Botox

Botox® is widely used as a facial filler to diminish wrinkles, providing a more youthful appearance, however, its applications extend beyond aesthetics. Botox has medicinal uses, treating conditions like excessive sweating, neck spasms, migraines, and an overactive bladder. Surprisingly, it can be used to treat endometriosis. If you're curious about how and where Botox is injected for this purpose, let's clarify what it can do. Botox is a brand name for a drug derived from botulinum toxin, which blocks nerve cells sending signals between muscles and the brain. This is how it smooths wrinkles, it 'freezes' muscles, stopping them from moving, contracting and spasming. Moreover, it can inhibit the release of chemical messages involved in transmitting pain signals to the brain. Pain can be caused by spasming pelvic floor muscles, and Botox offers a solution to prevent these painful spasms from occurring. In a 2006 study, researchers monitored women for two years who experienced chronic pelvic pain and pelvic floor muscle spasms after providing either Botox or a placebo saline solution injection into their pelvic floor muscles as a form of treatment.[1] The results revealed Botox reduced pressure in the pelvic floor muscles more effectively than the placebo, suggesting its potential usefulness for individuals who do not respond to physical therapy for these issues. Interestingly, the study found that the placebo group also experienced a significant reduction in painful sex, highlighting the role of the nervous system in remembering and amplifying pain — meaning when we associate something with a memory of pain, our bodies can frustratingly magnify the pain due to the pre-emptive assumption. The saline solution still offered support in pain relief due to this pain mechanism because receiving the placebo allowed the patients to change the narrative, believing they received a helpful treatment to curb their pain.

In 2019, a small study was conducted on thirteen women with endometriosis who experienced pelvic floor muscle spasms.[2] They were treated with Botox injections into the affected area, and within two months, all participants reported decreased pain, with some even stating their pain was now non-existent. Half of the women were able to reduce pain medication use as a result. Chronic pelvic pain is often linked to endometriosis, sometimes persisting after surgical or hormonal treatments. This pain can be caused by pelvic floor muscle spasms, whereby spasms occur when pressure is applied, replicating this discomfort. Injecting Botox into these muscles can temporarily halt their ability to contract as the toxin disrupts the communication between nearby nerves and the brain. Consequently, pain stemming from spasming pelvic floor muscles is significantly reduced or eliminated. If you are experiencing pain for this reason, Botox may offer an effective treatment option. Centres providing this service typically conduct a thorough examination to ensure the treatment will benefit you and confirm whether the pelvic floor muscles are the source of your pain.

Botox is approved by the U.S. Food and Drug Administration (FDA) and the UK's Medicines and Healthcare Products Regulatory Agency (MHRA) for specific medical uses, such as urological conditions. For the treatment of endometriosis-related pain, Botox is currently used off-label, meaning it hasn't been specifically approved for this purpose by regulatory bodies. Using drugs off-label is common practice in medicine and does not automatically imply the treatment is unsafe. For a drug to gain approval for conditions, large, well-controlled clinical trials must demonstrate the benefits, its effectiveness, any side effects, and the appropriate dose required. This is critical for Botox, as botulinum toxin is one of the most poisonous biological substances known, so whilst it's generally considered safe when used correctly, the lowest dose should be used to achieve results.[3] Another treatment option for relieving pelvic floor muscle pain is physiotherapy, which is safer and devoid of the side effects associated with Botox. A physical therapist can examine the musculoskeletal system to determine the root cause of muscle spasms, potentially addressing the underlying issue rather than just the symptoms as Botox does. It's also important to consider Botox injections temporarily reduce the strength of your pelvic floor muscles. Strong pelvic floor muscles are crucial for stabilising your core and supporting essential bodily functions, including bladder control and sexual health. Weakened pelvic floor muscles can lead to problems such as urinary incontinence, reduced sexual sensation, and difficulty achieving orgasm. You may know the importance of doing pelvic floor exercises from the public discourse around women doing their Kegel exercises. However, for those with overly tight pelvic floor muscles from years of chronic pelvic pain, reducing muscle strength might actually be beneficial, but this decision should be made on a case-by-case basis in consultation with a healthcare provider.

The duration of Botox's effects varies from person to person. Typically, relief can last between 10-12 weeks or up to six months in some cases. Thereafter, you can receive another injection if you feel it was effective in managing your symptoms. Whilst Botox has shown benefits in reducing pelvic floor muscle spasms and pain, the studies conducted so far have involved a limited number of participants. There's not enough research to truly understand the long-term effectiveness and potential side effects. Ongoing studies are being carried out, so let's watch this space. Botox may be a great tool for improving quality of life and reducing reliance on opioid pain medications. If you're considering gynaecological Botox, always seek out an experienced and qualified practitioner to ensure the treatment is tailored to your specific needs.

Bioidentical Hormones

Bioidentical hormones have garnered media attention as a potential solution for managing the symptoms of menopause, but they also have a role in treating endometriosis. These hormones are artificial, carefully designed to mimic the molecular structure of hormones produced naturally in the human body, such as testosterone, oestrogen, and progesterone. This sets them apart from traditional synthetic hormones used in medical treatments, which, while intended to replicate the effects of natural hormones, are structurally different at the molecular level. This slight dissimilarity can lead to variations in how the body metabolises and responds to them, affecting how they interact with hormone receptors and the way in which they are processed by enzymes or other biochemical processes. Ultimately, these slight differences can lead to variations in the body's response to these hormones, influencing their effectiveness and side effects. Traditional hormones are derived from various sources, including plants and animals, or are synthetic compounds. For example, these drugs may originate from animal urine or be manufactured entirely in a lab. In contrast, bioidentical hormones are typically derived from plant sources like soy or yam, which are then modified in a laboratory to create a structure identical to human hormones. This appeals to some people who believe bioidentical hormones may be better tolerated and, therefore, yield fewer side effects, as they are more 'natural' than conventional synthetic hormones. However, to clarify, the safety and efficacy of bioidentical hormones are still subject to ongoing debate and research. They are not without their own set of risks and so should be prescribed and monitored by a qualified healthcare professional.

Hormonal treatments, such as the Mirena® coil or birth control pills, are frequently recommended for alleviating endometriosis symptoms. However, concerns about the long-term use of hormone treatments and their side effects may cause some patients to seek alternatives, which is where bioidentical oestrogen and progesterone may offer a possible treatment option. Similar to traditional hormone methods, they are not a cure, but they can provide effective treatment in alleviating symptoms and managing the condition's progression. The goal is to create a hormonal environment that is less likely to facilitate the growth of endometriosis. In traditional hormone treatments, progesterone is often used in combination with oestrogen to suppress ovulation, which, in turn, reduces local oestrogen production by the ovaries. This is a well-established approach to managing endometriosis by countering the effects of oestrogen, thus diminishing some of the symptoms. Elevated oestrogen levels, sometimes in conjunction with low progesterone or progesterone resistance, are common. Maintaining healthy progesterone levels plays a crucial role in preventing excessive tissue growth by opposing the impact of high oestrogen levels, which can assist in the development of lesions. Progesterone also helps reduce pain associated with PMS and inflammation. Its calming effects on the body can help mood, sleep, and libido, as well as reduce anxiety. If you are struggling with the side effects of traditional hormone treatments but are afraid or unsure about coming off your treatment or are seeking options with greater tolerability, bioidentical hormones may be worth exploring. Although please be aware that the terminology surrounding bioidentical hormones conveys the notion they are natural and, therefore, holistic, gentle, and devoid of side effects — signifying they're better for you. Yet bioidentical hormones lack a standardised definition and fall under an umbrella term, so there are a range of hormone sources and manufacturing processes involved in each product on the market. Just because they're deemed natural doesn't mean they haven't also been commercially processed to become bioidentical. They have also been changed from their natural state to achieve their identical structure.

An array of bioidentical hormone preparations are available, including pills, creams, gels, patches, and injections. Some over-the-counter products, like bioidentical progesterone creams, are sold online without a prescription. It's crucial to emphasise that self-prescribing hormonal products can be dangerous; they should always be prescribed by a physician who can ensure the products have undergone rigorous testing for both efficacy and safety. Currently, no definitive evidence supports the broad claim that bioidentical hormones are inherently safer or cause fewer side effects than traditional synthetic hormones. This is especially important in the context of endometriosis, which is hormone-dependent, so more research is needed to evaluate its effectiveness and safety for this specific condition. This is noteworthy as one of the potential advantages of bioidentical hormones is that they can be tailored to individual needs. The particular hormone regimen, dosage, and duration of treatment can be customised based on a patient's unique medical history, age, and reproductive goals. But without substantial scientific support, it's difficult to fully assess the risks, benefits, and proper dosage for bioidentical hormone therapy, particularly in treating a complex condition like endometriosis, which must also consider the disease severity and symptomatology of the individual. If you are considering bioidentical hormones, it's imperative you have an open and informed conversation with your healthcare provider. This will help you weigh the potential risks, benefits, and side effects of this treatment. While these hormones may help manage symptoms, their side effects may not be suitable for everyone, and the effectiveness of each product will vary from person to person. Regular monitoring by a healthcare provider is needed to assess how well the treatment is working and to detect any adverse effects early on. Both traditional synthetic hormones and bioidentical hormones have their pros and cons. The decision between the two should be based on individual preferences, health concerns, and guidance from a qualified healthcare professional. Some individuals prefer bioidentical hormones due to their structural similarity to our hormones and personalised doses. In contrast, others may opt for traditional synthetic hormones, which have a longer history of use and more established clinical data. Ultimately, the choice should be made after carefully considering the individual's health and hormone replacement needs.

Cannabis and CBD

Cannabis, a plant known by many names, marijuana, dope, or weed, is undergoing a significant transformation in how it's perceived and utilised, particularly in medicine. In the early 1970s, cannabis was classified in the UK and US as a Class B or Class 1 drug, respectively, meaning possession, sale, and use were illegal. The landscape changed in 1996, when California became the first state to legalise medical marijuana. Later, in 2012, Colorado and Washington legalised recreational cannabis, with other states following suit. The movement in America's views towards marijuana gained momentum. Several countries around the world began to reform their cannabis laws. As of 2025, recreational cannabis is still outlawed in the UK. However, steps have been made towards a more lenient approach to medicinal cannabis. In 2018, the UK government legalised cannabis-based products for medicinal use in limited circumstances, allowing doctors to prescribe cannabis when other treatment options had been exhausted and where clinical evidence supported a potential benefit for the patient's condition. Within this timeframe, there was also a surge in the popularity of CBD products on the market due to their potential therapeutic properties. CBD is the abbreviated name for cannabidiol, one of the two major active chemicals in cannabis, the other is tetrahydrocannabinol, or THC for short. THC is the main psychoactive found in cannabis and is responsible for the 'high' sensation or euphoria people experience. Whilst CBD is a major active compound, it's essential to clarify it's *not* psychoactive, so it won't produce a 'high' sensation.

CBD

CBD's popularity is partly due to the lack of high received from using it, yet it remains a natural product marketed as remedying many ailments. It's widely available in all sorts of products, providing accessibility and interest to those who associate marijuana with illegal drug use, the unwanted smell, or smoking — all of which deter many people. Instead, CBD can be found in various forms, so there is a product to suit each person. Scientific studies have explored the use of CBD on a wide range of conditions and symptoms, from chronic pain and anxiety to multiple sclerosis and Parkinson's disease. Each of the exhaustive claims CBD is said to treat has varying levels of evidence behind it. One of the most well-established uses of CBD is for treating certain forms of epilepsy, with a prescription drug containing pure CBD approved for use in the U.S. and UK. In the context of endometriosis, CBD studies show promise as it may be effective in pain management and treating inflammation, sleep, anxiety, and depression. CBD is said to have analgesic effects, meaning it's capable of relieving pain, although this depends on the dose and route of application, such as whether ingested or applied to the skin as a topical cream. CBD also boasts anti-inflammatory and antioxidant properties, all of which have a potential role in the management of endometriosis. An in vivo study on rats demonstrated CBD significantly reduced the size of endometriosis lesions, displaying antioxidant effects, diminished inflammation, and lowered the presence of mast cells in the spinal cord.[1] The spinal cord is a crucial component of the central nervous system, and an increased presence of mast cells can contribute to neurogenic inflammation and central sensitisation, thus CBD's ability to reduce this is of interest. Another rat-model study concluded that CBD suppressed endometriosis, but this requires further studies on humans to clarify if the same could be possible.[2] If you are interested in using CBD, ensure it's a high-quality product from a reputable supplier and start with a lower dose so you can work your way up if needed. Ways to try CBD for endo include infused creams rubbed onto your skin in the location of pain, such as on your hips to aid pelvic pain or on your knees to reduce joint pain. If you want to ingest CBD, you can buy gummies which are sweetened to cover the taste and come in standardised amounts per serving, making it easy to track your intake. Tinctures are available, which you put under your tongue for faster absorption and allow you to control the dose. If painful sex is a problem, CBD-infused intimate products, such as lubes, can help relax pelvic muscles and relieve discomfort.

Cannabis

Cannabis used as a whole product may be preferential to CBD alone, as it's just one of the active compounds out of hundreds found in cannabis. In the same way, taking turmeric over curcumin supplements can be recommended to ensure you are not removing any helpful components — the same logic applies. The NHS is limited to only prescribing cannabis for a select group of patients on a case-by-case basis. You can only access a prescription for approved uses, including rare types of epilepsy, multiple sclerosis, or nausea and vomiting from chemotherapy. To obtain cannabis for medicinal purposes beyond these approved uses, such as for endometriosis, it will typically require a private healthcare prescription. The survey data on cannabis use is promising, with many women reporting improvement in pain not only from endometriosis but various gynaecological conditions.[3] This can be attributed to the body's endocannabinoid system, which comprises a network of receptors that interact with cannabinoids like CBD and THC, resembling a lock-and-key system that facilitates changes in the body. These receptors are widely distributed throughout the body, including the pelvis and reproductive organs, where endo pain predominantly occurs. When cannabinoids bind to the receptors in our muscles, they induce a relaxant effect, helping to alleviate muscle tension and spasms contributing to pain. This mechanism renders cannabis particularly effective for managing period pains, as the uterus contracts during the normal physiological process of shedding its lining; however, in endometriosis, contractions may be stronger or more painful due to a variety of reasons. Receptors are also found in the central nervous system, and their activation when cannabinoids bind can influence the perception of pain. Consequently, cannabis use can lead to a reduction in pain intensity, providing relief for individuals. Furthermore, immune cells possess cannabinoid receptors, and although CBD does not directly bind these receptors, they still interact and communicate with them, which can yield anti-inflammatory effects. Cannabinoids may also help regulate the immune response and reduce inflammation that way, further alleviating pain from endometriosis.

An American study found 26 of the 113 women surveyed used cannabis as a treatment for endometriosis, with the majority using it weekly.[4] They reported improvements in pain, cramping, muscle spasms, anxiety, sleep disturbances, libido, and irritability — highlighting the various ways cannabis can be effective in the symptom profile of endo. Cannabis also has anti-sickness properties, making it useful for nausea and vomiting. In New Zealand, a study on 213 women found 80% of them were illicit cannabis users, and 61% reported nausea or vomiting was improved from cannabis use.[5] Nevertheless, a review of the available literature in 2021 on the effect of cannabis-based products on the female reproductive system and endometriosis found that although the effects of animal studies show benefits, it's hard to derive the impact of this in humans.[6] The existing research on humans was predominantly conducted through surveys. This type of study can show evidence of patterns and trends; it can highlight areas that warrant further research, allowing for interest and funding for studies, yet despite these benefits, they're considered a weak study design and not prescribed as credible evidence due to possible bias. Owing to a lack of clear evidence on the benefits, National Guidance cannot recommend cannabis-based products for endometriosis, as they cannot recommend something without substantial credible data. This endorses the need for more research as the data that exists is encouraging, especially as the current treatment options for endo affect fertility or have undesirable side effects, preventing long-term use. There is a considerable need for treatments without these factors, and cannabis might provide that for some people. Until more research is undertaken to discern the advantages and risks of cannabis for endo, it's hard to know if the benefits outweigh the cons, which is essential before a drug can be recommended to the public.

While it shows strengths as a treatment, cannabis can produce a high, which may not be suitable for everyone, and that factor alone will put many off entirely. In regions where cannabis is legal, selecting high-quality products from reputable companies is crucial. They should be lab-tested and organic to ensure safety and minimise potential harm. Please note that cannabis is not without risk; psychosis, schizophrenia, and mood disturbances are concerns, particularly with long-term use. This is likely due to THC, and although the danger is not clear, it's generally considered the higher the THC content in a product, the greater the risk. It's also worth bearing in mind the risk of psychosis varies depending on how cannabis is used. For instance, when cannabis is applied to the skin through balms or topical products, there is no associated risk of psychosis because THC cannot enter the bloodstream in significant quantities. In contrast, smoking, vaping, or ingestion has a higher associated risk. Furthermore, how cannabis is used can also affect the results; inhalation may be the best for reducing pain (particularly pelvic pain), whilst oral forms such as gummies could be a superior method for improving mood and gastrointestinal symptoms.[7] This may be due to the rapid ability for inhaled cannabis to take effect, enhancing its pain-reducing effects.

If you use cannabis as a self-management strategy but buy it illegally, reconsider getting a legal prescription instead. Illegally sold weed does not need to be tested and approved, so the quality, ingredients, and strength are unknown, making it the most dangerous form to use. The changing landscape of cannabis and the emergence of CBD products provide new potential avenues for managing endometriosis and its symptoms. Still, everyone's response to treatments may vary, and more research is necessary to solidify their role in medical care. If you are interested in trying any of these, book a consultation with a medical cannabis clinic to learn more.

62

How to Deal with the Day-to-Day

Now that we've outlined various treatment methods and tools you can use to manage endometriosis, I hope you feel more equipped, knowing what's out there and what you can incorporate into your life. It's important not to wait for symptoms to worsen before seeking help or creating a plan of action. It's paramount to treat what you can as soon as you can. Endometriosis can be a progressive disease, so the earlier you take action, the better. Whether you've had surgical treatment or not, creating goals around the four pillars of health: diet, movement, sleep, and wellbeing — can make a significant difference in how you feel. These pillars don't require you to spend additional money to make a positive impact; they are accessible to all. While some treatments might come with a cost, you can integrate them when they are needed and attainable. Depending on your circumstances and the assistance you require, the NHS offers valuable resources like physiotherapy, pain management, and psychological therapies. These services can significantly enhance your quality of life if you are dealing with chronic pain or mental health challenges. Nevertheless, self-management is still key, as it's unrealistic to expect doctors to provide personalised advice and support for every aspect of this disease. This is partly due to the complexity of endometriosis, so everyone will have unique needs and different answers on how to resolve them effectively, but also because that would be very expensive, so it's impracticable for most people. If you continue to struggle, medications are also available to help relieve your symptoms. It's crucial to take charge of your health and find ways to improve your life despite the disease, especially if you are unable to access these services or if they are not specifically what you need.

Even if you're in a better place physically, there can still be an imprint that endometriosis leaves on you: fears of infertility, scars on your body, relationship issues, trauma, or simply feeling apprehensive that your endo will worsen or come back. As emotional and psychological impacts can linger, no matter where you are on your journey or which party you are in, build long and short-term strategies to attain the progress you are after. Start by setting manageable goals so you don't overwhelm yourself by trying to overhaul your life all at once (unless that works best for you). Typically, small, consistent steps toward change are more sustainable. For those in a bad spot or feeling lost, please know each step you take towards improving your life will help. It may feel like nothing is changing, but over time, even the minor improvements will add up, and there will be a day in a couple of months or even a year when you will look back at how far you have come and realise all those changes you made helped in some way or another. Recognise all your improvements and celebrate each victory no matter how small, to remind yourself that you do have control over your life and this disease cannot rob you of who you are. Endometriosis has the ability to knock you down, but it also shapes you into the person you are meant to be. Have hope that you can regain the life you want.

Living with endometriosis can be a daily challenge, but methods are out there which can help ease discomfort. A hot water bottle or a warm salt bath can be a delicious way to alleviate muscle pain and provide comfort when a flare-up strikes. Pairing this with a cup of warming tea, like chamomile or ginger, can further relax your body. Please be aware chronic use of hot water bottles on your skin can cause burn marks or irritation, so always wrap a hot water bottle in a cloth or cover and monitor your skin for changes.

Painful Sex

If you are struggling with painful sex, or maybe fear avoidance has started to creep in and affect your intimacy, it's essential to open up and talk about it to someone you trust — whether your partner, a friend, family member, or therapist. Honest and open conversation can help shed light on why fear is taking root, help clarify what you find painful, and allow you to understand the pain in a different way. It's natural not to want to engage in an activity that will hurt you or intensify existing pain. It's how humans are designed and it's great we have those mechanisms, but fear can worsen pain because your body is on high alert — which heightens the sensation. Pain is not just a physical experience; it's complex and influenced by cues from memory and emotion. Due to the nature of sex, the emotional weight of painful intercourse can be more significant than other types of pain, like burning yourself on a kettle where emotional ties are lower. These emotions lend to the way we view sex later when the pain has subsided. So you see, we are not only dealing with the physical component of painful sex but also the way it makes us feel to a higher degree. To effectively deal with pain, we need to identify why it exists and why we fear it. The 'Explaining Pain' concept of therapeutic intervention teaches us that pain is influenced by psychological, social, or environmental factors.[1] Addressing and working through these to understand how they are influencing your emotions or feelings towards painful sex can provide insight into how to manage and improve them. Examples to reflect on might include the events of a particularly awful experience, your partner's reaction to your pain and how that made you feel, pressures around the role of female sexuality, the mourning of the sex life you once had, or perhaps the disappointment of how sex is compared to how you envisioned it would be. Once you have pinpointed what other factors could be influencing your relationship with sex and addressed them by working through them, it may reduce your physical pain and even increase your desire. This is not to say the pain is all in your head, but it's vital to untangle this aspect for your overall healing.

Thereafter, you can move on to the physical aspect, where it's essential to decipher what exactly causes you pain. Understanding your body and identifying your specific pain triggers can help you find suitable positions that work for you so that you re-engage with sex whilst being mindful of your boundaries. Knowing your limits can be extremely empowering, allowing you to enjoy sex without crossing your pain thresholds. You might want to explore products like Ohnut®, a wearable ring placed on the end of the penis that helps control the depth of penetration, giving you more control to prevent pain and discomfort. If you struggle with all forms of penetration or if you have conditions like vulvodynia, vaginismus, or vestibulodynia, speak to a doctor about a referral to a specialist to see if they can help. Treatments might include physical therapy, medication, or counselling. Also, be mindful that many hormonal treatments recommended for endo, like the pill or GnRH agonist, can decrease sex drive or cause vaginal dryness — neither of which make for a good sex life and can also exacerbate painful intercourse. If you are affected by this, you could consider natural herbal remedies like ashwagandha or maca, which are regarded as aphrodisiacs, so they can support libido and increase your desire, but ensure you still use sufficient lubrication to ease discomfort. When choosing a lubricant, choose one that is paraben, glycine, petroleum, and fragrance-free, as well as pH-balanced and organic, where possible. If you prefer natural options, olive or coconut oil can be used, but ensure the olive oil is virgin (the irony didn't miss me) and the coconut oil is food-grade. If you use condoms for protection, be aware that natural oils can disintegrate the latex, making them ineffective at protection against pregnancy or sexually transmitted infections.

Finally, remember that intimacy isn't only about penetrative sex — kissing, cuddling, and other forms of closeness can be just as satisfying. What's more, sometimes it's normal not to want sex, and you shouldn't feel guilty about that. We all have patterns and cycles of sexual desire, and numerous factors can impact this. Our libido is individual, and we will all go through periods of high and low desire throughout life. Endometriosis can have compounding factors like pain, fatigue, and even embarrassment of our bodies when we are swollen and have scars, but these are all normal parts of the life experience which many people face in their own way. Intimacy can come in many ways, so try not to make sex the end goal or the elephant in the room if it's causing you distress. Try to communicate any issues you are dealing with to your partner instead of blocking them out, as opening out the discussion will provide them with the knowledge on how to support you, ensuring they too are not isolated — you never know, just by talking about it may improve how you are feeling. Whether you are single or in a committed relationship, always remember you deserve intimacy and to feel sexy and adored. Do not let yourself nor your partner get in the way of that.

Stress Management

Stress is a normal part of life and an emotion we cannot avoid, but maintaining healthy stress levels is crucial, even more so when you have endometriosis. We've all heard high stress levels aren't good for us, and earlier, we detailed how chronic stress causes inflammation. One way it does this is through increased cortisol and adrenaline levels. When these hormones remain elevated, it can be problematic. Prolonged stress can also release pro-inflammatory cytokines, disrupt the immune system, and even affect the gut microbiome — all of which can potentially trigger flare-ups, which we want to minimise. Managing stress is, therefore, vital. Luckily, there are various ways to do this, from exercise to supplements. Cortisol-lowering practices such as yoga, meditation, or getting enough sleep can reduce stress and inflammation. While engaging in hobbies like painting, sculpting, writing, hiking, or even watching feel-good movies can also help combat stress. Eating a low-inflammatory diet and taking care of your gut is also essential to include among your other stress-reducing strategies to keep the flare-ups at bay.

* * *

Managing endometriosis requires a holistic approach, ensuring your day-to-day life doesn't exacerbate your disease. You can achieve this by addressing your emotional health, managing stress, understanding your pain, and devising ways to improve symptoms. Most importantly, remember that you deserve to feel good in your body and to experience joy and intimacy.

63

Toxins to Avoid

A toxin is a term used to describe harmful substances that can have an adverse effect on living organisms, including humans, animals, and the environment. They come from a range of sources and cause a variety of health issues depending on the type and level of exposure. Toxins can be natural, produced by plants or animals yet are poisonous to humans, or synthetic toxins are man-made, often resulting from industrial processes. There has been substantial headway in the understanding of toxins and their detrimental effects on human health. One notable case highlighting their potential danger is Johnson and Johnson's baby powder lawsuit, which resulted in a $8.9 billion settlement after it was revealed the product contained asbestos, a known carcinogen, leading to the development of cancer in the plaintiffs. In the EU, strict regulations require all product ingredients to be listed in descending order of their quantity. This enables consumers to make informed choices if they don't wish to use certain ingredients. The EU also has an extensive list of banned chemicals due to their potential health concerns, particularly in cosmetic products. In contrast, the U.S. Food and Drug Administration (FDA) does not mandate the same level of regulation, allowing many chemicals banned in Europe to remain on the market. This deviation in standards is evident not only in cosmetic and personal care products but also in food safety, environmental standards, and pesticide and herbicide use. This is important to be aware of;

do not assume if a product is on the shelves, it's safe to use. Considering the vast rise in people who seem to be struggling with endometriosis compared to generations before, one question to ask is whether all the chemicals and products we use now and, therefore, the toxins we are exposed to are a driving factor behind this growth. If the toxins we outline inspire you to reduce your exposure due to the prospective health risks, apps like 'Think Dirty®' are a great resource to help you make purchasing decisions through easy-to-understand toxin ratings on household, personal care, and beauty products.

BPA

BPA is a common synthetic chemical due to its desirable characteristic of producing a hard and clear plastic. It's popularly used in food packaging and containers, such as reusable water bottles. However, BPA has been subject to potential health concerns, especially as research emerged that BPA can leach into food and beverages, exposing humans to it. BPA is considered an endocrine disruptor, a name for chemicals that can interfere with the endocrine system, which is in charge of creating and releasing hormones. These chemicals can block hormone receptors, prohibiting the ability of hormones to carry out their intended duties. They can also mimic hormones, leading to improper signalling in the body. If hormone production is altered or their release into the blood is prevented, hormones cannot travel to the areas of the body they are required, which can have various knock-on effects on how the body functions. Due to the vast role of hormones in regulating many biological processes in the body, endocrine disruptors can cause imbalances that lead to reproductive, developmental, neurological, and immune effects in humans. They also serve as a possible risk factor for developing endometriosis.[1]

BPA specifically, mimics oestrogen, allowing it to bind to the body's receptors, disrupting processes related to oestrogen regulation.[2] BPA can, therefore, lead to hormone imbalances and is associated with health issues

— primarily reproductive problems, developmental effects, or breast and prostate cancer.[3] As of 2024, France is the only country to ban the chemical entirely, while in the UK, EU, and U.S., BPA is still legal, with restricted use in manufacturing products intended for infants and young children. Whilst this is great for protecting children, adults should also avoid BPA due to posed health risks, especially those with hormone-dependent conditions. Fortunately, marketing makes this much easier, with many companies highlighting their products are BPA-free. If you are looking to buy new food packaging, such as food storage containers or a coffee cup, always ensure the product is BPA-free. If existing products in your house are not BPA-free, you may want to consider replacing them to reduce exposure.

Dioxin

As detailed in Part 1, dioxin plays a possible role in the pathogenesis of endometriosis. They are a group of highly toxic environmental pollutants formed primarily as byproducts of certain industrial processes such as pesticide and herbicide production. Once dioxins are formed, they take a long time to break down, so can accumulate in the environment and food chain, where they persist for years or even decades. Classed as endocrine disruptors, they are associated with adverse effects on the reproductive and immune systems, causing inflammation, oxidative stress, and DNA damage[4] — promoting the argument this chemical is one to avoid. In 2001, international agreements were established to develop goals and regulations to reduce dioxin production due to their adverse effects on human health and the environment. Despite a significant reduction achieved, they still pose a significant health risk due to their long-lasting presence in the environment, making them harder to avoid. Dioxins can accumulate in fat, so consuming fatty animal meats is considered one of the primary routes for human exposure.[5] If you eat meat, try choosing leaner cuts to limit animal fat consumption. Smaller fish should have less dioxin accumulated in their body, so good seafood options include sardines, clams, and scallops. You can also incorporate more fruits, vegetables, grains, and non-animal sources of protein, such as beans or tofu, to reduce your exposure. Unfortunately, dioxins have been found in tampons and sanitary towels as a by-product of chlorine-bleaching, a process intended to clean the fibres of impurities. Due to the health risks, many manufacturers have switched to alternative methods to prevent dioxin production or instead produce them in trace amounts, which apparently pose no health risks to us. You can research if your favourite tampon brand is dioxin-free or look at their packaging. Whilst we should try to reduce our exposure, it's probably not required to boycott tampons, particularly if they are your favourite form of menstrual product. Exposure to dioxin via tampons is approximately 13,000-240,000 times less than the amount found in food sources.[6] If you still don't want to take the risk, alternative methods such as menstrual cups or reusable pads can be used. Reusable fabric pads, the kind you put in the washing machine once you've used them, are especially great for days when you are unsure if you will bleed, namely the days at the beginning or end of your period or if you spot regularly. Not only does this prevent the use of sanitary products that were never needed in the end, but it also limits toxins, saves you money, and reduces the environmental footprint of sanitary products going to landfill sites.

Polybrominated Diphenyl Ethers (PBDEs)

PBDEs are a class of synthetic flame-retardant chemicals used in an array of products, from electrical equipment to furniture, to prevent them from catching fire easily. PBDEs are endocrine disruptors tied to reproductive, neurological, developmental, and immune system issues, with a notable relationship for causing thyroid disruption or kidney and liver damage. Research has also linked PBDEs to an increased risk of endometriosis, suggesting another why reason the disease can run in families.[7] Genetics are not always the cause of recurring health patterns. An alternative contributing factor is that children will have many of the same environmental exposures as their parents, making adverse effects more likely to accumulate in groups of people. Due to health concerns, many countries banned these chemicals or implemented phase-outs to reduce the amount found in the environment. However, PBDEs are like dioxins wherein they leach out of products, enter the environment, and then accumulate as they break down slowly — meaning they can be found in our air, water, soil, food, and animal feed years later. Despite being banned for almost a decade, a study by Indiana University in the U.S. found PBDEs were still passing through the umbilical cord to foetuses and suggested newborn babies had higher circulating levels of the PBDEs than their mothers.[8] Due to their persistence in the environment, humans are primarily exposed to PBDEs through contaminated food, i.e., fish and meat products.[9] They accumulate in fat tissue, so avoiding high consumption of fatty meat and large fatty fish is preferable. It's also important to look at your home environment as products manufactured before the ban may still contain PBDEs, so they are a risk factor for exposure. Consider your mattress, sofa, and outer plastic casings on old electronics, and if they were purchased prior to 2004, research into whether they contain PBDEs. If you cannot find an answer, it may be worthwhile purchasing PBDE-free replacements. You lay on your mattress every night, so the exposure risk could be high, and certainly not something you want in your house, possibly making you sick.

Triclocarban & Triclosan

Triclosan & triclocarban are man-made chemicals designed to act as antibacterial and antifungal agents when added to consumer products such as soaps, toothpaste, body washes, clothing, furniture, toys, and kitchen appliances. The intention was to prevent bacterial and fungal growth, reducing the risk of infections spreading to the consumer while maintaining product freshness and prolonging shelf life. Unfortunately, there are several health concerns surrounding the chemicals, including their potential to act as endocrine disruptors, linking them to hormonal imbalances with potential implications for reproduction and development.[10] Triclosan and triclocarban are also persistent toxins that take a long time to break down, so their accumulation in the environment can pose a risk to humans and the ecosystem.

In relation to endometriosis, a study found women with the disease had significantly higher triclosan levels in their blood compared to women without the condition[11] and that the level of exposure correlated with the severity of the disease. This means that patients with stage 4 endometriosis had higher levels in comparison to those with stage 2 or 3. This finding raises significant concerns and underscores the importance of avoiding exposure to such chemicals. As antibacterial agents, their presence in the human body is a concern as our microbiome influences our health. Their ability to disrupt the microbiome may contribute to issues with allergies or thyroid function.[12] Evidence also suggests widespread exposure to triclosan and triclocarban contributes to the development of antibiotic-resistant bacteria, making it harder for doctors to treat bacterial infections.[13] Due to these concerns, many countries banned or reduced the use of these chemicals. In 2014, the United States banned triclosan & triclocarban (alongside several other chemicals with similar anti-microbial properties) from over-the-counter consumer antiseptic wash products, including hand soaps and body washes. Similarly, the EU imposed a partial ban — triclocarban is only allowed in cosmetic products up to 0.2%, whilst toothpaste will have to bear the warning "Not to be used for children under 6 years of age".[13] To avoid the risks associated, it may be best to ensure your hygiene products don't contain these chemicals as they are not entirely banned. Certain companies have removed these chemicals from their products to meet consumer demands, whilst other environmentally friendly companies have never used them for these reasons. Please always do your research to find the latest information.

Parabens

Parabens are preservatives found in many beauty and hygiene products, preventing the growth of bacteria, mould, and yeast. Parabens have received much attention and scrutiny in the 2020's, leading to huge waves in marketing and accessibility to paraben-free beauty products. The problem is that parabens are considered endocrine disruptors, and research shows that they mimic oestrogen, so exert oestrogenic effects on the body.[14] This is increasingly problematic with prolonged exposure to these chemicals. As they are in an abundance of beauty and personal care products (as well as processed foods and pharmaceuticals), women have a particularly high risk of exposure without knowing it. This can lead to hormonal imbalances, increasing the risk of hormone-dependent cancer such as breast cancer.[15] Due to paraben's oestrogenic effects, there are concerns regarding their ability to interfere with reproductive health, possibly having a role in infertility.[16] The current literature has contrasting results on whether this is true, but it may depend on the specific paraben and dose exposed to. In my opinion, the existing research provides a clear incentive to avoid these chemicals where possible until we get more answers. The research community has also considered the impact of paraben exposure and endometriosis. One study found women who used more personal care products were indeed exposed to a greater number of parabens, as reflected in their urine samples. The study also found that higher exposure to certain chemicals was associated with a higher risk of endometriosis.[17] Understanding risks associated with parabens is valuable as they are currently legal and widely used, although regulatory agencies in the U.S., EU, and UK have set concentration limits on products. You can reduce your exposure by sourcing paraben-free products where possible. If this is not clearly advertised on the product, you can check the label for ingredients such as methylparaben, propylparaben, butylparaben, and ethylparaben. You can write these down on your phone so you have them whenever you need.

Phthalates

Phthalates are chemicals used in hundreds of products due to their wide variety of uses. They are added to plastics like food wrap or vinyl flooring to make them more flexible and durable, but they are also found in health and personal care products like perfumes, cosmetics, and moisturisers. Concerns have been raised over their safety due to their ability to leach, posing human health risks. Phthalates are also endocrine disruptors, and exposure is associated with hormonal imbalances through reducing testosterone levels in men and women.[18] Testosterone is a key hormone for everyone throughout their lifespan. Reduced levels can cause alterations in the development and function of the reproductive system and our overall health. Science seems to have a better understanding of the effects of phthalates on men than on women. Yet considering women's exposure to phthalates in both variety and quantity is typically far greater due to the healthcare products used, this is concerning. Evidence suggests phthalates can negatively impact ovarian function, impair the growth of follicles, and decrease hormone production by ovarian cells.[19] There's even research linking phthalates exposure to endometriosis, with several papers indicating phthalates can cause inflammation and oxidative stress — both of which are required for the pathogenesis of endometriosis.[20] Phthalates directly caused the proliferation of endometriosis cells in vitro, meaning in a petri dish or test tube.[21] While patients with stage 3 or 4 endometriosis had significantly high levels of detectable phytates (particularly DEHP and MEHP) in their blood and peritoneal fluid samples.[22] Due to health concerns regarding exposure, certain phthalates are restricted or banned, particularly in children's toys and cosmetics in the EU and UK. However, many others are still legal in a multitude of products, especially in industrial and manufacturing processes, albeit the restrictions vary between countries. To understand your personal exposure, check whether the products you frequently use contain phthalates, and it may be worthwhile gradually transitioning all your beauty and healthcare products to ones that are phthalate-free. You can check the listed ingredients — often written as acronyms like DEP, DBP, and DEHP. To further prevent exposure, try not to microwave food in plastic containers and wash your hands frequently to remove any phthalates that have leached onto your skin.

64

Medical Research

Research into understanding and potentially curing endometriosis is ongoing, offering hope of future treatments and a promising outlook for the disease in the years to come. Here are some exciting projects you may want to know more about.

NPSR1 Gene Research

Critical research efforts are being led by institutions such as The University of Oxford, Baylor College of Medicine, University of Wisconsin-Madison, and Bayer AG to deepen our understanding of genetic factors behind endometriosis. In 2021, a significant breakthrough was made when these researchers identified a rare variant of a gene called NPSR1, which increases the risk of developing stage 3 or 4 endometriosis.[1] Most women carrying this rare variant exhibited more aggressive forms of the disease. In seeking a form of non-hormonal and non-invasive treatment (unlike those that exist today), scientists discovered this gene could be used as a potential drug target, so they are exploring drug formulations that inhibit this gene whilst understanding its possible impact. Initial experiments conducted on mice, where the NPRS1 gene was inhibited, showed reduced inflammation and abdominal pain, signalling this discovery has the potential for future non-hormonal treatment options. While these results are promising, animal studies only mimic certain aspects of human disease. Without being able to cover the full spectrum of how endometriosis works in humans, more research is needed to determine whether this discovery could lead to innovative treatments for us, particularly in those with stage 3 or 4 with this gene.

AMY109: A New Antibody Treatment

In early 2022, a Japanese drug manufacturer called Chugai Pharmaceutical Company announced a new antibody treatment, unofficially named AMY109, which successfully shrunk endometriosis lesions in primates.[2] AMY109 works by binding and blocking Interleukin-8 (IL-8), a signalling molecule with a major role in inflammation,[3] commonly upregulated in those with endometriosis and associated with disease progression.[2] Therefore, preventing this molecule from inducing inflammation should positively impact the disease. In the study, AMY109 was injected into the subcutaneous tissue of primates with endometriosis once a month. The treatment resulted in a lower inflammatory immune response with reduced fibrosis, adhesions, and lesion size. This marks a significant upgrade to hormonal therapies that exist today, which can only slow or stop the growth of lesions rather than reverse it. Additionally, AMY109 comes without the adverse side effects typically associated with hormonal therapies, such as weight gain and hot flushes. This research has reached the next stage and is being investigated in humans in the UK. With more research, scientists will determine if AMY109 can be utilised as a disease-modifying therapy for endometriosis.

Dichloroacetate (DCA)

Endo is a complex condition, and its aetiology or the causes of its development can be multifactorial, so multiple aspects of the disease need to be studied to understand various forms of treatment. One characteristic is that it shares similar behaviours to cancer. In this instance, we are referring to an altered cellular metabolism. Usually, cells generate energy in the mitochondria through oxidative phosphorylation, a highly efficient method for the cell. Cancer cells, however, adopt a less efficient but rapid energy production method called aerobic glycolysis, producing energy without oxygen and generating lactate as a byproduct. This metabolic switch in how cancer cells produce energy supports their rapid growth. Research indicates endometriosis cells also alter their energy production, likewise moving to aerobic glycolysis and producing lactate. Lactate is considered a key factor for driving cell invasion, angiogenesis, and immune suppression — all vital to the growth of tumours.[4] Endometriosis switching its energy production in a similar way is thought to contribute to the survival and growth of lesions. Understanding the parallels to cancer is important, as one of the challenges with endometriosis is that even with surgery, disease recurrence is high. Therefore, drawing insights from cancer research helps develop strategies to treat endo. A study discovered that using a substance called Dichloroacetate (DCA) could correct the altered energy production in endometriosis cells.[5] DCA is already licensed to treat various cancers, so its safety for humans is established. This is great as it can help fast-track studies like this. Laboratory experiments demonstrated treatment reduced lactate production in endometriosis cells. Subsequently, DCA was given to mice with endometriosis, resulting in diseased tissue reducing in size. DCA prevents an enzyme called pyruvate dehydrogenase kinase from working, causing cells to produce less lactate. This means DCA might be capable of stopping the growth of cells and the production of new blood vessels, which in turn reduces tumour growth. It may also influence immune cells to promote tissue repair, so it has the potential to benefit various aspects of endometriosis. The promising results from the prospective use of DCA have led to a handful of EPiC studies untaken by The University of Edinburgh, Aberdeen, and Birmingham to investigate the use of this drug in patients with endometriosis. The EPiC2 study, a randomised, double-blind, placebo-controlled feasibility trial, represents the highest level of research, so the results which are expected in 2026 will provide critical evidence into whether DCA is a viable treatment option — maybe bringing us closer to a new therapeutic approach.

Salivary & Blood MicroRNA Testing

MicroRNAs are a family of small molecules crucial for regulating protein synthesis within cells. They are involved in controlling gene expression and play a role in various biological processes, including disease mechanisms. Notably, specific microRNA has emerged as potential biomarkers for diagnosing diseases, including endometriosis. MicroRNAs can be detected in saliva and blood, prompting scientific exploration into whether endo can be diagnosed using a non-invasive blood or mouth swab test. Despite numerous studies previously investigating endometriosis blood markers, there was a lack of conclusive data, perpetuating the reliance on surgery for diagnosis. However, advancements in technology, specifically Artificial Intelligence (AI) and Machine Learning (ML), have revolutionised the analysis of microRNA, enabling the possibility of developing highly accurate blood tests which differentiate between people with and without endometriosis, serving as a replacement for diagnostic surgery.[6] AI modelling has also demonstrated promising results for future saliva-based testing by analysing saliva samples to identify endometriosis. One study identified 109 microRNAs exhibiting strong or consistent patterns with endo, indicating their potential to serve as disease biomarkers.[7] These advancements could revolutionise the diagnostic landscape, overcoming previous limitations in research and offering a more precise, non-invasive, and reliable diagnostic method. Nevertheless, several unresolved concerns necessitate further research, such as determining whether microRNA tests can accurately detect disease stages, identify changes across the menstrual cycle, and maintain accuracy across different ethnic groups and in patients undergoing hormone treatments. Despite these challenges, ongoing research has the potential to overcome these hurdles and transform the way endometriosis is managed in clinical practice, ultimately reducing the current statistics of patients waiting far too long for a diagnosis. Until this data is confirmed and approved, microRNA testing won't be widely accessible, although some countries may already offer this.

IMAGENDO®: AI-Powered Diagnostic Imaging

Another exciting application of AI in endometriosis research is in medical imaging. Currently, the first-line diagnostic procedure is to provide patients with an ultrasound scan. Yet endometriosis is often difficult to detect through all types of scans, requiring highly qualified and specialised radiographers to discern its pattern to diagnose. Even then, false negatives are possible as scans cannot rule out the condition. Consequently, diagnostic surgery is still often required for confirmation. IMAGENDO® is an AI system that seeks to enhance diagnostic accuracy by combining and analysing data from ultrasound and MRI tests to discern patterns of endometriosis that may be undetectable to the human eye.[8] By harnessing AI technology, IMAGENDO® seeks to enhance the precision of non-invasive diagnostics, detecting subtle or complex patterns in ultrasound and MRI scans. Such advancements hold the potential for more accurate, rapid, and non-invasive means of diagnosis, potentially sparing patients without the condition from having unnecessary diagnostic surgeries whilst streamlining healthcare resources and allocating treatment for those who truly genuinely need it.

DETECT: Imaging Angiogenesis in Endometriosis

Researchers at the University of Oxford are attempting to go beyond the detection of structural and anatomical changes seen using ultrasound and MRI by detecting functional changes in the DETECT study.[9] This is particularly important for superficial endometriosis, where lesions are often subtle and missed on standard imaging. As we have discussed, angiogenesis, the process of developing new blood vessels, is a vital process for growing lesions, especially in the early phases. The DETECT study seeks to visualise angiogenesis using SPECT-CT and a marker called ^{99m}Tc-maraciclatide. This marker has previously shown success in detecting inflammation and angiogenesis in other diseases, such as rheumatoid arthritis and various cancers and is now being applied to endometriosis too. New diagnostic approaches such as this, are needed to mitigate the current limitations in non-invasive diagnostics and to reduce the diagnostic delay seen across the globe.

65

(Not) The End

"In all things, it is better to have hope than to despair."
– Johann Wolfgang Von Goethe

As we conclude this journey, my greatest wish is that you have discovered something valuable within these pages — whether that's information you didn't have before or a deeper explanation for questions you've often wondered about. From breaking down what research has discovered to date to strategising ways to manage your health, we have covered a lot of ground so that you have the understanding you are entitled to. Endo Warriors are a collective of resilient, powerful people, and I believe each of you deserves to find greater peace, trust, and confidence in your body as well as hope in your future.

Endometriosis affects us all differently, so each journey is unique. Even so, a common theme is the ability of the disease to make us feel like we have hit the brakes on our lives. It might require us to slow down at work, withdraw from our social lives, or even put kinks in our plans for parenthood. The various sacrifices can touch every corner of our lives. Therefore, time and patience are often required to establish your new 'normal' so that you can work through these issues. You are not alone in your fears or worries, and the endometriosis community is always here to offer support where possible. No matter your situation and the challenges you need to navigate, I hope you have the insight and guidance you need to help you move forward and live with the disease. Science is steadily moving towards better answers, so with time and the right tools, we should all see improvements.

The first step is *believing* you can transform your life. Faith in your ability to heal and optimism about your future are invaluable assets on this journey. You might have challenging days, months, or moments that get you down because they remind you that you have a disease, but how you move through these is up to you. This is not to say you are not allowed to get upset or face the reality of your condition at times. It's natural to feel low or angry at the world; acknowledging these emotions is also part of the process. On tougher days, please do what you need to get through it, whether that's taking a rest to recuperate or having a cry. But try to end each day with the commitment that when you wake up in the morning, you will get up and try again to work on your future health. No matter how small that act may be, and *even* if you still wake up feeling groggy and sore. The foundation of true change is choosing to believe in your body's capacity to heal; even when progress seems incremental, as each day is an opportunity. Embrace a holistic approach to your health, which emphasises there are many factors can enhance your wellbeing. We shouldn't just focus on our physical health; we also need to include the mental, emotional, spiritual, and social aspects. Incorporating this mentality endorses there are many ways we can work on our healing so knowing this makes it easier to make each day count.

Parts of this book may have felt heavy because it needed to reflect how this disease can touch numerous aspects of people's lives. But within that reality, I hope it also brought positivity and the realisation there is always something that can be done. With hindsight, I can look back over the years and see all the ways this disease affected my life, and what it stole from me, but I can also recognise each of the steps I took, the education I garnered, and the tools I used to reclaim my life. I am grateful for each part that got me to where I am today. You deserve a life that you enjoy. Endometriosis does not define you, nor should it have the power to take away what you love about life. There is a whole lot more life to live, so getting in control of your endo, building your toolkit, and believing that change is possible is essential.

Though a cure doesn't currently exist, it's possible to reach a state of remission, where symptoms are minimised or disappear. This might occur after surgery, pregnancy or menopause — however, this isn't always the case, or flare-ups may still appear nonetheless. Another way to work towards remission is by employing a scientific experience on yourself to determine the symptoms you would like to address, understand what aggravates them, what provides relief and how to resolve them. The tools outlined in this book can help on this journey. Don't forget to incorporate the four pillars of health – diet, movement, sleep and well-being when developing your strategies for a holistic approach. Consider whether additional therapies are required or worth exploring to target specific symptoms. Another facet of your experiment should be lowering inflammation. Not only is chronic inflammation detrimental to your overall health, but it also encourages endometriosis to progress. Several methods have been included within the book to accomplish this. Reducing inflammation can lead to more energy and less pain — two very important ingredients to getting your life back.

When setting your goals, decipher what resonates and appeals to you, and remember to see the process as rewarding and fun. Embrace the mindset that each step has the potential to bring you closer to a better day in the future to look forward to. For example, if you integrate a supplement into your routine, feel optimistic about this change and imagine how it will help you. This is because placebo studies show that what you consciously believe in impacts your healing. Having high expectations of recovery is more likely to yield positive results. If you know you can improve how you feel, that faith will drive positive action; if not, that belief can also impact your experience. This also means believing in the powerful connection between the mind, body, and spirit. These aspects are interconnected, as each affects the others in profound ways. When you nurture your mental wellness, it positively impacts your physical health and vice versa. Your spirit, representing your beliefs, values, and emotions, is also integral to your physical and mental health. We can harmonise these three aspects by choosing tools we believe will help our wellbeing.

This is your path; you have the freedom to choose how you want to live it. Although we may need to make some adjustments along the way, you *can* accomplish your goals. Ideally, each person should develop their toolkit so that when they experience a flare, they know how to manage it, feel reassured it will pass, and when it does, they can get back to living their life with minimal symptoms. Your toolkit is there to help you live the life you want.

On your journey, celebrate each win you get. Be patient, stay positive, and acknowledge that the extra effort you have to make sometimes is inspiring. I wish you all the strength, luck, and unwavering perseverance as you move forward on your journey to reclaim your life.

You should never feel in the dark about your disease, so if this book took some of the darkness away, then it served its purpose.

With love,
    Alice

References

PART 1

The Beginning

[1] - UK Clinical Research Collaboration 2023. UK Health Research Analysis 2022. https://hrcsonline.net/wp-content/uploads/2024/04/UK_Health_Research_Analysis_Report_2022_web_v1-1-postpub.pdf.

2 - Public Health England. Survey reveals women experience severe reproductive health issues. GOV.UK. https://www.gov.uk/government/news/survey-reveals-women-experience-severe-reproductive-health-issues. Published June 26, 2018. Accessed 24th July 2024

3 - Women's health strategy for England. GOV.UK. https://www.gov.uk/government/publications/womens-health-strategy-for-england/womens-health-strategy-for-england. Published August 23, 2022. Accessed 24th July 2024

4 - Endometriosis UK. "Dismissed, Ignored and Belittled": The Long Road to Endometriosis Diagnosis in the UK.; 2024. https://www.endometriosis-uk.org/sites/default/files/2024-03/Endometriosis%20UK%20diagnosis%20survey%202023%20report%20March.pdf.

Introduction

1 - Eskenazi B, Warner ML. EPIDEMIOLOGY OF ENDOMETRIOSIS. Obstetrics and Gynecology Clinics of North America. 1997;24(2):235-258. doi:10.1016/s0889-8545(05)70302-8

2 - Sung H, Ferlay J, Siegel RL, et al. Global Cancer Statistics 2020: GLOBOCAN estimates of incidence and mortality worldwide for 36 cancers in 185 countries. *CA: A Cancer Journal for Clinicians.* 2021;71(3):209-249.

doi:10.3322/caac.21660

3 - Mahase E. Type 1 diabetes: Global prevalence is set to double by 2040, study estimates. *The BMJ*. September 2022:o2289. doi:10.1136/bmj.o2289

4. Guo J, Garratt A, Hill A. Worldwide rates of diagnosis and effective treatment for cystic fibrosis. *Journal of Cystic Fibrosis*. 2022;21(3). doi:https ://doi.org/10.1016/j.jcf.2022.01.009

5. Rei C, Williams T, Feloney M. Endometriosis in a man as a rare source of abdominal pain: A case Report and Review of the literature. *Case Reports in Obstetrics and Gynecology*. 2018;2018:1-6. doi:10.1155/2018/2083121

6 - Simoens S, Dunselman GAJ, Dirksen CD, et al. The burden of endometriosis: costs and quality of life of women with endometriosis and treated in referral centres. *Human Reproduction*. 2012;27(5):1292-1299. doi:10.1093/humrep/des073

7 - Sperschneider ML, Hengartner MP, Schwartz AK, et al. Does endometriosis affect professional life? A matched case-control study in Switzerland, Germany and Austria. *BMJ Open*. 2019;9(1):e019570. doi:10.1136/bmjopen-2017-019570

8 - Gunawardena S, Dior UP, Cheng C, Healey M. New Diagnosis of Endometriosis is Less Common in Women over Age Forty Presenting with Pelvic Pain. *Journal of Minimally Invasive Gynecology*. 2021;28(4):891-898.e1. doi:10.1016/j.jmig.2020.08.012

9 - Bougie O, Yap MaI, Sikora L, Flaxman T, Singh S. Influence of race/eth-nicity on prevalence and presentation of endometriosis: a systematic review and meta-analysis. *BJOG an International Journal of Obstetrics & Gynaecology*. 2019;126(9):1104-1115. doi:10.1111/1471-0528.15692

10 - Zhang L, Losin E a R, Ashar YK, Koban L, Wager TD. Gender biases in estimation of others' pain. *Journal of Pain*. 2021;22(9):1048-1059. doi:10.10 16/j.jpain.2021.03.001

11 - Hoffman KM, Trawalter S, Axt JR, Oliver MN. Racial bias in pain assessment and treatment recommendations, and false beliefs about biological differences between blacks and whites. *Proceedings of the National Academy of Sciences*. 2016;113(16):4296-4301. doi:10.1073/pn as.1516047113

12 - Mvondo MA, Ekenfack JD, Essono SM, et al. Soy intake since the prepubertal age may contribute to the pathogenesis of endometriosis in adulthood. *Journal of Medicinal Food*. 2019;22(6):631-638. doi:10.1089/jmf. 2018.0160

13 - Szczęsna D, Wieczorek K, Jurewicz J. An exposure to endocrine active persistent pollutants and endometriosis — a review of current epidemiological studies. *Environmental Science and Pollution Research*. 2022;30(6):13974-13993. doi:10.1007/s11356-022-24785-w

14 - Tang Y, Zhao M, Lin L, et al. Is body mass index associated with the incidence of endometriosis and the severity of dysmenorrhoea: a case–control study in China? *BMJ Open*. 2020;10(9):e037095. doi:10.1136/bmjopen-2020-037095

15 - Sharfman A. Childbearing for women born in different years, England and Wales - Office for National Statistics. https://www.ons.g ov.uk/peoplepopulationandcommunity/birthsdeathsandmarriages/conce ptionandfertilityrates/bulletins/childbearingforwomenbornindifferentye arsenglandandwales/2020. Published January 27, 2022

History of Endometriosis

1 - Knapp VJ. How old is endometriosis? Late 17th- and 18th-century European descriptions of the disease. *Fertil Steril*. 1999;72(1):10-14. doi:10.1016/s0015-0282(99)00196-x

2 - Shroen D. Disputatio inauguralis medica de ulceribus uteri. Jena: Krebs, 1690:6–17.

3 - Broughton W. Dissertatio medica inauguralis de ulcere uteri. Edin-burgh: Hamilton and Balfour, 1755:16–22.

4 - Hoctin P. Dissertatio medica inauguralis de inflammatione uteri. Lou-vain: Coster, 1779:1–16.

5 - Russel WW: Aberrant portions of the müllerian duct found in an ovary. Johns Hopkins Hospital Bull 1899;10:8-10.

6 - Rokitansky K. Uber uterusdrusen neubildung. *Ztchr Gesselsch Arzte Wein*. 1860;16:577.

7 - von Rokitansky KF. *Ueber uterusdrüsen-neubildung in uterus-und*

ovarial-sarcomen. Druck von Carl Ueberreuter; 1860. 6 p

8 - Sampson J.A. Metastatic or embolic endometriosis, due to the men-strual dis- semination of endometrial tissue into the venous circulation. *Am. J. Pathol.* 1927;3:93.

9 - Sampson J.A. Peritoneal endometriosis due to the menstrual dis-semination of endometrial tissue into the peritoneal cavity. *Am. J. Obstet. Gynecol.* 1927;14:422–469. doi: 10.1016/S0002-9378(15)30003-X

10 - Hippocrates. Hippocrates: Diseases of Women: Vol. XI. Harvard University Press. 1995

11 - Nezhat C, Nezhat F, Nezhat C. Endometriosis: ancient disease, ancient treatments. *Fertility and Sterility.* 2012;98(6):S1-S62. doi:10.10 16/j.fertnstert.2012.08.001

My story

1 - All Party Parliamentary Group appg onEndometriosis. Endometriosis in the UK: time for change: APPG on Endometriosis Inquiry Report 2020. Endometriosis-UK. https://www.endometriosis-uk.org/sites/defa ult/files/files/Endometriosis%20APPG%20Report%20Oct%202020.pdf. Published 2020. Accessed February 28, 2024.

What Is Endometriosis?

1 - Asante A, Taylor RN. Endometriosis: the role of neuroangiogenesis. *Annual Review of Physiology.* 2011;73(1):163-182. doi:10.1146/annurev-physiol-012110-142158

2 - Zondervan KT, Becker CM, Missmer SA. Endometriosis. *New England Journal of Medicine.* 2020;382(13):1244-1256. doi:10.1056/nejmra1810764

What is Inflammation?

1 - Ahn SH, Monsanto SP, Miller C, Singh SS, Thomas R, Tayade C. Pathophysiology and immune dysfunction in endometriosis. *BioMed Research International.* 2015;2015:1-12. doi:10.1155/2015/795976

2 - Taylor HS, Kotlyar AM, Flores VA. Endometriosis is a chronic sys-

temic disease: clinical challenges and novel innovations. *The Lancet.* 2021;397(10276):839-852. doi:10.1016/s0140-6736(21)00389-5

What Are Adhesions?

1 - El-Kader AIA, Gonied A, Mohamed ML, Mohamed S. Impact of Endometriosis-Related Adhesions on Quality of Life among Infertile Women. *PubMed.* 2019;13(1):72-76. doi:10.22074/ijfs.2019.5572

2 - Abd El-Kader AI, Gonied AS, Lotfy Mohamed M, Lotfy Mohamed S. Impact of Endometriosis-Related Adhesions on Quality of Life among Infertile Women. *Int J Fertil Steril.* 2019;13(1):72-76. doi:10.22074/ijfs.2019.5572

3 - Tabibian N, Swehli E, Boyd A, Umbreen A, Tabibian JH. Abdominal adhesions: A practical review of an often overlooked entity. *Annals of Medicine and Surgery.* 2017;15:9-13. doi:10.1016/j.amsu.2017.01.021

What Are the Types of Endometriosis?

1 - Horne A, Daniels J, Hummelshøj L, Cox E, Cooper K. Surgical removal of superficial peritoneal endometriosis for managing women with chronic pelvic pain: time for a rethink? *BJOG: An International Journal of Obstetrics and Gynaecology.* 2019;126(12):1414-1416. doi:10.1111/1471-0528.15894

2 - Hoyle AT, Puckett Y. Endometrioma. StatPearls - NCBI Bookshelf. https://www.ncbi.nlm.nih.gov/books/NBK559230/. Published June 5, 2023.

3 - Evangelinakis N, Grammatikakis I, Salamalekis G, et al. Prevalence of acute hemoperitoneum in patients with endometriotic ovarian cysts: a 7-year retrospective study. *Clin Exp Obstet Gynecol.* 2009;36(4):254-255.

4 - D'Alterio MN, D'Ancona G, Raslan MA, Tinelli A, Daniilidis A, Angioni S. Management challenges of deep infiltrating endometriosis. *DOAJ (DOAJ: Directory of Open Access Journals).* April 2021. doi:10.22074/ijfs.2020.134689

5 - Koninckx P, Ussia A, Adamyan LV, Wattiez A, Gomel V, Dc M. Pathogenesis of endometriosis: the genetic/epigenetic theory. *Fertility and Sterility.* 2019;111(2):327-340. doi:10.1016/j.fertnstert.2018.10.013

6 - Nisolle M, Donnez J. Peritoneal endometriosis, ovarian endometrio-

sis, and adenomyotic nodules of the rectovaginal septum are three different entities. *Fertility and Sterility.* 1997;68(4):585-596. doi:10.1016/s0015-0282(97)00191-x

7 - Benagiano G, Bianchi P, Guo S. Endometriosis in adolescent and young women. *Minerva Obstetrics and Gynecology.* 2021;73(5). doi:10.23736/s2724-606x.21.04764-x

8 - Gross and Histological Appearance of Endometriotic Lesions. AMI 2018 Meeting. https://meetingarchive.ami.org/2018/project/gross-and-h istological-appearance-of-endometriotic-lesions/. Published 2017.

What Causes Endometriosis?

1 – Sampson JA. Peritoneal endometriosis due to the menstrual dissemination of endometrial tissue into the peritoneal cavity. Am J Obstet Gynecol 1927; 14:422-69.

2 – Halme J, Hammond MG, Hulka JF, Raj SG, Talbert LM. Retrograde menstruation in healthy women and in patients with endometriosis. *Obstet Gynecol.* 1984;64(2):151-154.

3 – Liu DT, Hitchcock A. Endometriosis: its association with retrograde menstruation, dysmenorrhoea and tubal pathology. *Br J Obstet Gynaecol.* 1986;93(8):859-862. doi:10.1111/j.1471-0528.1986.tb07995.x

4 – Tal A, Tal R, Pluchino N, Taylor HS. Endometrial cells contribute to preexisting endometriosis lesions in a mouse model of retrograde menstruation . Biol Reprod. 2019;100(6):1453-1460. Doi:10.1093/biol re/ioz039

5 – Meyer R. Uber den staude der frage der adenomyosites adenomyoma in allgemeinen und adenomyometritis sarcomastosa. Zentralb Gynakol 1919; 36:745.

6 – Burney RO, Giudice L. Pathogenesis and pathophysiology of endometriosis. *Fertility and Sterility.* 2012;98:511–519

7 – Sourial S, Tempest N, Hapangama DK. Theories on the pathogenesis of endometriosis. *International Journal of Reproductive Medicine.* 2014;2014:1-9. doi:10.1155/2014/179515

8 - Andres MP, Arcoverde FVL, Souza CCC, Fernandes LFC, Abrão MS, Kho

RM. Extrapelvic Endometriosis: A Systematic Review. *Journal of Minimally Invasive Gynecology.* 2020;27(2):373-389. doi:10.1016/j.jmig.2019.10.004

9 – Halban J. Metastatic hysteroadenosis. *Wien iln Wochenschr.* 1924;37:1205–6.

10 – Laila F. Jerman, Alison J. Hey-Cunningham, The Role of the Lymphatic System in Endometriosis: A Comprehensive Review of the Literature, *Biology of Reproduction*, Volume 92, Issue 3, 1 March 2015, 64, 1–10, https://doi.org/10.1095/biolreprod.114.124313

11 - Wang Y, Nicholes K, Shih IM. The Origin and Pathogenesis of Endometriosis. *Annu Rev Pathol.* 2020;15:71-95. Doi:10.1146/annurev-pathmechdis-012419-032654

12 - Signorile PG, Viceconte R, Baldi A. New Insights in Pathogenesis of Endometriosis. Front Med (Lausanne). 2022 Apr 28;9:879015. Doi: 10.3389/fmed.2022.879015. PMID: 35572957; PMCID: PMC9095948.

13 - Smolarz B, Szyłło K, Romanowicz H. Endometriosis: Epidemiology, Classification, Pathogenesis, Treatment and Genetics (Review of Literature). *Int J Mol Sci.* 2021;22(19):10554. Published 2021 Sep 29. doi:10.3390/ijms221910554

14 - Hansen KA, Eyster KM. Genetics and Genomics of Endometriosis. *Clinical Obstetrics and Gynecology.* 2010;53(2):403-412. doi:10.1097/grf.obo 13e3181db7ca1

15 - Di W, Guo S. The search for genetic variants predisposing women to endometriosis. *Current Opinion in Obstetrics & Gynecology.* 2007;19(4):395-401. doi:10.1097/gco.0b013e328235a5b4

16 - Dyson MT, Bulun SE. Cutting SRC-1 down to size in endometriosis. *Nature Medicine.* 2012;18(7):1016-1018. doi:10.1038/nm.2855

17 - Bulun SE, Fang Z, Imir G, et al. Aromatase and endometriosis. *Semin Reprod Med.* 2004;22(1):45-50. doi:10.1055/s-2004-823026

18 - Zhang P, Wang G. Progesterone resistance in endometriosis: current evidence and putative mechanisms. *International Journal of Molecular Sciences.* 2023;24(8):6992. doi:10.3390/ijms24086992

19 - McGlade EA, Miyamoto A, Winuthayanon W. Progesterone and Inflammatory Response in the Oviduct during Physiological and Pathological

Conditions. *Cells.* 2022;11(7):1075. doi:10.3390/cells11071075

20 - Patel, BG, Rudnicki, M, Yu, J, Shu, Y, Taylor, RN. Progesterone resistance in endometriosis: origins, consequences and interventions. *Acta Obstet Gynecol Scand* 2017; 96: 623– 632.

21 - Herington JL, Bruner-Tran KL, Lucas JA, Osteen KG. Immune interactions in endometriosis. *Expert Review of Clinical Immunology.* 2011;7(5):611-626. doi:10.1586/eci.11.53

22 - García-Gómez E, Vázquez-Martínez ER, Reyes-Mayoral C, Cruz-Orozco O, Camacho-Arroyo I, Cerbón M. Regulation of inflammation pathways and inflammasome by sex steroid hormones in endometriosis. *Frontiers in Endocrinology.* 2020;10. doi:10.3389/fendo.2019.00935

23 - Grandi G, Mueller C, Papadia A, et al. Inflammation influences steroid hormone receptors targeted by progestins in endometrial stromal cells from women with endometriosis. *Journal of Reproductive Immunology.* 2016;117:30-38. doi:10.1016/j.jri.2016.06.004

24 - Christodoulakos G, Augoulea A, Lambrinoudaki I, Sioulas V, Creatsas G. Pathogenesis of endometriosis: The role of defective 'immunosurvei llance.' *The European Journal of Contraception & Reproductive Health Care.* 2007;12(3):194-202. doi:10.1080/13625180701387266

25 - Miyashira, C. H., Oliveira, F. R., Andres, M. P., Gingold, J. A., & Abrão, M. S. (2022). The microbiome and endometriosis. *Reproduction and Fertility,* 3(3), R163–R175. https://doi.org/10.1530/raf-21-0113

26 - Khan KN, Fujishita A, Hiraki K, et al. Bacterial contamination hypothesis: a new concept in endometriosis. *Reproductive Medicine and Biology.* 2018;17(2):125-133. doi:10.1002/rmb2.12083

27 - Puca, J. & Hoyne, G. F. Microbial dysbiosis and disease pathogenesis of endometriosis, could there be a link?. *Allied J. Med. Res.* 1(1), 1–9 (2016).

28 - Tai FW, Chang CY, Chiang JH, Lin WC, Wan L. Association of Pelvic Inflammatory Disease with Risk of Endometriosis: A Nationwide Cohort Study Involving 141,460 Individuals. *J Clin Med.* 2018;7(11):379. Published 2018 Oct 24. Doi:10.3390/jcm7110379

29 - Bouquet de Jolinière J, Ayoubi JM, Lesec G, et al. Identification of displaced endometrial glands and embryonic duct remnants in female

fetal reproductive tract: possible pathogenetic role in endometriotic and pelvic neoplastic processes. *Front Physiol.* 2012;3:444. Published 2012 Dec 3. Doi:10.3389/fphys.2012.00444

30 - Nezhat C., Nezhat F., Nezhat C. Endometriosis: ancient disease, ancient treatments. *Fertil. Steril.* 2012;98(6 Supplement):S1–S62.

31 - Rathna R, Varjani S, Nakkeeran E. Recent developments and prospects of dioxins and furans remediation. *Journal of Environmental Management.* 2018;223:797-806. doi:10.1016/j.jenvman.2018.06.095

32 - Guo SW, Simsa P, Kyama CM, et al. Reassessing the evidence for the link between dioxin and endometriosis: from molecular biology to clinical epidemiology. *Mol Hum Reprod.* 2009;15(10):609-624. doi:10.1093/moleh r/gap075

33 - World Health Organization: WHO. Dioxins. https://www.who.int/n ews-room/fact-sheets/detail/dioxins-and-their-effects-on-human-hea lth. Published November 29, 2023.

What are the Stages of Endometriosis?

1 – Medicine NAS for R. Revised American Society for Reproductive Medicine classification of endometriosis: 1996. *Fertility and Sterility.* 1997;67(5):817-821. doi:10.1016/s0015-0282(97)81391-x

2 – Brosens I, Brosens JJ. Redefining endometriosis: Is deep endometriosis a progressive disease? *Human Reproduction.* 2000;15(1):1-3. doi:10.109 3/humrep/15.1.1

3 – Acién P, Velasco I. Endometriosis: a disease that remains enigmatic. *ISRN Obstetrics and Gynecology (Print).* 2013;2013:1-12. doi:10.1155/2013/24 2149

4 – Nirgianakis K, Ma L, McKinnon B, Mueller MD. Recurrence Patterns after Surgery in Patients with Different Endometriosis Subtypes: A Long-Term Hospital-Based Cohort Study. *J Clin Med.* 2020;9(2):496. Published 2020 Feb 11. doi:10.3390/jcm9020496

What Are the Symptoms of Endometriosis

1 - Yang X, Xu X, Lin L, et al. Sexual function in patients with endometrio-

sis: a prospective case–control study in China. *Journal of International Medical Research.* 2021;49(4):030006052110043. doi:10.1177/03000605211 004388

2 - Brott NR, Le JK. Mittelschmerz. [Updated 2022 May 8]. In: Stat-Pearls [Internet]. Treasure Island (FL): StatPearls Publishing; 2022 Jan-. Available from: https://www.ncbi.nlm.nih.gov/books/NBK549822/

3 - Sinaii N, Cleary SD, Ballweg ML, Nieman LK, Stratton P. High rates of autoimmune and endocrine disorders, fibromyalgia, chronic fatigue syndrome and atopic diseases among women with endometriosis: a survey analysis. *Human Reproduction.* 2002;17(10):2715-2724. doi:10.1093/humre p/17.10.2715

4 - Nyholt DR, Gillespie NG, Merikangas KR, Treloar SA, Martin NG, Montgomery GW. Common genetic influences underlie comorbidity of migraine and endometriosis. *Genet Epidemiol.* 2009;33(2):105-113. doi:10.100 2/gepi.20361

5 - Maroun, P., Cooper, M. J. W., Reid, G. D., & Keirse, M. J. N. C. (2009). Relevance of gastrointestinal symptoms in endometriosis. *Australian and New Zealand Journal of Obstetrics and Gynaecology,* 49(4), 411–414. https://d oi.org/10.1111/j.1479-828x.2009.01030.x

6 - Griffiths AN, Koutsouridou RN, Penketh RJ. Predicting the presence of rectovaginal endometriosis from the clinical history: a retrospective observational study. *J Obstet Gynaecol.* 2007;27(5):493-495. doi:10.1080/0 1443610701405721

7 - Ek M, Roth B, Ekström P, Valentin L, Bengtsson M, Ohlsson B. Gastrointestinal symptoms among endometriosis patients—A case-cohort study. *BMC Women S Health.* 2015;15(1). doi:10.1186/s12905-015-0213-2

8 - Ramin-Wright A, Schwartz ASK, Geraedts K, et al. Fatigue – a symptom in endometriosis. *Human Reproduction.* 2018;33(8):1459-1465. doi:10.1093/humrep/dey115

9 - Boneva RS, Lin JS, Wieser F, et al. Endometriosis as a Comorbid Condition in Chronic Fatigue Syndrome (CFS): Secondary Analysis of Data From a CFS Case-Control Study. *Front Pediatr.* 2019;7:195. Published 2019 May 21. doi:10.3389/fped.2019.00195

10 - Friedl F, Riedl D, Fessler S, et al. Impact of endometriosis on quality of life, anxiety, and depression: an Austrian perspective. *Arch Gynecol Obstet.* 2015;292(6):1393-1399. doi:10.1007/s00404-015-3789-8

11 - Brasil DL, Montagna E, Trevisan CM, La Rosa VL, Laganà AS, Barbosa CP, et al. Psychological stress levels in women with endometriosis: systematic review and meta-analysis of observational studies. Minerva Med 2020;111:90-102. DOI: 10.23736/S0026-4806.19.06350-X

12 - Counsellor VS. Endometriosis. A clinical and surgical review. *Am J Obstet Gynecol.* 1938;36:877.

Bowel Endometriosis

1 - Charatsi D, Koukoura O, Ntavela IG, et al. Gastrointestinal and urinary tract endometriosis: A review on the commonest locations of extrapelvic endometriosis. *Advances in Medicine.* 2018;2018:1-11. doi:10.1155/2018/346 1209

Rectovaginal Endometriosis

1 - Abesadze E, Chiàntera V, Sehouli J, Mechsner S. Post-operative management and follow-up of surgical treatment in the case of rectovaginal and retrocervical endometriosis. *Archives of Gynecology and Obstetrics.* 2020;302(4):957-967. doi:10.1007/s00404-020-05686-0

2 - Foti PV, Farina R, Palmucci S, et al. Endometriosis: clinical features, MR imaging findings and pathologic correlation. *Insights Into Imaging.* 2018;9(2):149-172. doi:10.1007/s13244-017-0591-0

3 - Signorile PG, Campioni M, Vincenzi B, D'Avino A, Baldi A. Rectovaginal septum endometriosis: an immunohistochemical analysis of 62 cases. *In Vivo.* 2009;23(3):459-464.

4 - Moawad NS, Caplin A. Diagnosis, management, and long-term outcomes of rectovaginal endometriosis. *Int J Womens Health.* 2013;5:753-763. Published 2013 Nov 8. doi:10.2147/IJWH.S37846

5 Byrne D, Curnow T, Smith P on behalf of BSGE Endometriosis Centres, *et al*Laparoscopic excision of deep rectovaginal endometriosis in BSGE endometriosis centres: a multicentre prospective cohort study*BMJ Open*

2018;8:e018924. doi:10.1136/bmjopen-2017-018924

Extragenital Endometriosis

1 - Nezhat C, Li A, Falik R, et al. Bowel endometriosis: diagnosis and management. *Am J Obstet Gynecol.* 2018;218(6):549-562. doi:10.1016/j.ajo g.2017.09.023

2 - Andres MP, Arcoverde FVL, Souza CCC, Fernandes LFC, Abrão MS, Kho RM. Extrapelvic Endometriosis: A Systematic Review. *Journal of Minimally Invasive Gynecology.* 2020;27(2):373-389. doi:10.1016/j.jmig.2019.10.004

3 - Leonardi M, Espada M, Kho RM, et al. Endometriosis and the urinary tract: From diagnosis to surgical treatment. *Diagnostics.* 2020;10(10):771. doi:10.3390/diagnostics10100771

4 - Nawaz MM, Masood Y, Usmani AS, Basheer MI, Sheikh UN, Mir K. Renal endometriosis: A benign disease with malignant presentation. *Urology Case Reports.* 2022;43:102110. doi:10.1016/j.eucr.2022.102110

5 - Nezhat C, Paka C, Gomaa M, Schipper E. Silent loss of kidney seconary to ureteral endometriosis. *JSLS.* 2012;16(3):451-455. doi:10.4293/1086808 12x13462882736213

6 - Nezhat C, Lindheim SR, Backhus L, et al. Thoracic Endometriosis Syndrome: A Review of Diagnosis and Management. *JSLS.* 2019;23(3):e201 9.00029. doi:10.4293/JSLS.2019.00029

7 - Nezhat C, King LP, Paka C, Odegaard J, Beygui R. Bilateral thoracic endometriosis affecting the lung and diaphragm. *JSLS.* 2012;16(1):140-142. doi:10.4293/108680812X13291597716384

Tilted Uterus

1 - Raissi D, Yu BQ, Han Q. Uterine anteversion after uterine fibroid embolization. *Radiology Case Reports.* 2018;13(6):1150-1153. doi:10.1016/j.r adcr.2018.08.009

2 - Tissot M, Lecointre L, Faller E, Afors K, Akladios C, Audebert A. Clinical presentation of endometriosis identified at interval laparoscopic tubal sterilization: Prospective series of 465 cases. *Journal of Gynecology Obstetrics and Human Reproduction.* 2017;46(8):647-650. doi:10.1016/j.jog

oh.2017.05.003

3 - Egbase PE, Al-Sharhan M, Grudzinskas JG. Influence of position and length of uterus on implantation and clinical pregnancy rates in IVF and embryo transfer treatment cycles. *Human Reproduction.* 2000;15(9):1943-1946. doi:10.1093/humrep/15.9.1943

Frozen Pelvis

1 - El-Kader AIA, Gonied AS, Mohamed ML, Mohamed SL. Impact of Endometriosis-Related Adhesions on Quality of Life among Infertile Women. *PubMed.* 2019;13(1):72-76. doi:10.22074/ijfs.2019.5572

2 - Frozen pelvis in advanced endometriosis. Seckin Endometriosis Center. https://drseckin.com/frozen-pelvis/. Published September 26, 2023.

3 - Molloy DW, Martin M, Speirs AL, et al. Performance of patients with a "frozen pelvis" in an in vitro fertilization program. *Fertility and Sterility.* 1987;47(3):450-455. doi:10.1016/s0015-0282(16)59054-2

4 - Diamond MP, Freeman ML. Clinical implications of postsurgical adhesions. *Human Reproduction Update.* 2001;7(6):567-576. doi:10.1093/humupd/7.6.567

Adenomyosis

1 - Mishra I, Melo P, Easter C, Sephton V, Dhillon-Smith R, Coomarasamy A. Prevalence of adenomyosis in women with subfertility: systematic review and meta-analysis. *Ultrasound in Obstetrics and Gynecology.* 2023;62(1):23-41. doi:10.1002/uog.26159

2 - Sztachelska M, Ponikwicka-Tyszko D, Martínez-Rodrigo L, et al. Functional Implications of Estrogen and Progesterone Receptors Expression in Adenomyosis, Potential Targets for Endocrinological Therapy. *J Clin Med.* 2022;11(15):4407. Published 2022 Jul 28. doi:10.3390/jcm11154407

3 - Naftalin J, Hoo W, Pateman K, Mavrelos D, Holland T, Jurkovic D. How common is adenomyosis? A prospective study of prevalence using transvaginal ultrasound in a gynaecology clinic. *Human Reproduction.* 2012;27(12):3432-3439. doi:10.1093/humrep/des332

4 - Harada T, Khine YM, Kaponis A, Nikellis T, Decavalas G, Taniguchi F. The impact of adenomyosis on women's fertility. *Obstetrical & Gynecological Survey*. 2016;71(9):557-568. doi:10.1097/ogx.0000000000000346

5 - Gunther R, Walker C. Adenomyosis. StatPearls - NCBI Bookshelf. https://www.ncbi.nlm.nih.gov/books/NBK539868/. Published June 12, 2023.

6 - Upson K, Missmer SA. Epidemiology of Adenomyosis. *Seminars in Reproductive Medicine*. 2020;38(02/03):089-107. doi:10.1055/s-0040-1718920

7 - Adenomyosis - Symptoms & causes - Mayo Clinic. Mayo Clinic. https://www.mayoclinic.org/diseases-conditions/adenomyosis/symptoms-causes/syc-20369138. Published April 6, 2023. Accessed 9th December 2024.

8 - Peric H, Fraser IS. The symptomatology of adenomyosis. *Best Practice & Research in Clinical Obstetrics & Gynaecology*. 2006;20(4):547-555. doi:10.1016/j.bpobgyn.2006.01.006

9 - Dueholm M, Lundorf E. Transvaginal ultrasound or MRI for diagnosis of adenomyosis. *Curr Opin Obstet Gynecol*. 2007;19(6):505-512. doi:10.1097/GCO.0b013e3282f1bf00

Biochemistry of Endometriosis

1 - Laschke MW, Elitzsch A, Vollmar B, Menger MD. In vivo analysis of angiogenesis in endometriosis-like lesions by intravital fluorescence microscopy. *Fertil Steril*. 2005;84 Suppl 2:1199-1209. doi:10.1016/j.fertnstert.2005.05.010

2 - Losordo DW, Isner JM. Estrogen and angiogenesis: A review. *Arterioscler Thromb Vasc Biol*. 2001;21(1):6-12. doi:10.1161/01.atv.21.1.6

3 - Mori T, Ito F, Koshiba A, et al. Local estrogen formation and its regulation in endometriosis. *Reprod Med Biol*. 2019;18(4):305-311. Published 2019 Jun 18. doi:10.1002/rmb2.12285

4 - Zeitoun KM, Bulun SE. Aromatase: a key molecule in the pathophysiology of endometriosis and a therapeutic target. *Fertil Steril*. 1999;72(6):961-969. doi:10.1016/s0015-0282(99)00393-3

5 - Dyson MT, Bulun SE. Cutting SRC-1 down to size in endometriosis. *Nature Medicine*. 2012;18(7):1016-1018. doi:10.1038/nm.2855

6 - Reis FM, Coutinho LM, Vannuccini S, Batteux F, Chapron C, Petraglia F. Progesterone receptor ligands for the treatment of endometriosis: the mechanisms behind therapeutic success and failure. Hum Reprod Update. 2020 Jun 18;26(4):565-585. doi: 10.1093/humupd/dmaa009. PMID: 32412587; PMCID: PMC7317284.

7 - Donnez J, Dolmans MM. Endometriosis and Medical Therapy: From Progestogens to Progesterone Resistance to GnRH Antagonists: A Review. J Clin Med. 2021 Mar 5;10(5):1085. doi: 10.3390/jcm10051085. PMID: 33807739; PMCID: PMC7961981.

8 - Gibbons T, Rahmioglu N, Zondervan KT, Becker CM. Crimson clues: advancing endometriosis detection and management with novel blood biomarkers. *Fertility and Sterility*. 2024;121(2):145-163. doi:10.1016/j.fertns tert.2023.12.018

9 - Karimi-Zarchi M, Dehshiri-Zadeh N, Sekhavat L, Nosouhi F. Correlation of CA-125 serum level and clinico-pathological characteristic of patients with endometriosis. *Int J Reprod Biomed*. 2016;14(11):713-718.

10 - Niloff JM, Knapp RC, Schaetzl E, Reynolds C, Bast RC Jr. CA125 antigen levels in obstetric and gynecologic patients. *Obstet Gynecol*. 1984;64(5):703-707.

11 - Burghaus S, Drazic P, Wölfler M, et al. Multicenter evaluation of blood-based biomarkers for the detection of endometriosis and adenomyosis: A prospective non-interventional study. *International Journal of Gynecology & Obstetrics*. 2023;164(1):305-314. doi:10.1002/ijgo.15062

12 - Mann J, Truswell AS. *Essentials of human nutrition*. Oxford University Press; 2017.

13 - NDNS: results from years 9 to 11 (2016 to 2017 and 2018 to 2019). GOV.UK. https://www.gov.uk/government/statistics/ndns-results-from-years-9-to-11-2016-to-2017-and-2018-to-2019. Published December 11, 2020.

14 - Scientific Advisory Committee on Nutrition. (2010). *Iron and Health 2010*. https://assets.publishing.service.gov.uk/government/uploads/syste

m/uploads/attachment_data/file/339309/SACN_Iron_and_Health_Rep ort.pdf . Accessed 22nd March 2023

15 - Cho HY, Park ST, Park SH. Red blood cell indices as an effective marker for the existence and severity of endometriosis (STROBE). *Medicine (Baltimore)*. 2022;101(42):e31157. doi:10.1097/MD.0000000000031157

16 - S. Defrère, J.C. Lousse, R. González-Ramos, S. Colette, J. Donnez, A. Van Langendonckt, Potential involvement of iron in the pathogenesis of peritoneal endometriosis, *Molecular Human Reproduction*, Volume 14, Issue 7, July 2008, Pages 377–385, https://doi.org/10.1093/molehr/gan033

17 - Donnez J, Cacciottola L. Endometriosis: An Inflammatory Disease That Requires New Therapeutic Options. *Int J Mol Sci.* 2022;23(3):1518. Published 2022 Jan 28. doi:10.3390/ijms23031518

Microbiology

1 - Flandroy L, Poutahidis T, Berg G, et al. The impact of human activities and lifestyles on the interlinked microbiota and health of humans and of ecosystems. *Sci Total Environ*. 2018;627:1018-1038. doi:10.1016/j.scitotenv. 2018.01.288

2 - Sevelsted A., Stokholm J., Bønnelykke K., Bisgaard H. Cesarean section and chronic immune disorders. *Pediatrics*. 2015;135:e92–e98. doi: 10.1542/peds.2014-0596.

3 - Dominguez-Bello MG, De Jesus-Laboy KM, Shen N, et al. Partial restoration of the microbiota of cesarean-born infants via vaginal micro-bial transfer. *Nat Med*. 2016;22(3):250-253. doi:10.1038/nm.4039

4 - María Remes Troche J, Coss Adame E, Ángel Valdovinos Díaz M, et al. *Lactobacillus acidophilus* LB: a useful pharmabiotic for the treatment of digestive disorders. *Therap Adv Gastroenterol*. 2020;13:1756284820971201. Published 2020 Nov 24. doi:10.1177/1756284820971201

5 - Marshall B. Helicobacter pylori—a Nobel pursuit?. *Can J Gastroenterol*. 2008;22(11):895-896. doi:10.1155/2008/459810

6 - Jiang I, Yong PJ, Allaire C, Bedaiwy MA. Intricate Connections between the Microbiota and Endometriosis. *Int J Mol Sci*. 2021;22(11):5644. Published 2021 May 26. doi:10.3390/ijms22115644

7 - Miyashira CH, Oliveira FR, Andres MP, Gingold JA, Abrão MS. The microbiome and endometriosis. *Reproduction & Fertility.* 2022;3(3):R163-R175. doi:10.1530/raf-21-0113

8 - Leonardi M, Hicks C, El-Assaad F, El-Omar E, Condous G. Endometriosis and the microbiome: a systematic review. *BJOG.* 2020;127(2):239-249. doi:10.1111/1471-0528.15916

9 - Khan K.N., Fujishita A., Masumoto H., Muto H., Kitajima M., Masuzaki H., Kitawaki J. Molecular Detection of Intrauterine Microbial Colonization in Women with Endometriosis. *Eur. J. Obstet. Gynecol. Reprod. Biol.* 2016;199:69–75. doi: 10.1016/j.ejogrb.2016.01.040

10 - Laschke MW, Menger MD. The gut microbiota: a puppet master in the pathogenesis of endometriosis?. *Am J Obstet Gynecol.* 2016;215(1):68.e1-68.e684. doi:10.1016/j.ajog.2016.02.036

11 - Baker J.M., Al-Nakkash L., Herbst-Kralovetz M.M. Estrogen–Gut Microbiome Axis: Physiological and Clinical Implications. *Maturitas.* 2017;103:45–53. doi: 10.1016/j.maturitas.2017.06.025.

12 - Qi X, Yun C, Pang Y, Qiao J. The impact of the gut microbiota on the reproductive and metabolic endocrine system. *Gut Microbes.* 2021;13(1). doi:10.1080/19490976.2021.1894070

13 - COJOCARU, M. (2010). ENDOMETRIOSIS AND THE HUMAN MICRO-BIOME. *Journal of Clinical Sexology,* 3(2). https://www.journalofclinicalsex ology.com/wp-content/uploads/2020/08/ENDOMETRIOSIS-AND-THE-HUMAN-MICROBIOME.pdf

14 - Chadchan SB, Naik SK, Popli P, et al. Gut microbiota and microbiota-derived metabolites promotes endometriosis. *Cell Death Discovery.* 2023;9(1). doi:10.1038/s41420-023-01309-0

15 - Khan KN, Fujishita A, Hiraki K, et al. Bacterial contamination hypothesis: a new concept in endometriosis. *Reprod Med Biol.* 2018;17(2):125-133. Published 2018 Jan 18. doi:10.1002/rmb2.12083

16 - Khodaverdi S, Mohammadheigi R, Khaledi M, et al. Beneficial Effects of Oral Lactobacillus on Pain Severity in Women Suffering from Endometriosis: A Pilot Placebo-Controlled Randomized Clinical Trial. *Int J Fertil Steril.* 2019;13(3):178-183. doi:10.22074/ijfs.2019.5584

17 - Itoh H, Uchida M, Sashihara T, Ji ZS, Li J, Tang Q, et al. Lactobacillus gasseri Oll2809 is effective especially on the menstrual pain and dysmenorrhea in endometriosis patients: Randomized, double-blind, placebo-controlled study. *Cytotechnology* (2011) 63(2):153–61. doi: 10.1007/s10616-010-9326-5

18 - Kyono K, Hashimoto T, Kikuchi S, Nagai Y, Sakuraba Y. A pilot study and case reports on endometrial microbiota and pregnancy outcome: An analysis using 16S rRNA gene sequencing among IVF patients, and trial therapeutic intervention for dysbiotic endometrium. *Reprod Med Biol.* 2018;18(1):72-82. Published 2018 Oct 25. doi:10.1002/rmb2.12250

19 - Venkatesan P. Bacterial infection linked to endometriosis. *The Lancet Microbe.* 2023;4(10):e768. doi:10.1016/s2666-5247(23)00221-5

20 - Muraoka A, Suzuki M, Hamaguchi T, et al. *Fusobacterium* infection facilitates the development of endometriosis through the phenotypic transition of endometrial fibroblasts. *Sci Transl Med.* 2023;15(700):eadd1531. doi:10.1126/scitranslmed.add1531

21 - Jess T, Frisch M, Jørgensen KT, *et al*Increased risk of inflammatory bowel disease in women with endometriosis: a nationwide Danish cohort study*Gut* 2012;**61:**1279-1283.

The Nervous System

1 - Maddern J, Grundy L, Castro J, Brierley SM. Pain in endometriosis. *Frontiers in Cellular Neuroscience.* 2020;14. doi:10.3389/fncel.2020.590823

2 - Lumley MA, Cohen JL, Borszcz GS, et al. Pain and emotion: a biopsychosocial review of recent research. *Journal of Clinical Psychology.* 2011;67(9):942-968. doi:10.1002/jclp.20816

Comorbidities

1 - Rogers, J. *McCance & Huether Pathophysiology: The Biologic Basis for Disease in Adults and Children.* Elsevier Health Sciences. 2022

2 - Maroun P, Cooper MJ, Reid GD, Keirse MJ. Relevance of gastrointestinal symptoms in endometriosis. *Aust N Z J Obstet Gynaecol.* 2009;49(4):411-414. doi:10.1111/j.1479-828X.2009.01030.x

3 - Chiaffarino F, Cipriani S, Ricci E, et al. Endometriosis and inflammatory bowel disease: A systematic review of the literature. *Eur J Obstet Gynecol Reprod Biol.* 2020;252:246-251. doi:10.1016/j.ejogrb.2020.06.051

4 - Cornish JA, Tan E, Simillis C, Clark SK, Teare J, Tekkis PP. The risk of oral contraceptives in the etiology of inflammatory bowel disease: a meta-analysis. *Am J Gastroenterol.* 2008;103(9):2394-2400. doi:10.1111/j.1572-0241.2008.02064.x

5 - Ananthakrishnan AN, Higuchi LM, Huang ES, et al. Aspirin, non-steroidal anti-inflammatory drug use, and risk for Crohn disease and ulcerative colitis: a cohort study. *Ann Intern Med.* 2012;156(5):350-359. doi:10.7326/0003-4819-156-5-201203060-00007

6 - Berkowitz L, Schultz BM, Salazar GA, Pardo-Roa C, Sebastián VP, Álvarez-Lobos MM and Bueno SM (2018) Impact of Cigarette Smoking on the Gastrointestinal Tract Inflammation: Opposing Effects in Crohn's Disease and Ulcerative Colitis. *Front. Immunol.* 9:74. doi: 10.3389/fimmu.2018.00074

7 - Galvez-Sánchez CM, Duschek S, Reyes Del Paso GA. Psychological impact of fibromyalgia: current perspectives. *Psychol Res Behav Manag.* 2019;12:117-127. Published 2019 Feb 13. doi:10.2147/PRBM.S178240

8 - Jahan F, Nanji K, Qidwai W, Qasim R. Fibromyalgia syndrome: an overview of pathophysiology, diagnosis and management. *Oman Med J.* 2012;27(3):192-195. doi:10.5001/omj.2012.44

9 - Shafrir AL, Palmor MC, Fourquet J, et al. Co-occurrence of immune-mediated conditions and endometriosis among adolescents and adult women. *Am J Reprod Immunol.* 2021;86(1):e13404. doi:10.1111/aji.13404

10 - King's College London. "Fibromyalgia likely the result of autoimmune problems." ScienceDaily. ScienceDaily, 1 July 2021. Available from www.sciencedaily.com/releases/2021/07/210701120703.htm>. Accessed 29th March 2023

11 - Ruschak, I., Montesó-Curto, P., Rosselló, L., Aguilar Martín, C., Sánchez-Montesó, L., & Toussaint, L. (2023). Fibromyalgia Syndrome Pain in Men and Women: A Scoping Review. Healthcare (Basel, Switzerland), 11(2), 223. https://doi.org/10.3390/healthcare11020223

12 - *Possible Causes | Myalgic Encephalomyelitis/Chronic Fatigue Syndrome (ME/CFS) | CDC.* 2018. Available from https://www.cdc.gov/me-cfs/about/possible-causes.html. Accessed 29th March 2023

13 - Boneva RS, Lin JS, Wieser F, et al. Endometriosis as a Comorbid Condition in Chronic Fatigue Syndrome (CFS): Secondary Analysis of Data From a CFS Case-Control Study. *Front Pediatr.* 2019;7:195. Published 2019 May 21. doi:10.3389/fped.2019.00195

14 - Al-Shaiji TF, Alshammaa DH, Al-Mansouri MM, Al-Terki AE. Association of endometriosis with interstitial cystitis in chronic pelvic pain syndrome: Short narrative on prevalence, diagnostic limitations, and clinical implications. *Qatar Med J.* 2021;2021(3):50. Published 2021 Oct 7. doi:10.5339/qmj.2021.50

15 - Dukowicz AC, Lacy BE, Levine GM. Small intestinal bacterial overgrowth: a comprehensive review. *Gastroenterol Hepatol (N Y).* 2007;3(2):112-122.

16 - Losurdo G, D'Abramo FS, Indellicati G, Lillo C, Ierardi E, Di Leo A. The influence of small intestinal bacterial overgrowth in digestive and Extra-Intestinal disorders. *International Journal of Molecular Sciences.* 2020;21(10):3531. doi:10.3390/ijms21103531

17 - Chen B, Kim JJW, Zhang Y, Du L, Dai N. Prevalence and predictors of small intestinal bacterial overgrowth in irritable bowel syndrome: a systematic review and meta-analysis. *Journal of Gastroenterology.* 2018;53(7):807-818. doi:10.1007/s00535-018-1476-9

18 - NICE, When should I suspect polycystic ovary syndrome?, 2022, Available at https://cks.nice.org.uk/topics/polycystic-ovary-syndrome/diagnosis/when-to-suspect/. Accessed 29th March 2023

19 - Amisi CA. Markers of insulin resistance in Polycystic ovary syndrome women: An update. *World J Diabetes.* 2022;13(3):129-149. doi:10.4239/wjd.v13.i3.129

20 - Lu KT, Ho YC, Chang C, Lan K, Wu CC, Su Y. Evaluation of Bodily Pain Associated with Polycystic Ovary Syndrome: A Review of Health-Related Quality of Life and Potential Risk Factors. *Biomedicines.* 2022;10(12):3197. doi:10.3390/biomedicines10123197

21 - Gupta KK, Gupta VK, Naumann RW. Ovarian cancer: screening and future directions. *International Journal of Gynecological Cancer*. 2019;29(1):195-200. doi:10.1136/ijgc-2018-000016

22 - Cancer Research UK. Breast cancer statistics. Cancer Research UK. https://www.cancerresearchuk.org/health-professional/cancer-statistics/statistics-by-cancer-type/breast-cancer. Published January 30, 2024.

23 - Kim HS, Kim TH, Chung HH, Song YS. Risk and prognosis of ovarian cancer in women with endometriosis: a meta-analysis. *British Journal of Cancer*. 2014;110(7):1878-1890. doi:10.1038/bjc.2014.29

24 - Somigliana E, Vigano' P, Parazzini F, Stoppelli S, Giambattista E, Vercellini P. Association between endometriosis and cancer: a comprehensive review and a critical analysis of clinical and epidemiological evidence. *Gynecol Oncol*. 2006;101(2):331-341. doi:10.1016/j.ygyno.2005.11.033

25 - Kvaskoff M, Horne A, Missmer SA. Informing women with endometriosis about ovarian cancer risk. *The Lancet*. 2017;390(10111):2433-2434. doi:10.1016/s0140-6736(17)33049-0

26 - Anglesio MS, Papadopoulos N, Ayhan A, et al. Cancer-Associated Mutations in Endometriosis without Cancer. *N Engl J Med*. 2017;376(19):1835-1848. doi:10.1056/NEJMoa1614814

27 - Wilson, M.R., Reske, J.J., Holladay, J. *et al.* ARID1A and PI3-kinase pathway mutations in the endometrium drive epithelial transdifferentiation and collective invasion. *Nat Commun* **10**, 3554 (2019). https://doi.org/10.1038/s41467-019-11403-6

28 - Brilhante AV, Augusto KL, Portela MC, et al. Endometriosis and Ovarian Cancer: an Integrative Review (Endometriosis and Ovarian Cancer). *Asian Pac J Cancer Prev*. 2017;18(1):11-16. Published 2017 Jan 1. doi:10.22034/APJCP.2017.18.1.11

29 - Dahiya A, Sebastian A, Thomas A, George R, Thomas V, Peedicayil A. Endometriosis and malignancy: The intriguing relationship. *Int J Gynaecol Obstet*. 2021;155(1):72-78. doi:10.1002/ijgo.13585

30 - Ferris JS, Daly MB, Buys SS, Genkinger JM, Liao Y, Terry MB. Oral contraceptive and reproductive risk factors for ovarian cancer within sisters in the breast cancer family registry. *British Journal of Cancer*.

2014;110(4):1074-1080. doi:10.1038/bjc.2013.803

31 - Kvaskoff M, Mu F, Terry KL, et al. Endometriosis: a high-risk population for major chronic diseases?. *Hum Reprod Update*. 2015;21(4):500-516. doi:10.1093/humupd/dmv013

32 - Poeta do Couto C, Policiano C, Pinto FJ, Brito D, Caldeira D. Endometriosis and cardiovascular disease: A systematic review and meta-analysis. *Maturitas*. 2023;171:45-52. doi:10.1016/j.maturitas.2023.04.001

33 - Rippe JM. Lifestyle strategies for risk factor reduction, prevention, and treatment of cardiovascular disease. *American Journal of Lifestyle Medicine*. 2018;13(2):204-212. doi:10.1177/1559827618812395

34 - DiBenedetti D, Soliman AM, Gupta C, Surrey ES. Patients' perspectives of endometriosis-related fatigue: qualitative interviews. *J Patient Rep Outcomes*. 2020;4(1):33. Published 2020 May 6. doi:10.1186/s41687-020-00200-1

35 - Bungum HF, Vestergaard C, Knudsen UB. Endometriosis and type 1 allergies/immediate type hypersensitivity: a systematic review. *Eur J Obstet Gynecol Reprod Biol*. 2014;179:209-215. doi:10.1016/j.ejogrb.2014.04.025

36 - Herington JL, Bruner-Tran KL, Lucas JA, Osteen KG. Immune interactions in endometriosis. *Expert Rev Clin Immunol*. 2011;7(5):611-626. doi:10.1586/eci.11.53

37 - McCallion A, Nasirzadeh Y, Lingegowda H, et al. Estrogen mediates inflammatory role of mast cells in endometriosis pathophysiology. *Front Immunol*. 2022;13:961599. Published 2022 Aug 9. doi:10.3389/fimmu.2022.961599

38 - Zaitsu M, Narita S, Lambert K, et al. Estradiol activates mast cells via a non-genomic estrogen receptor-α and calcium influx. *Molecular Immunology*. 2007;44(8):1977-1985. doi:10.1016/j.molimm.2006.09.030

39 - Maintz L, Novak N. Histamine and histamine intolerance. *Am J Clin Nutr*. 2007;85(5):1185-1196. doi:10.1093/ajcn/85.5.1185

40 - Eriksson NE, Formgren H, Svenonius E. Food hypersensitivity in patients with pollen allergy. *Allergy*. 1982;37(6):437-443. doi:10.1111/j.1398-9995.1982.tb02323.x

41 - Yuk J, Kim YJ, Yi KW, Kim T, Hur JY, Shin JH. High rate of nickel

allergy in women with endometriosis: A 3-year population-based study. *Journal of Obstetrics and Gynaecology Research.* 2015;41(8):1255-1259. doi:10.1111/jog.12707

42 - Sharma AD. Low nickel diet in dermatology. *Indian J Dermatol.* 2013;58(3):240. doi:10.4103/0019-5154.110846

43 - Borghini R, Porpora MG, Casale R, et al. Irritable Bowel Syndrome-Like Disorders in Endometriosis: Prevalence of Nickel Sensitivity and Effects of a Low-Nickel Diet. An Open-Label Pilot Study. *Nutrients.* 2020;12(2):341. Published 2020 Jan 28. doi:10.3390/nu12020341

44 - Lamb K, Nichols TR. Endometriosis: a comparison of associated disease histories. *Am J Prev Med.* 1986;2(6):324-329.

45 - Zervou MI, Vlachakis D, Papageorgiou L, Eliopoulos E, Goulielmos GN. Increased risk of rheumatoid arthritis in patients with endometriosis: genetic aspects. *Rheumatology (Oxford).* 2022;61(11):4252-4262. doi:10.1093/rheumatology/keac143

46 - CTG labs - NCBI. Pilot Study of the IL-1 Antagonist Anakinra for the Treatment of Endometriosis Related Symptoms, ClinicalTrials.gov. https://clinicaltrials.gov/study/NCT03991520.

47 - Myles J. Lewis, Ali S. Jawad, The effect of ethnicity and genetic ancestry on the epidemiology, clinical features and outcome of systemic lupus erythematosus, *Rheumatology*, Volume 56, Issue suppl_1, April 2017, Pages i67–i77, https://doi.org/10.1093/rheumatology/kew399

48 - Ferrari-Souza JP, Pedrotti MT, Moretto EE, Farenzena LP, Crippa LG, Cunha-Filho JS. Endometriosis and Systemic Lupus Erythematosus: Systematic Review and Meta-analysis. *Reprod Sci.* 2023;30(4):997-1005. doi:10.1007/s43032-022-01045-3

49 - Coloma JL, Martínez-Zamora, Tàssies D, et al. Serological autoimmune profile of systemic lupus erythematosus in deep and non-deep endometriosis patients. *J Reprod Immunol.* 2023;156:103827. doi:10.1016/j.jri.2023.103827

50 - Chen F-Y, Chen S-W, Chen X, Huang J-Y, Ye Z, Wei JC-C. Hydroxychloroquine might reduce risk of incident endometriosis in patients with systemic lupus erythematosus: A retrospective population-based cohort

study. *Lupus*. 2021;30(10):1609-1616. doi:10.1177/09612033211031009

51 - Press Release: New BBC research wake-up call to provide better care | Endometriosis UK. https://www.endometriosis-uk.org/press-release-new-bbc-research-wake-call-provide-better-care.

52 - Laganà AS, La Rosa VL, Rapisarda AMC, et al. Anxiety and depression in patients with endometriosis: impact and management challenges. *Int J Womens Health*. 2017;9:323-330. Published 2017 May 16. doi:10.2147/IJWH.S119729

53 - Liebermann C, Kohl Schwartz AS, Charpidou T, et al. Maltreatment during childhood: a risk factor for the development of endometriosis?. *Hum Reprod*. 2018;33(8):1449-1458. doi:10.1093/humrep/dey111

54 - Coelho R, Viola TW, Walss-Bass C, Brietzke E, Grassi-Oliveira R. Childhood maltreatment and inflammatory markers: a systematic review. *Acta Psychiatr Scand*. 2014;129(3):180-192. doi:10.1111/acps.12217

55 - Redlich R, Opel N, Förster K, Engelen J, Dannlowski U. Structural neuroimaging of maltreatment and inflammation in depression. In: *Elsevier eBooks*. ; 2018:287-300. doi:10.1016/b978-0-12-811073-7.00016-7

56 - Lousse JC, Van Langendonckt A, Defrere S, Ramos RG, Colette S, Donnez J. Peritoneal endometriosis is an inflammatory disease. *Front Biosci (Elite Ed)*. 2012;4(1):23-40. Published 2012 Jan 1. doi:10.2741/e358

57 - Bouayed J, Rammal H, Soulimani R. Oxidative stress and anxiety: relationship and cellular pathways. *Oxid Med Cell Longev*. 2009;2(2):63-67. doi:10.4161/oxim.2.2.7944

58 - Asante A, Taylor RN. Endometriosis: the role of neuroangiogenesis. *Annu Rev Physiol*. 2011;73:163-182. doi:10.1146/annurev-physiol-012110-142158

59 - Bashir ST, Redden C, Raj K, et al. Endometriosis leads to central nervous system-wide glial activation in a mouse model of endometriosis. *Journal of Neuroinflammation*. 2023;20(1). doi:10.1186/s12974-023-02713-0

60 - Skovlund CW, Mørch LS, Kessing LV, Lange T, Lidegaard Ø. Association of Hormonal Contraception With Suicide Attempts and Suicides. *Am*

J Psychiatry. 2018;175(4):336-342. doi:10.1176/appi.ajp.2017.17060616

61 - Xie J, Kvaskoff M, Li Y, et al. Severe teenage acne and risk of endometriosis. *Hum Reprod.* 2014;29(11):2592-2599. doi:10.1093/humrep /deu207

62 - Yang Q, Ciebiera M, Bariani MV, et al. Comprehensive review of uterine fibroids: developmental origin, pathogenesis, and treatment. *Endocrine Reviews.* 2021;43(4):678-719. doi:10.1210/endrev/bnab039

63 - Giuliani E, As-Sanie S, Marsh EE. Epidemiology and management of uterine fibroids. *Int J Gynaecol Obstet.* 2020;149(1):3-9. doi:10.1002/ijgo. 13102

64 - Uimari O, Järvelä I, Ryynänen M. Do symptomatic endometriosis and uterine fibroids appear together?. *J Hum Reprod Sci.* 2011;4(1):34-38. doi:10.4103/0974-1208.82358

65 - Barjon K, Mikhail LN. Uterine Leiomyomata. [Updated 2022 Aug 8]. In: StatPearls [Internet]. Treasure Island (FL): StatPearls Publishing; 2023 Jan-. Available from: https://www.ncbi.nlm.nih.gov/books/NBK546680/

Fertility

1 - Horne A, Pearson C. *Endometriosis: The Experts' Guide to Treat, Manage and Live Well with Your Symptoms.* Random House; 2018.

2 - endometriosis.org. Myths and misconceptions in endometriosis – Endometriosis.org. Copyright 2005-2011 endometriosis.org. https://endo metriosis.org/resources/articles/myths/.

3 - Endometriosis and Fertility - Brigham and Women's Hospital. https://www.brighamandwomens.org/obgyn/infertility-reproductive-surgery/endometriosis/endometriosis-and-fertility.

4 - Bonavina G, Taylor HS. Endometriosis-associated infertility: From pathophysiology to tailored treatment. *Frontiers in Endocrinology.* 2022;13. doi:10.3389/fendo.2022.1020827

5 - Frangež HB, Bokal EV, Štimpfel M, et al. Reproductive outcomes after laparoscopic surgery in infertile women affected by ovarian endometriomas, with or without in vitro fertilisation: results from the SAFE (surgery and ART for endometriomas) trial. *Journal of Obstetrics and Gynaecology.*

2021;42(5):1293-1300. doi:10.1080/01443615.2021.1959536

6 - Kumar N, Singh AK. Trends of male factor infertility, an important cause of infertility: A review of literature. *Journal of Human Reproductive Sciences*. 2015;8(4):191. doi:10.4103/0974-1208.170370

7 - NICE. Recommendations | Endometriosis: diagnosis and management | Guidance | NICE. https://www.nice.org.uk/guidance/ng73/chapter/Recommendations. Published September 6, 2017.

8 - Becker CM, Bokor A, Heikinheimo O, et al. ESHRE guideline: endometriosis. *Human Reproduction Open*. 2022;2022(2). doi:10.1093/hropen/hoac009

9 - NICE. Fertility problems: assessment and treatment. NICE 2016. https://www.nice.org.uk/guidance/cg156/resources/fertility-problems-assessment-and-treatment-35109634660549. Published 2017. Accessed February 26, 2024.

10 - Website N. Intrauterine insemination (IUI). nhs.uk. https://www.nhs.uk/conditions/artificial-insemination/. Published November 3, 2023.

11 - New HFEA report shows dramatic reduction in twin births from IVF | HFEA. https://www.hfea.gov.uk/about-us/news-and-press-releases/2022/new-hfea-report-shows-dramatic-reduction-in-twin-births-from-ivf/#:~:text=The%20number%20of%20multiple%20births,of%20IVF%20births%20were%20twins.

12 - Press release: Age is the key factor for egg freezing success says new HFEA report, as overall treatment numbers remain low | HFEA. https://www.hfea.gov.uk/about-us/news-and-press-releases/2018/press-release-age-is-the-key-factor-for-egg-freezing-success-says-new-hfea-report-as-overall-treatment-numbers-remain-low/.

13 - Irani M, Zaninović N, Rosenwaks Z, Xu K. Does maternal age at retrieval influence the implantation potential of euploid blastocysts? *American Journal of Obstetrics and Gynecology*. 2019;220(4):379.e1-379.e7. doi:10.1016/j.ajog.2018.11.1103

Is Endometriosis Preventable and What Are the Risk Factors?

1 - Stefansson H, Geirsson RT, Steinthorsdottir V, et al. Genetic factors

contribute to the risk of developing endometriosis. *Human Reproduction.* 2002;17(3):555-559. doi:10.1093/humrep/17.3.555

2 - Marcellin L, Santulli P, Pinzauti S, et al. Age at menarche does not correlate with the endometriosis phenotype. *PLoS One.* 2019;14(7):e0219497. Published 2019 Jul 23. doi:10.1371/journal.pone.0219497

3 - Treloar SA, Bell TA, Nagle CM, Purdie DM, Green AC. Early menstrual characteristics associated with subsequent diagnosis of endometriosis. *Am J Obstet Gynecol.* 2010;202(6):534.e1-534.e5346. doi:10.1016/j.ajog.2009.10.857

4 - Wei M, Cheng Y, Bu H, Zhao Y, Zhao W. Length of menstrual cycle and risk of endometriosis. *Medicine.* 2016;95(9):e2922. doi:10.1097/md.0000000000002922

5 - Matalliotakis I, Çakmak H, Fragouli Y, Goumenou AG, Mahutte NG, Arıcı A. Epidemiological characteristics in women with and without endometriosis in the Yale series. *Archives of Gynecology and Obstetrics.* 2007;277(5):389-393. doi:10.1007/s00404-007-0479-1

6 - NICE. *Endometriosis: What are the causes and risk factors?* NICE. https://cks.nice.org.uk/topics/endometriosis/background-information/causes-risk-factors/. 2020.

7 - Pillet MCL, Schneider A, Borghese B, et al. Deep infiltrating endometriosis is associated with markedly lower body mass index: a 476 case-control study. *Human Reproduction.* 2011;27(1):265-272. doi:10.1093/humrep/der346

8 - Pantelis A, Machairiotis N, Lapatsanis DP. The Formidable yet Unresolved Interplay between Endometriosis and Obesity. *ScientificWorldJournal.* 2021;2021:6653677. Published 2021 Apr 20. doi:10.1155/2021/6653677

9 - Holdsworth-Carson SJ, Dior U, Colgrave EM, et al. The association of body mass index with endometriosis and disease severity in women with pain. *Journal of Endometriosis and Pelvic Pain Disorders.* 2018;10(2):79-87. doi:10.1177/2284026518773939

10 - Hong J, Yi KW. What is the link between endometriosis and adiposity? *Obstetrics & Gynecology Science.* 2022;65(3):227-233. doi:10.5468/ogs.2134

3

11 - Shah DK, Correia KF, Vitonis AF, Missmer SA. Body size and endometriosis: results from 20 years of follow-up within the Nurses' Health Study II prospective cohort. *Hum Reprod.* 2013;28(7):1783-1792. doi:10.1093/humrep/det120

Menopause

1 - Becker CM, Bokor A, Heikinheimo O, et al. ESHRE guideline: endometriosis. *Human Reproduction Open.* 2022;2022(2). doi:10.1093/hropen/hoac009

2 - Secosan C, Balulescu L, Brasoveanu S, et al. Endometriosis in Menopause—Renewed attention on a controversial disease. *Diagnostics.* 2020;10(3):134. doi:10.3390/diagnostics10030134

Endometriosis in Infants, Children and Adolescents

1 – Drosdzol A, Skrzypulec V. Endometrioza w ginekologii dzieciecej i dziewczecej [Endometriosis in pediatric and adolescent gynecology]. *Ginekol Pol.* 2008;79(2):133-136.

2 - Schuster M, Mackeen D. Fetal endometriosis: a case report. *Fertility and Sterility.* 2015;103(1):160-162. doi:10.1016/j.fertnstert.2014.09.045

3 - Hirsch MS, Dhillon-Smith R, Cutner A, Yap M, Creighton SM. The Prevalence of Endometriosis in Adolescents with Pelvic Pain: A Systematic Review. *Journal of Pediatric and Adolescent Gynecology.* 2020;33(6):623-630. doi:10.1016/j.jpag.2020.07.011

4 - Brosens I, Gordts S, Benagiano G. Endometriosis in adolescents is a hidden, progressive and severe disease that deserves attention, not just compassion. *Hum Reprod.* 2013;28(8):2026-2031. doi:10.1093/humrep/det243

5 - Dun EC, Kho KA, Morozov VV, Kearney S, Zurawin JL, Nezhat CH. Endometriosis in adolescents. *JSLS.* 2015;19(2):e2015.00019. doi:10.4293/JSLS.2015.00019

Endometriosis in Biological Males and Transgender Men

1 - Balgobind S, Menon V, McKenzie P, Gupta R, Canagasingham B, O'Toole SA. The bleeding obvious – a case of male endometriosis. *Pathology.* 2019;51:S71-S72. doi:10.1016/j.pathol.2018.12.168

2 - Rei C, Williams T, Feloney M. Endometriosis in a Man as a Rare Source of Abdominal Pain: A Case Report and Review of the Literature. *Case Rep Obstet Gynecol.* 2018;2018:2083121. Published 2018 Jan 31. doi:10.1155/2018 /2083121

3 - Beckman EN, Pintado SO, Leonard GL, Sternberg WH. Endometriosis of the prostate. *Am J Surg Pathol.* 1985;9(5):374-379. doi:10.1097/00000478-198505000-00008

4 - Pinkert TC, Catlow CE, Straus R. Endometriosis of the urinary bladder in a man with prostatic carcinoma. *Cancer.* 1979;43(4):1562-1567. doi:10.1002/1097-0142(197904)43:4<1562::aid-cncr2820430451>3.0.co;2 -w

5 - Jabr FI, Mani V. An unusual cause of abdominal pain in a male patient: Endometriosis. *Avicenna J Med.* 2014;4(4):99-101. doi:10.4103/2231-0770.140660

6 - González RS, Vnencak-Jones CL, Shi C, Fadare O. Endomyometriosis ("Uterus - like mass") in an XY Male: Case Report With Molecular Confirmation and Literature Review. *International Journal of Surgical Pathology.* 2014;22(5):421-426. doi:10.1177/1066896913501385

7 - Simsek G, Bulus H, Tas A, Koklu S, Yilmaz SB, Coskun A. An unusual cause of inguinal hernia in a male patient: endometriosis. *Gut Liver.* 2012;6(2):284-285. doi:10.5009/gnl.2012.6.2.284

8 - Okita F, Abrao M, Lara LAS, Andres MP, Cunha C, Oliviera Brito LG. Endometriosis in Transgender Men – a Systematic Review with Metanalysis. *Journal of Minimally Invasive Gynecology.* 2021;28(11):S103-S104. doi:https://doi.org/10.1016/j.jmig.2021.09.140

PART 2

1 - Wolthuis A, Meuleman C, Tomassetti C, D'Hooghe T, De Buck Van

Overstraeten A, D'Hoore A. Bowel endometriosis: Colorectal surgeon's perspective in a multidisciplinary surgical team. *World Journal of Gastroenterology*. 2014;20(42):15616. doi:10.3748/wjg.v20.i42.15616

2 - Dun EC, Kho KA, Morozov V, Kearney S, Zurawin J, Nezhat CH. Endometriosis in adolescents. *JSLS*. 2015;19(2):e2015.00019. doi:10.4293/jsls.2015.00019

PART 3

Introduction

1 - NHS. *Information for you about Laparoscopic Excision of Endometriosis*. NHS North Bristol. 2017 https://www.nbt.nhs.uk/sites/default/files/attachments/Information%20for%20you%20about%20Laparoscopic%20Excision%20of%20Endometriosis_NBT003081.pdf. Accessed 28th May 2023

2 - Guo S. Recurrence of endometriosis and its control. *Human Reproduction Update*. 2009;15(4):441–461. doi:10.1093/humupd/dmp007

3 - Nirgianakis K, Ma L, McKinnon B, Mueller MD. Recurrence Patterns after Surgery in Patients with Different Endometriosis Subtypes: A Long-Term Hospital-Based Cohort Study. *Journal of Clinical Medicine*. 2020;9(2):496. doi:10.3390/jcm9020496

Pain Medication

1 - NICE, Ibuprofen, Available at https://bnf.nice.org.uk/drugs/ibuprofen/. Accessed 31st May 2023

Hormone Treatment:

1 - Donnez J, Dolmans MM. Endometriosis and Medical Therapy: From Progestogens to Progesterone Resistance to GnRH Antagonists: A Review. *J Clin Med*. 2021;10(5):1085. Published 2021 Mar 5. doi:10.3390/jcm10051085

2 - Zhang P, Wang G. Progesterone Resistance in Endometriosis: Current Evidence and Putative Mechanisms. *Int J Mol Sci*. 2023;24(8):6992. Published 2023 Apr 10. doi:10.3390/ijms24086992

Surgery

1 - Misal, M., Scott, D., Girardo, M., & Wasson, M. (2021). Histologic-Proven Recurrence of Endometriosis after Previous Ablation Vs. Excision Surgery. *Journal of Minimally Invasive Gynecology*, 28(11), S108–S109. https://doi.org/10.1016/j.jmig.2021.09.156

2 - Selçuk I, Bozdağ G. Recurrence of endometriosis; risk factors, mechanisms and biomarkers; review of the literature. *J Turk Ger Gynecol Assoc.* 2013;14(2):98-103. Published 2013 Jun 1. doi:10.5152/jtgga.2013.523 85

3 - Rizk, B., Turki, R., Lotfy, H., Ranganathan, S., Zahed, H., Freeman, A. R., Shilbayeh, Z., Sassy, M., Shalaby, M., & Malik, R. (2015). Surgery for endometriosis-associated infertility: do we exaggerate the magnitude of effect?. *Facts, views & vision in ObGyn*, 7(2), 109–118.

4 - Pundir J, Omanwa K, Kovoor E, Pundir V, Lancaster G, Barton-Smith P. Laparoscopic Excision Versus Ablation for Endometriosis-associated Pain: An Updated Systematic Review and Meta-analysis. *J Minim Invasive Gynecol.* 2017;24(5):747-756. doi:10.1016/j.jmig.2017.04.008

5 - Redwine D. B. (1991). Conservative laparoscopic excision of endometriosis by sharp dissection: life table analysis of reoperation and persistent or recurrent disease. *Fertility and sterility*, 56(4), 628–634. https://doi.org/10.1016/s0015-0282(16)54591-9

Bowel Surgery

1 - Wang G, Tokushige N, Russell P, Dubinovsky S, Markham R, Fraser IS. Hyperinnervation in intestinal deep infiltrating endometriosis. *J Minim Invasive Gynecol.* 2009;16(6):713-719. doi:10.1016/j.jmig.2009.07.012.

2 - Wolthuis AM, Meuleman C, Tomassetti C, D'Hooghe T, de Buck van Overstraeten A, D'Hoore A. Bowel endometriosis: colorectal surgeon's perspective in a multidisciplinary surgical team. *World J Gastroenterol.* 2014;20(42):15616-15623. doi:10.3748/wjg.v20.i42.15616

Urological Surgery:

1 - Vercellini P, Pisacreta A, Pesole A, Vicentini S, Stellato G,

Crosignani PG. Is ureteral endometriosis an asymmetric disease?. *BJOG*. 2000;107(4):559-561. doi:10.1111/j.1471-0528.2000.tb13279.x

Hysterectomy

1 - Amarin Z. Hysterectomy: past, present and future. In: *IntechOpen eBooks.* ; 2022. doi:10.5772/intechopen.103086

2 - Murphy AA. Clinical aspects of endometriosis. *Annals of the New York Academy of Sciences.* 2002;955(1):1-10. doi:10.1111/j.1749-6632.2002.tb02760.x

3 - Sandström A, Bixo M, Johansson M, Bäckström T, Türkmen Ş. Effect of hysterectomy on pain in women with endometriosis: a population-based registry study. *BJOG: An International Journal of Obstetrics and Gynaecology.* 2020;127(13):1628-1635. doi:10.1111/1471-0528.16328

4 - King NR, Zeccola A, Wang L, Harris J, Foley CE. The impact of patient age on regret following hysterectomy. *American Journal of Obstetrics & Gynecology.* 2023;228(3). https://www.ajog.org/article/S0002-9378(22)02319-5/abstract.

Fertility and Surgery

1 - Horne PA, Pearson C. *Endometriosis: The Experts' Guide to Treat, Manage and Live Well with Your Symptoms.* National Geographic Books; 2018.

2 - Dückelmann AM, Taube E, Abesadze E, Chiantera V, Sehouli J, Mechsner S. When and how should peritoneal endometriosis be operated on in order to improve fertility rates and symptoms? The experience and outcomes of nearly 100 cases. *Arch Gynecol Obstet.* 2021;304(1):143-155. doi:10.1007/s00404-021-05971-6

3 - Rizk B, Turki R, Lotfy H, et al. Surgery for endometriosis-associated infertility: do we exaggerate the magnitude of effect?. *Facts Views Vis Obgyn.* 2015;7(2):109-118.

4 - Endometriosis UK. *Endometriosis, Fertility and Pregnancy.* https://www.endometriosis-uk.org/sites/default/files/2023-02/Endometriosis%20UK%20-%20Endometriosis%2C%20Fertility%20and%20Pregnancy%20Jan%202023.pdf.

5 - Leone Roberti Maggiore U, Scala C, Venturini PL, Remorgida V, Ferrero S. Endometriotic ovarian cysts do not negatively affect the rate of spontaneous ovulation. *Hum Reprod.* 2015;30(2):299-307. doi:10.1093/hu mrep/deu308

6 - Carrillo LIV, Seidman DS, Cittadini E, Meirow D. The role of fertility preservation in patients with endometriosis. *Journal of Assisted Reproduction and Genetics.* 2016;33(3):317-323. doi:10.1007/s10815-016-0646-z

7 - Ferrero S, Scala C, Tafi E, Racca A, Venturini PL, Maggiore ULR. Impact of large ovarian endometriomas on the response to superovulation for in vitro fertilization: A retrospective study. *European Journal of Obstetrics & Gynecology and Reproductive Biology.* 2017;213:17-21. doi:10.1016/j.ejogrb.2 017.04.003

8 - Alshehre SM, Narice BF, Fenwick MA, Metwally M. The impact of endometrioma on in vitro fertilisation/intra-cytoplasmic injection IVF/ICSI reproductive outcomes: a systematic review and meta-analysis. *Arch Gynecol Obstet.* 2021;303(1):3-16. doi:10.1007/s00404-020-05796-9

9 - Lapointe M, Pontvianne M, Faller E, et al. Impact of surgery for colorectal endometriosis on postoperative fertility and pregnancy outcomes. *J Gynecol Obstet Hum Reprod.* 2022;51(4):102348. doi:10.101 6/j.jogoh.2022.102348

10 - Iversen ML, Seyer-Hansen M, Forman A. Does surgery for deep infiltrating bowel endometriosis improve fertility? A systematic review. *Acta Obstetricia Et Gynecologica Scandinavica.* 2017;96(6):688-693. doi:10.11 11/aogs.13152

11 - Uccella S, Cromi A, Agosti M, et al. Fertility rates, course of pregnancy and perinatal outcomes after laparoscopic ureterolysis for deep endometriosis: A long-term follow-up study. *Journal of Obstetrics and Gynaecology.* 2016;36(6):800-805. doi:10.3109/01443615.2016.1154512

12 - Fabio Barra and others, Ureteral endometriosis: a systematic review of epidemiology, pathogenesis, diagnosis, treatment, risk of malignant transformation and fertility, *Human Reproduction Update*, Volume 24, Issue 6, November-December 2018, Pages 710–730, https://doi.org/10.1093/hu mupd/dmy027

13 - Becker CM, Bokor A, Heikinheimo O, et al. ESHRE guideline: endometriosis. *Human Reproduction Open.* 2022;2022(2). doi:10.1093/hropen/hoac009

14 - Chavarro JE, Rich-Edwards JW, Rosner BA, Willett WC. Diet and lifestyle in the prevention of ovulatory disorder infertility. *Obstet Gynecol.* 2007;110(5):1050-1058. doi:10.1097/01.AOG.0000287293.25465.e1

15 - Chavarro JE, Rich-Edwards JW, Rosner BA, Willett WC. Iron intake and risk of ovulatory infertility. *Obstet Gynecol.* 2006;108(5):1145-1152. doi:10.1097/01.AOG.0000238333.37423.ab

16 - Chavarro JE, Rich-Edwards JW, Rosner BA, Willett WC. Protein intake and ovulatory infertility. *Am J Obstet Gynecol.* 2008;198(2):210.e1-210.e2107. doi:10.1016/j.ajog.2007.06.057

The Four Pillars of Health - Nutrition

1 - Michaels M, Madsen K. Immunometabolism and microbial metabolites at the gut barrier: Lessons for therapeutic intervention in inflammatory bowel disease. *Mucosal Immunology.* 2023;16(1):72-85. doi:10.1016/j.mucimm.2022.11.001

2 - Wiertsema SP, Van Bergenhenegouwen J, Garssen J, Knippels LMJ. The Interplay between the Gut Microbiome and the Immune System in the Context of Infectious Diseases throughout Life and the Role of Nutrition in Optimizing Treatment Strategies. *Nutrients.* 2021;13(3):886. doi:10.339 0/nu13030886

Myth #1 - Food has No Role in Managing Endometriosis

1 - Xiao Y, Xia J, Li L, et al. Associations between dietary patterns and the risk of breast cancer: a systematic review and meta-analysis of observational studies. *Breast Cancer Research.* 2019;21(1). doi:10.1186/s13058-019-1096-1

2 - Tsubura A, Uehara N, Kiyozuka Y, Shikata N. Dietary factors modifying breast cancer risk and relation to time of intake. *Journal of Mammary Gland Biology and Neoplasia.* 2005;10(1):87-100. doi:10.1007/s10911-005-2543-4

3 - Tomio K, Kawana K, Taguchi A, et al. Omega-3 polyunsaturated fatty acids suppress the cystic lesion formation of peritoneal endometriosis in transgenic mouse models. *PLOS ONE*. 2013;8(9):e73085. doi:10.1371/journ al.pone.0073085

4 - Tomio K, Kawana K, Taguchi A, et al. Omega-3 polyunsaturated fatty acids suppress the cystic lesion formation of peritoneal endometriosis in transgenic mouse models. *PLOS ONE*. 2013;8(9):e73085. doi:10.1371/journ al.pone.0073085

5 - Attaman J, Stanic AK, Kim M, Lynch MJ, Rueda BR, Styer AK. The Anti-Inflammatory impact of omega-3 polyunsaturated fatty acids during the establishment of Endometriosis-Like lesions. *American Journal of Reproductive Immunology*. 2014;72(4):392-402. doi:10.1111/aji.12276

6 - Missmer SA, Chavarro JE, Malspeis S, et al. A prospective study of dietary fat consumption and endometriosis risk. *Human Reproduction*. 2010;25(6):1528-1535. doi:10.1093/humrep/deq044

7 - Marcinkowska A, Górnicka M. The role of dietary fats in the development and treatment of endometriosis. *Life*. 2023;13(3):654. doi:10.3390/li fe13030654

8 - Netsu S, Konno R, Odagiri K, Soma M, Fujiwara H, Suzuki M. Oral eicosapentaenoic acid supplementation as possible therapy for endometriosis. *Fertility and Sterility*. 2008;90(4):1496-1502. doi:10.1016/j.fer tnstert.2007.08.014

9 - Habib N, Buzzaccarini G, Centini G, et al. Impact of lifestyle and diet on endometriosis: a fresh look to a busy corner. *Przeglad Menopauzalny*. 2022;21(2):124-132. doi:10.5114/pm.2022.116437

10 - Rahbar N, Asgharzadeh N, Ghorbani R. Effect of omega-3 fatty acids on intensity of primary dysmenorrhea. *International Journal of Gynecology & Obstetrics*. 2012;117(1):45-47. doi:10.1016/j.ijgo.2011.11.019

11 - Donnez J, Binda MM, Donnez O, Dolmans MM. Oxidative stress in the pelvic cavity and its role in the pathogenesis of endometriosis. *Fertility and Sterility*. 2016;106(5):1011-1017. doi:10.1016/j.fertnstert.2016.07.1075

12 - Carvalho L, Samadder AN, Agarwal A, Fernandes LM, Abrão MS. Oxidative stress biomarkers in patients with endometriosis: systematic

review. *Archives of Gynecology and Obstetrics.* 2012;286(4):1033-1040. doi:10.1007/s00404-012-2439-7

13 - Marcinkowska A, Górnicka M. The role of dietary fats in the development and treatment of endometriosis. *Life.* 2023;13(3):654. doi:10.3390/life13030654

14 - Arab A, Karimi E, Vingrys K, Kelishadi MR, Mehrabani S, Askari G. Food groups and nutrients consumption and risk of endometriosis: a systematic review and meta-analysis of observational studies. *Nutrition Journal.* 2022;21(1). doi:10.1186/s12937-022-00812-x

15 - Jurkiewicz-Przondziono J, Lemm M, Kwiatkowska-Pamuła A, Ziółko E, Wójtowicz M. Influence of diet on the risk of developing endometriosis. *Ginekologia Polska.* 2017;88(2):96-102. doi:10.5603/gp.a2017.0017

16 - Brinkman M, Baglietto L, Krishnan K, et al. Consumption of animal products, their nutrient components and postmenopausal circulating steroid hormone concentrations. *European Journal of Clinical Nutrition.* 2009;64(2):176-183. doi:10.1038/ejcn.2009.129

17 - Wang Y, Uffelman C, Hill E, et al. The Effects of red meat intake on inflammation biomarkers in Humans: A Systematic Review and Meta-Analysis of Randomized Controlled Trials. *Current Developments in Nutrition.* 2022;6:994. doi:10.1093/cdn/nzac068.023

18 - Yamamoto A, Harris HR, Vitonis AF, Chavarro JE, Missmer SA. A prospective cohort study of meat and fish consumption and endometriosis risk. *American Journal of Obstetrics and Gynecology.* 2018;219(2):178.e1-178.e10. doi:10.1016/j.ajog.2018.05.034

19 - Ashrafi M, Jahangiri N, Sadatmahalleh SJ, Aliani F, Akhoond MR. Diet and the risk of endometriosis in Iranian women: a Case-Control Study. *DOAJ (DOAJ: Directory of Open Access Journals).* 2020;14(3):193-200. doi:10.22074/ijfs.2020.44378

20 - Trabert B, Peters U, De Roos AJ, Scholes D, Holt VL. Diet and risk of endometriosis in a population-based case–control study. *British Journal of Nutrition.* 2010;105(3):459-467. doi:10.1017/s0007114510003661

21 - Parazzini F, Chiaffarino F, Surace M, et al. Selected food intake and risk of endometriosis. *Human Reproduction.* 2004;19(8):1755-1759.

doi:10.1093/humrep/deh395

Myth #2 - You Have to Be Vegan

1 - Barnard ND, Holtz D, Schmidt N, et al. Nutrition in the prevention and treatment of endometriosis: A review. *Frontiers in Nutrition.* 2023;10. doi:10.3389/fnut.2023.1089891

2 - Menzel J, Biemann R, Longree A, et al. Associations of a vegan diet with inflammatory biomarkers. *Scientific Reports.* 2020;10(1). doi:10.1038/s41598-020-58875-x

3 - Malekinejad H, Rezabakhsh A. Hormones in Dairy Foods and Their Impact on Public Health - A Narrative Review Article. *Iran J Public Health.* 2015;44(6):742-758.

4 - Qi X, Zhang W, Ge M, et al. Relationship between dairy products intake and risk of endometriosis: A Systematic Review and Dose-Response Meta-Analysis. *Frontiers in Nutrition.* 2021;8. doi:10.3389/fnut.2021.701860

5 - Endocrinology NLD&. Iodine deficiency in the UK: grabbing the low-hanging fruit. *The Lancet Diabetes & Endocrinology.* 2016;4(6):469. doi:10.1016/s2213-8587(16)30055-9

6 - Teas J, Hurley TG, Hébert JR, Franke AA, Sepkovic DW, Kurzer MS. Dietary seaweed modifies oestrogen and phytoestrogen metabolism in healthy postmenopausal women. *The Journal of Nutrition.* 2009;139(5):939-944. doi:10.3945/jn.108.100834

7 - Skibola CF. The effect of Fucus vesiculosus, an edible brown seaweed, upon menstrual cycle length and hormonal status in three pre-menopausal women: a case report. *BMC Complement Altern Med.* 2004;4:10. Published 2004 Aug 4. doi:10.1186/1472-6882-4-10

Myth #3 - You Need to Go Gluten-Free

1 - Marziali M, Venza M, Lazzaro S, Lazzaro A, Micossi C, Stolfi VM. Gluten-free diet: a new strategy for management of painful endometriosis related symptoms?. *Minerva Chir.* 2012;67(6):499-504.

2 - Mills DS. A conundrum: wheat and gluten avoidance and its implication with endometriosis patients. *Fertility and Sterility.* 2011;96(3):S139.

doi:10.1016/j.fertnstert.2011.07.540

3 - Schwartz N, Afeiche MC, Terry KL, et al. Glycemic index, glycemic load, fiber, and gluten intake and risk of laparoscopically confirmed endometriosis in premenopausal women. *The Journal of Nutrition.* 2022;152(9):2088-2096. doi:10.1093/jn/nxac107

Myth #4 - Soy is Bad for Endometriosis

1 - Mueller SO, Simon S, Chae K, Metzler M, Korach KS. Phytoestrogens and their human metabolites show distinct agonistic and antagonistic properties on estrogen receptor (ER) and ER in human cells. *Toxicological Sciences.* 2004;80(1):14-25. doi:10.1093/toxsci/kfh147

2 - Dyson MT, Bulun SE. Cutting SRC-1 down to size in endometriosis. *Nature Medicine.* 2012;18(7):1016-1018. doi:10.1038/nm.2855

3 - Harris HA, Bruner-Tran KL, Zhang X, Osteen KG, Lyttle CR. A selective estrogen receptor-β agonist causes lesion regression in an experimentally induced model of endometriosis. *Human Reproduction.* 2005;20(4):936-941. doi:10.1093/humrep/deh711

4 - Marquardt RM, Kim TH, Shin JH, Guo SW. Progesterone and estrogen signaling in the endometrium: What goes wrong in endometriosis? *International Journal of Molecular Sciences.* 2019;20(15):3822. doi:10.3390/ijms20153822

5 - Bartiromo L, Schimberni M, Villanacci R, et al. Endometriosis and phytoestrogens: Friends or foes? A Systematic review. *Nutrients.* 2021;13(8):2532. doi:10.3390/nu13082532

6 - Vahid Dastjerdi M, Eslami B, Alsadat Sharifi M, et al. Effect of Soy Isoflavone on Hot Flushes, Endometrial Thickness, and Breast Clinical as well as Sonographic Features. *Iran J Public Health.* 2018;47(3):382-389.

7 - Tsuchiya M, Miura T, Hanaoka T, et al. Effect of soy isoflavones on endometriosis. *Epidemiology.* 2007;18(3):402-408. doi:10.1097/01.ede.0000257571.01358.f9

8 - Yen C, Kim M, Lee C. Epidemiologic factors associated with endometriosis in East Asia. *Gynecology and Minimally Invasive Therapy.* 2019;8(1):4. doi:10.4103/gmit.gmit_83_18

9 - Upson K, Sathyanarayana S, Scholes D, Holt VL. Early-life factors and endometriosis risk. *Fertility and Sterility*. 2015;104(4):964-971.e5. doi:10.1016/j.fertnstert.2015.06.040

10 - Glazier MG, Bowman MA. A review of the evidence for the use of phytoestrogens as a replacement for traditional estrogen replacement therapy. *Archives of Internal Medicine*. 2001;161(9):1161. doi:10.1001/archin te.161.9.1161

11 - Liu J, Yuan F, Gao J, et al. Oral isoflavone supplementation on endometrial thickness: a meta-analysis of randomized placebo-controlled trials. *Oncotarget*. 2016;7(14):17369-17379. doi:10.18632/oncotarget.7959

Food to Support the Microbiome

1 - Barber TM, Kabisch S, Pfeiffer AFH, Weickert MO. The health benefits of dietary fibre. *Nutrients*. 2020;12(10):3209. doi:10.3390/nu12103209

2 - Zengul A, Demark-Wahnefried W, Barnes S, et al. Associations between Dietary Fiber, the Fecal Microbiota and Estrogen Metabolism in Postmenopausal Women with Breast Cancer. *Nutrition and Cancer*. 2020;73(7):1108-1117. doi:10.1080/01635581.2020.1784444

3 - Holt VL, Trabert B, Upson K. Endometriosis. In: *Elsevier eBooks*. ; 2013:271-284. doi:10.1016/b978-0-12-384978-6.00018-2

4 - Pouille CL, Ouaza S, Roels E, et al. Chicory: Understanding the effects and effectors of this functional food. *Nutrients*. 2022;14(5):957. doi:10.339 0/nu14050957

5 - Kumar VP, Prashanth KVH, Venkatesh YP. Structural analyses and immunomodulatory properties of fructo-oligosaccharides from onion (Allium cepa). *Carbohydrate Polymers*. 2015;117:115-122. doi:10.1016/j.carb pol.2014.09.039

6 - Zhang N, Xue-Song H, Zeng Y, Wu X, Peng X. Study on prebiotic effectiveness of neutral garlic fructan in vitro. *Food Science and Human Wellness*. 2013;2(3-4):119 123. doi:10.1016/j.fshw.2013.07.001

7 - Van Den Abbeele P, Ghyselinck J, Marzorati M, et al. In vitro evaluation of prebiotic properties of a commercial artichoke inflorescence extract revealed bifidogenic effects. *Nutrients*. 2020;12(6):1552. doi:10.339

0/nu12061552

8 - Wirngo FE, Lambert MNT, Jeppesen PB. The physiological effects of dandelion (Taraxacum officinale) in type 2 diabetes. *The Review of Diabetic Studies.* 2016;13(2-3):113-131. doi:10.1900/rds.2016.13.113

9 - Public Health England. SACHIN's sugars and health recommendations: why 5%? GOV.UK. https://www.gov.uk/government/publications/sacns-sugars-and-health-recommendations-why-5. Published July 17, 2015.

10 - Ma X, Fang N, Liang H, et al. Excessive intake of sugar: An accomplice of inflammation. *Frontiers in Immunology.* 2022;13. doi:10.3389/fimmu.2022.988481

11 - Ranneh Y, Akim AM, Hamid HA, et al. Honey and its nutritional and anti-inflammatory value. *BMC Complementary Medicine and Therapies.* 2021;21(1). doi:10.1186/s12906-020-03170-5

12 - Sarkari R. High Intake of Sugar and the Balance between Pro- and Anti-Inflammatory Gut Bacteria. *Nutrients.* 2020;12(5):1348. doi:10.3390/nu12051348

13 - Ahmed SH, Guillem K, Vandaele Y. Sugar addiction. *Current Opinion in Clinical Nutrition and Metabolic Care.* 2013;16(4):434-439. doi:10.1097/mco.0b013e328361c8b8

14 - Lephart ED, Naftolin F. Oestrogen action and gut microbiome metabolism in dermal health. *Dermatology and Therapy.* 2022;12(7):1535-1550. doi:10.1007/s13555-022-00759-1

15 - Madison AA. Stress, depression, diet, and the gut microbiota: human–bacteria interactions at the core of psychoneuroimmunology and nutrition. *Current Opinion in Behavioral Sciences.* 2019;28:105-110. doi:10.1016/j.cobeha.2019.01.011

16 - Nijs J, Yılmaz ST, Elma Ö, et al. Nutritional intervention in chronic pain: an innovative way of targeting central nervous system sensitization? *Expert Opinion on Therapeutic Targets.* 2020;24(8):793-803. doi:10.1080/14728222.2020.1784142

Low Inflammatory Diet

1 - Ma X, Fang N, Liang H, et al. Excessive intake of sugar: An accomplice of inflammation. *Frontiers in Immunology.* 2022;13. doi:10.3389/fimmu.20 22.988481

2 - Asensi MT, Napoletano A, Sofi F, Dinu M. Low-Grade Inflammation and Ultra-Processed Foods Consumption: A review. *Nutrients.* 2023;15(6):1546. doi:10.3390/nu15061546

3 - Zhu F, Du B, Xu B. Anti-inflammatory effects of phytochemicals from fruits, vegetables, and food legumes: A review. *Critical Reviews in Food Science and Nutrition.* 2017;58(8):1260-1270. doi:10.1080/10408398.2016.1 251390

4 - Xu Y, Wan Q, Feng J, Li D, Li K, Zhou Y. Whole grain diet reduces systemic inflammation. *Medicine.* 2018;97(43):e12995. doi:10.1097/md.00 00000000012995

5 - Liu P, Maharjan R, Wang Y, et al. Association between dietary inflammatory index and risk of endometriosis: A population-based analysis. *Frontiers in Nutrition.* 2023;10. doi:10.3389/fnut.2023.1077915

6 - Malik V, Hu FB. The role of sugar-sweetened beverages in the global epidemics of obesity and chronic diseases. *Nature Reviews Endocrinology.* 2022;18(4):205-218. doi:10.1038/s41574-021-00627-6

7 - Gazvani MR, Smith L, Haggarty P, Fowler PA, Templeton A. High ω-3:ω-6 fatty acid ratios in culture medium reduce endometrial-cell survival in combined endometrial gland and stromal cell cultures from women with and without endometriosis. *Fertility and Sterility.* 2001;76(4):717-722. doi:10.1016/s0015-0282(01)01991-4

8 - Yamamoto A, Harris HR, Vitonis AF, Chavarro JE, Missmer SA. A prospective cohort study of meat and fish consumption and endometriosis risk. *American Journal of Obstetrics and Gynecology.* 2018;219(2):178.e1-178.e10. doi:10.1016/j.ajog.2018.05.034

9 - Jungbauer A, Medjakovic S. Anti-inflammatory properties of culinary herbs and spices that ameliorate the effects of metabolic syndrome. *Maturitas.* 2012;71(3):227-239. doi:10.1016/j.maturitas.2011.12.009

10 - Jiang T. Health benefits of culinary herbs and spices. *Journal of AOAC INTERNATIONAL.* 2019;102(2):395-411. doi:10.5740/jaoacint.18-0418

11 - Oteng A, Kersten S. Mechanisms of Action of trans Fatty Acids. *Advances in Nutrition*. 2020;11(3):697-708. doi:10.1093/advances/nmz125

12 - WHO REPLACE trans fat. https://www.who.int/teams/nutrition-and-food-safety/replace-trans-fat#:~:text=Increased%20intake%20of%20trans%20fat,each%20year%20around%20the%20world. Published January 29, 2024.

13 - Ma X, Fang N, Liang H, et al. Excessive intake of sugar: An accomplice of inflammation. *Frontiers in Immunology*. 2022;13. doi:10.3389/fimmu.2022.988481

14 - Christ A, Lauterbach MA, Latz E. Western diet and the immune system: an inflammatory connection. *Immunity*. 2019;51(5):794-811. doi:10.1016/j.immuni.2019.09.020

15 - Parazzini F, Chiaffarino F, Surace M, et al. Selected food intake and risk of endometriosis. *Human Reproduction*. 2004;19(8):1755-1759. doi:10.1093/humrep/deh395

16 - Uribarri J, Cai W, Peppa M, et al. Circulating glycotoxins and dietary advanced glycation endproducts: two links to inflammatory response, oxidative stress, and aging. *The Journals of Gerontology: Series A*. 2007;62(4):427-433. doi:10.1093/gerona/62.4.427

17 - Gao J, Guo X, Wei W, et al. The association of fried meat consumption with the gut microbiota and fecal metabolites and its impact on glucose homoeostasis, intestinal endotoxin levels, and systemic inflammation: a Randomized Controlled-Feeding trial. *Diabetes Care*. 2021;44(9):1970-1979. doi:10.2337/dc21-0099

18 - DiNicolantonio JJ, O'Keefe J. The Importance of Maintaining a Low Omega-6/Omega-3 Ratio for Reducing the Risk of Autoimmune Diseases, Asthma, and Allergies. *Mo Med*. 2021;118(5):453-459.

Vegetables & Fruit

1 - Harris HR, Eke AC, Chavarro JE, Missmer SA. Fruit and vegetable consumption and risk of endometriosis. *Hum Reprod*. 2018;33(4):715-727. doi:10.1093/humrep/dey014

2 - C Wang SQ, Cheng LS, Liu Y, Wang JY, Jiang W. Indole-3-Carbinol (I3C)

and its Major Derivatives: Their Pharmacokinetics and Important Roles in Hepatic Protection. *Curr Drug Metab.* 2016;17(4):401-409. doi:10.2174/138 9200217666151210125105

3 - Thomson CA, Ho E, Strom MB. Chemopreventive properties of 3,3'-diindolylmethane in breast cancer: evidence from experimental and human studies. *Nutr Rev.* 2016;74(7):432-443. doi:10.1093/nutrit/nuw010

4 - Lord RS, Bongiovanni B, Bralley JA. Estrogen metabolism and the diet-cancer connection: rationale for assessing the ratio of urinary hydroxylated estrogen metabolites. *Altern Med Rev.* 2002;7(2):112-129.

5 - Thomson CA, Ho E, Strom M. Chemopreventive properties of 3,3'-diindolylmethane in breast cancer: evidence from experimental and human studies. *Nutrition Reviews.* 2016;74(7):432-443. doi:10.1093/n utrit/nuw010

6 - Parazzini F, Chiaffarino F, Surace M, et al. Selected food intake and risk of endometriosis. *Human Reproduction.* 2004;19(8):1755-1759. doi:10.1093/humrep/deh395

7 - Harris HR, Eke AC, Chavarro JE, Missmer SA. Fruit and vegetable consumption and risk of endometriosis. *Hum Reprod.* 2018;33(4):715-727. doi:10.1093/humrep/dey014

8 - Trabert B, Peters U, De Roos AJ, Scholes D, Holt VL. Diet and risk of endometriosis in a population-based case-control study. *Br J Nutr.* 2011;105(3):459-467. doi:10.1017/S0007114510003661

9 - Polak G, Banaszewska B, Filip M, Radwan M, Wdowiak A. Environmental Factors and Endometriosis. *Int J Environ Res Public Health.* 2021;18(21):11025. Published 2021 Oct 20. doi:10.3390/ijerph182111025

10 - Darling AM, Chavarro JE, Malspeis S, Harris HR, Missmer SA. A prospective cohort study of Vitamins B, C, E, and multivitamin intake and endometriosis. *J Endometr.* 2013;5(1):17-26. doi:10.5301/je.500015

Organic Food

1 - Crinnion WJ. Organic foods contain higher levels of certain nutrients, lower levels of pesticides, and may provide health benefits for the consumer. *Altern Med Rev.* 2010;15(1):4-12.

2 - Davis H, Magistrali A, Butler G, Stergiadis S. Nutritional Benefits from Fatty Acids in Organic and Grass-Fed Beef. *Foods*. 2022;11(5):646. doi:10.3390/foods11050646

3 - Średnicka-Tober D, Barański M, Seal C, et al. Composition differences between organic and conventional meat: a systematic literature review and meta-analysis. *Br J Nutr*. 2016;115(6):994-1011. doi:10.1017/S0007114 515005073

FODMAP Diet

1 - Shepherd S, Lomer M, Gibson PR. Short-Chain carbohydrates and functional gastrointestinal disorders. *The American Journal of Gastroen-terology*. 2013;108(5):707-717. doi:10.1038/ajg.2013.96

2 - Moore JS, Gibson PR, Perry RE, Burgell R. Endometriosis in patients with irritable bowel syndrome: Specific symptomatic and demographic profile, and response to the low FODMAP diet. *Australian and New Zealand Journal of Obstetrics and Gynaecology*. 2017;57(2):201-205. doi:10.1111/ajo.1 2594

3 - Armour M, Middleton A, Lim S, Sinclair J, Varjabedian D, Smith C. Dietary Practices of Women with Endometriosis: A Cross-Sectional Survey. *Journal of Alternative and Complementary Medicine*. 2021;27(9):771-777. doi:10.1089/acm.2021.0068

4 - Nanayakkara WS, Skidmore P, O'Brien L, Wilkinson T, Gearry RB. Efficacy of the low FODMAP diet for treating irritable bowel syndrome: the evidence to date. *Clinical and Experimental Gastroenterology*. June 2016:131. doi:10.2147/ceg.s86798

5 - *Low FODMAP Diet - FODMAP Foods*. Gastroenterology Consultants of San Antonio. Retrieved July 19, 2023, from https://www.gastroconsa.com/wp-content/uploads/2019/09/Low-FODMAP-Diet-FODMAP-Foods-Upd ated.pdf

Histamine & Allergies

1 - Schink M, Konturek PC, Herbert S, et al. Different nutrient intake and prevalence of gastrointestinal comorbidities in women with endometriosis.

PubMed. 2019;70(2). doi:10.26402/jpp.2019.2.09

2 - McCallion A, Nasirzadeh Y, Lingegowda H, et al. Estrogen mediates inflammatory role of mast cells in endometriosis pathophysiology. *Frontiers in Immunology.* 2022;13. doi:10.3389/fimmu.2022.961599

3 - Zaitsu M, Narita S, Lambert K, et al. Estradiol activates mast cells via a non-genomic estrogen receptor-α and calcium influx. *Molecular Immunology.* 2007;44(8):1977-1985. doi:10.1016/j.molimm.2006.09.030

4 - Zhu T, Ding S, Li T, Zhu L, Huang X, Zhang X. Estrogen is an important mediator of mast cell activation in ovarian endometriomas. *Reproduction.* 2018;155(1):73-83. doi:10.1530/rep-17-0457

5 - Graziottin. *Mast cells and their role in sexual pain disorders: Goldstein A. Pukall C. Goldstein I. (Eds), Female Sexual Pain Disorders: Evaluation and Management, p. 176-179.* Blackwell Publishing; 2009. https://www.fondaz ionegraziottin.org/ew/ew_articolo/1820%20-%20mast%20cells%20and %20SPD.pdf.

6 - Hart DA. Targeting mast cells as a viable therapeutic option in endometriosis. *European Medical Journal.* August 2017:76-83. doi:10.3359 0/emjreprohealth/10314034

Alcohol

1 - World Health Organization: WHO. No level of alcohol consumption is safe for our health. *WHO.* https://www.who.int/europe/news/item/0 4-01-2023-no-level-of-alcohol-consumption-is-safe-for-our-health. Published January 4, 2023.

2 - Wu D, Cederbaum AI. Alcohol, oxidative stress, and free radical damage. *Alcohol Res Health.* 2003;27(4):277-284.

3 - Spencer RL, Hutchison KE. Alcohol, aging, and the stress response. *Alcohol Res Health.* 1999;23(4):272-283.

4 - Bishehsari F, Magno E, Swanson G, et al. Alcohol and Gut-Derived Inflammation. *Alcohol Res.* 2017;38(2):163-171.

5 - Lowe P, Gyöngyösi B, Satishchandran A, et al. Reduced gut microbiome protects from alcohol-induced neuroinflammation and alters intestinal and brain inflammasome expression. *Journal of Neuroinflammation.*

2018;15(1). doi:10.1186/s12974-018-1328-9

6 - De Angelis C, Nardone A, Garifalos F, et al. Smoke, alcohol and drug addiction and female fertility. *Reproductive Biology and Endocrinology.* 2020;18(1). doi:10.1186/s12958-020-0567-7

7 - McDonald JA, Goyal A, Terry MB. Alcohol intake and breast cancer risk: Weighing the Overall evidence. *Current Breast Cancer Reports.* 2013;5(3):208-221. doi:10.1007/s12609-013-0114-z

8 - Alcohol and Cancer risk fact sheet. Cancer.gov. https://www.cancer.gov/about-cancer/causes-prevention/risk/alcohol/alcohol-fact-sheet. Published July 14, 2021.

Supplements:

1 - Office of Dietary Supplements - Folate. https://ods.od.nih.gov/factsheets/Folate-HealthProfessional/.

2 - Mann J, Truswell AS. *Essentials of human nutrition.* Oxford University Press; 2017.

3 - Messalli EM, Schettino MT, Mainini G, et al. The possible role of zinc in the etiopathogenesis of endometriosis. *Clin Exp Obstet Gynecol.* 2014;41(5):541-546.

4 - Mier-Cabrera J, Aburto-Soto T, Burrola-Méndez S, et al. Women with endometriosis improved their peripheral antioxidant markers after the application of a high antioxidant diet. *Reprod Biol Endocrinol.* 2009;7:54. Published 2009 May 28. doi:10.1186/1477-7827-7-54

5 - Wong CP, Rinaldi NA, Ho E. Zinc deficiency enhanced inflammatory response by increasing immune cell activation and inducing IL6 promoter demethylation. *Mol Nutr Food Res.* 2015;59(5):991-999. doi:10.1002/mnfr.201400761

6 - Gammoh NZ, Rink L. Zinc in Infection and Inflammation. *Nutrients.* 2017;9(6):624. Published 2017 Jun 17. doi:10.3390/nu9060624

7 - Teimoori B, Ghasemi M, Hoseini ZS, Razavi M. The efficacy of zinc administration in the treatment of primary dysmenorrhea. *Oman Medical Journal.* 2016;31(2):107-111. doi:10.5001/omj.2016.21

8 - Onuma T, Mizutani T, Fujita Y, et al. Zinc deficiency is associated

with the development of ovarian endometrial cysts. *Am J Cancer Res.* 2023;13(3):1049-1066. Published 2023 Mar 15.

9 - Nasiadek M, Stragierowicz J, Klimczak M, Kilanowicz A. The role of zinc in selected female reproductive system disorders. *Nutrients.* 2020;12(8):2464. doi:10.3390/nu12082464

10 - Palmery M, Saraceno A, Vaiarelli A, Carlomagno G. Oral contraceptives and changes in nutritional requirements. *Eur Rev Med Pharmacol Sci.* 2013;17(13):1804-1813.

11 - Viering D, De Baaij JHF, Walsh SB, Kleta R, Böckenhauer D. Genetic causes of hypomagnesemia, a clinical overview. *Pediatric Nephrology.* 2016;32(7):1123-1135. doi:10.1007/s00467-016-3416-3

12 - Pickering G, Mazur A, Trousselard M, et al. Magnesium Status and Stress: The Vicious Circle Concept revisited. *Nutrients.* 2020;12(12):3672. doi:10.3390/nu12123672

13 - Serefko A, Szopa A, Wlaź P, et al. Magnesium in depression. *Pharmacological Reports.* 2013;65(3):547-554. doi:10.1016/s1734-1140(13)71032-6

14 - Parazzini F, Di Martino M, Pellegrino P. Magnesium in the gynecological practice: a literature review. Magnesium in the gynecological practice: a literature review. *Magnes Res.* 2017;30(1):1-7. doi:10.1684/mrh.2017.0419

15 - Derbyshire E. Micronutrient intakes of British adults across Mid-Life: A secondary analysis of the UK National Diet and Nutrition Survey. *Frontiers in Nutrition.* 2018;5. doi:10.3389/fnut.2018.00055

16 - Nielsen FH. Magnesium deficiency and increased inflammation: current perspectives. *Journal of Inflammation Research.* 2018;Volume 11:25-34. doi:10.2147/jir.s136742

17 - Kapper C, Oppelt P, Ganhör C, et al. Minerals and the Menstrual Cycle: Impacts on Ovulation and Endometrial Health. *Nutrients.* 2024;16(7):1008. Published 2024 Mar 29. doi:10.3390/nu16071008

18 - Harris HR, Chavarro JE, Malspeis S, Willett WC, Missmer SA. Dairy-Food, calcium, magnesium, and vitamin D intake and endometriosis: A Prospective cohort study. *American Journal of Epidemiology.* 2013;177(5):420-430. doi:10.1093/aje/kws247

19 - Lima LG, Santos AAMD, Gueiber TD, Gomes RZ, Martins CM,

Chaikoski AC. Relation between Selenium and Female Fertility: A Systematic Review. Relação entre o selênio e a fertilidade feminina: Uma revisão sistemática. *Rev Bras Ginecol Obstet.* 2022;44(7):701-709. doi:10.1055/s-0042-1744288

20 - Bowden JF, Bender DA, Coulson WF, Symes EK. Increased uterine uptake and nuclear retention of [3H]oestradiol through the oestrous cycle and enhanced end-organ sensitivity to oestrogen stimulation in vitamin B6 deficient rats. *Journal of Steroid Biochemistry.* 1986;25(3):359-365. doi:10.1016/0022-4731(86)90248-7

21 - Wyatt KM, Dimmock PW, Jones PW, Shaughn O'Brien PM. Efficacy of vitamin B-6 in the treatment of premenstrual syndrome: systematic review. *BMJ.* 1999;318(7195):1375-1381. doi:10.1136/bmj.318.7195.1375

22 - Roshanzadeh G, Jahanian Sadatmahalleh S, Moini A, Mottaghi A, Rostami F. The relationship between dietary micronutrients and endometriosis: A case-control study. *Int J Reprod Biomed.* 2023;21(4):333-342. Published 2023 May 8. doi:10.18502/ijrm.v21i4.13272

23 - Brody S, Preut R, Schommer K, Schürmeyer TH. A randomized controlled trial of high dose ascorbic acid for reduction of blood pressure, cortisol, and subjective responses to psychological stress. *Psychopharmacology (Berl).* 2002;159(3):319-324. doi:10.1007/s00213-001-0929-6

24 - Kiondo P, Tumwesigye NM, Wandabwa J, Wamuyu-Maina G, Bimenya GS, Okong P. Plasma vitamin C assay in women of reproductive age in Kampala, Uganda, using a colorimetric method. *Trop Med Int Health.* 2012;17(2):191-196. doi:10.1111/j.1365-3156.2011.02907.x

25 - Henmi H, Endo T, Kitajima Y, Manase K, Hata H, Kudo R. Effects of ascorbic acid supplementation on serum progesterone levels in patients with a luteal phase defect. *Fertility and Sterility.* 2003;80(2):459-461. doi:10.1016/s0015-0282(03)00657-5

26 - Erten Ö, Ensarı TA, Dilbaz B, et al. Vitamin C is effective for the prevention and regression of endometriotic implants in an experimentally induced rat model of endometriosis. *Taiwanese Journal of Obstetrics & Gynecology.* 2016;55(2):251-257. doi:10.1016/j.tjog.2015.07.004

27 - Hoorsan H, Simbar M, Tehrani FR, et al. The effectiveness of

antioxidant therapy (vitamin C) in an experimentally induced mouse model of ovarian endometriosis. Women's Health. 2022;18. doi:10.1177/1745505 7221096218-

28 - Amini L, Chekini R, Nateghi MR, et al. The Effect of Combined Vitamin C and Vitamin E Supplementation on Oxidative Stress Markers in Women with Endometriosis: A Randomized, Triple-Blind Placebo-Controlled Clinical Trial. *Pain Research & Management*. 2021;2021:1-6. doi:10.1155/2021/5529741-

29 - Santanam N, Kavtaradze N, Murphy AA, Dominguez CE, Parthasarathy S. Antioxidant supplementation reduces endometriosis-related pelvic pain in humans. *Translational Research*. 2013;161(3):189-195. doi:10.1016/j.trsl.2012.05.001

30 - Abbas MA, Taha MO, Disi AM, Shomaf M. Regression of endometrial implants treated with vitamin D3 in a rat model of endometriosis. *European Journal of Pharmacology*. 2013;715(1-3):72-75. doi:10.1016/j.ejphar.2013.06. 016

31 - Yıldırım B, Güler ÖT, Akbulut M, Öztekin Ö, Sariiz G. 1–Alpha, 25–Di-hydroxyvitamin D3 regresses endometriotic implants in rats by inhibiting neovascularization and altering regulation of matrix metalloproteinase. *Postgraduate Medicine*. 2014;126(1):104-110. doi:10.3810/pgm.2014.01.2730

32 - La Fata G, Weber P, Mohajeri MH. Effects of Vitamin E on Cognitive Performance during Ageing and in Alzheimer's Disease. *Nutrients*. 2014;6(12):5453-5472. doi:10.3390/nu6125453

33 - Rizvi S, Raza ST, Ahmed F, Ahmad A, Abbas S, Mahdi F. The role of vitamin e in human health and some diseases. *Sultan Qaboos Univ Med J*. 2014;14(2):e157-e165.

34 – Zheng SL, Chen X, Chen Y, Wu Z, Chen XM, Li X. Antioxidant vitamins supplementation reduce endometriosis related pelvic pain in humans: a systematic review and meta-analysis. *Reproductive Biology and Endocrinology*. 2023;21(1). doi:10.1186/s12958-023-01126-1

35 - De Andrade AZ, Rodrigues JK, Dib LA, et al. Marcadores séricos de estresse oxidativo em mulheres inférteis com endometriose. *RBGO Gynecology & Obstetrics*. 2010;32(6):279-285. doi:10.1590/s0100-

72032010000600005

36 - Spencer LT, Mann CD, Metcalfe MS, et al. The effect of omega-3 FAs on tumour angiogenesis and their therapeutic potential. *European Journal of Cancer.* 2009;45(12):2077-2086. doi:10.1016/j.ejca.2009.04.026

37 - Missmer SA, Chavarro JE, Malspeis S, et al. A prospective study of dietary fat consumption and endometriosis risk. *Human Reproduction.* 2010;25(6):1528-1535. doi:10.1093/humrep/deq044

38 -Hopeman MM, Riley JK, Frolova AI, Jiang H, Jungheim ES. Serum Polyunsaturated Fatty Acids and Endometriosis. *Reprod Sci.* 2015;22(9):1083-1087. doi:10.1177/1933719114565030

39 - Gazvani MR, Smith L, Haggarty P, Fowler PA, Templeton A. High ω-3:ω-6 fatty acid ratios in culture medium reduce endometrial-cell survival in combined endometrial gland and stromal cell cultures from women with and without endometriosis. *Fertility and Sterility.* 2001;76(4):717-722. doi:10.1016/s0015-0282(01)01991-4

40 - Tomio K, Kawana K, Taguchi A, et al. Omega-3 polyunsaturated fatty acids suppress the cystic lesion formation of peritoneal endometriosis in transgenic mouse models. *PLOS ONE.* 2013;8(9):e73085. doi:10.1371/journal.pone.0073085

41 - Covens A, Christopher P, Casper RF. The effect of dietary supplementation with fish oil fatty acids on surgically induced endometriosis in the rabbit. *Fertility and Sterility.* 1988;49(4):698-703. doi:10.1016/s0015-0282(16)59842-2

42 - Hansen SO, Knudsen UB. Endometriosis, dysmenorrhoea and diet. *Eur J Obstet Gynecol Reprod Biol.* 2013;169(2):162-171. doi:10.1016/j.ejogrb.2013.03.028

43 - Morales-Prieto DM, Herrmann J, Osterwald H, et al. Comparison of dienogest effects upon 3,3'-diindolylmethane supplementation in models of endometriosis and clinical cases. *Reproductive Biology.* 2018;18(3):252-258. doi:10.1016/j.repbio.2018.07.002

44 - Jiang I, Yong PJ, Allaire C, Bedaiwy MA. Intricate Connections between the Microbiota and Endometriosis. *International Journal of Molecular Sciences.* 2021;22(11):5644. doi:10.3390/ijms22115644

45 - Itoh H, Uchida M, Sashihara T, et al. Lactobacillus gasseri OLL2809 is effective especially on the menstrual pain and dysmenorrhea in endometriosis patients: randomized, double-blind, placebo-controlled study. *Cytotechnology.* 2010;63(2):153-161. doi:10.1007/s10616-010-9326-5

46 - Khodaverdi S, Mohammadbeigi R, Khaledi M, et al. Beneficial Effects of Oral Lactobacillus on Pain Severity in Women Suffering from Endometriosis: A Pilot Placebo-Controlled Randomized Clinical Trial. *DOAJ (DOAJ: Directory of Open Access Journals).* 2019;13(3):178-183. doi:10.22 074/ijfs.2019.5584

47 - Chouzenoux S, Jeljeli M, Bourdon M, et al. A new strategy against endometriosis: Oral probiotic treatments. *Clinical Obstetrics, Gynecology and Reproductive Medicine.* 2021;7(1). doi:10.15761/cogrm.1000324

48 - Kumar LS, Pugalenthi LS, Ahmad M, Reddy S, Barkhane Z, Elmadi J. Probiotics in Irritable Bowel Syndrome: A review of their therapeutic role. *Cureus.* April 2022. doi:10.7759/cureus.24240

49 - Jackson LW, Schisterman EF, Dey-Rao R, Browne RW, Armstrong D. Oxidative stress and endometriosis. *Human Reproduction.* 2005;20(7):2014-2020. doi:10.1093/humrep/dei001

50 - Pınar N, Soylu Karapınar O, Özcan O, Özgür T, Bayraktar S. Effect of alpha-lipoic acid on endometrial implants in an experimental rat model. *Fundam Clin Pharmacol.* 2017;31(5):506-512. doi:10.1111/fcp.12293

51 - Leo D, Cagnacci A, Cappelli, Biasioli A, Leonardi D, Seracchioli R. Role of a natural integrator based on lipoic acid, palmitoiletanolamide and myrrh in the treatment of chronic pelvic pain and endometriosis. *Minerva Ginecologica.* 2019;71(3). doi:10.23736/s0026-4784.19.04384-3

52 - Caruso S, Iraci Sareri M, Casella E, Ventura B, Fava V, Cianci A. Chronic pelvic pain, quality of life and sexual health of women treated with palmitoylethanolamide and α-lipoic acid. *Minerva Ginecol.* 2015;67(5):413-419.

53 - Agostinis C, Zorzet S, De Leo R, Zauli G, De Seta F, Bulla R. The combination of N-Acetyl cysteine, Alpha-Lipoic acid, and bromelain shows high Anti-Inflammatory properties in NovelIn VivoandIn VitroModels of

Endometriosis. *Mediators of Inflammation*. 2015;2015:1-9. doi:10.1155/201 5/918089

54 - Di Nicuolo F, Castellani R, Nardone A, et al. Alpha-Lipoic acid plays a role in endometriosis: New evidence on Inflammasome-Mediated Interleukin Production, cellular adhesion and Invasion. *Molecules.* 2021;26(2):288. doi:10.3390/molecules26020288

55 - Foyouzi N, Berkkanoğlu M, Arıcı A, Kwintkiewicz J, Izquierdo DM, Dulęba AJ. Effects of oxidants and antioxidants on proliferation of endometrial stromal cells. *Fertility and Sterility*. 2004;82:1019-1022. doi:10.1016/j.fertnstert.2004.02.133

56 - Wu Y, Guo S. Inhibition of proliferation of endometrial stromal cells by trichostatin A, RU486, CDB-2914, N-Acetylcysteine, and ICI 182780. *Gynecologic and Obstetric Investigation*. 2006;62(4):193-205. doi:10.1159/0 00093975

57 - Ngô C, Chéreau C, Nicco C, Weill B, Chapron C, Batteux F. Reactive oxygen species controls endometriosis progression. *The American Journal of Pathology*. 2009;175(1):225-234. doi:10.2353/ajpath.2009.080804

58 - Pittaluga E, Costa G, Krasnowska EK, et al. More than antioxidant: N-acetyl-L-cysteine in a murine model of endometriosis. *Fertility and Sterility*. 2010;94(7):2905-2908. doi:10.1016/j.fertnstert.2010.06.038

59 - Porpora MG, Brunelli R, Costa G, et al. A promise in the treatment of endometriosis: an observational cohort study on ovarian endometrioma reduction by N-acetylcysteine. *Evid Based Complement Alternat Med.* 2013;2013:240702. doi:10.1155/2013/240702

60 - Anastasi E, Scaramuzzino S, Viscardi MF, et al. Efficacy of N-Acetylcysteine on Endometriosis-Related pain, size reduction of ovarian endometriomas, and fertility outcomes. *International Journal of Environmental Research and Public Health*. 2023;20(6):4686. doi:10.3390/ijerph20 064686

61 - Lete I, Mendoza N, De La Viuda E, Carmona F. Effectiveness of an antioxidant preparation with N-acetyl cysteine, alpha lipoic acid and bromelain in the treatment of endometriosis-associated pelvic pain: LEAP study. *European Journal of Obstetrics & Gynecology and Reproductive Biology*.

2018;228:221-224. doi:10.1016/j.ejogrb.2018.07.002

62 - Sharma I, Thakur A, Sharma A, Singh R, Kumar R, Sharma A. Phytoalexins: Implications in Plant Defense and Human Health. In: *Plant Secondary Metabolites.* ; 2022:329-353. doi:10.1007/978-981-16-4779-6_10

63 - Arablou T, Aryaeian N, Khodaverdi S, et al. The effects of resveratrol on the expression of VEGF, TGF-β, and MMP-9 in endometrial stromal cells of women with endometriosis. *Scientific Reports.* 2021;11(1). doi:10.1038/s41598-021-85512-y

64 - Mohammadi RK, Arablou T. Resveratrol and endometriosis: In vitro and animal studies and underlying mechanisms (Review). *Biomedicine & Pharmacotherapy.* 2017;91:220-228. doi:10.1016/j.biopha.2017.04.078

65 - Dull AM, Moga MA, Dimienescu OG, Sechel G, Burtea V, Anastasiu CV. Therapeutic Approaches of Resveratrol on Endometriosis via Anti-Inflammatory and Anti-Angiogenic Pathways. *Molecules.* 2019;24(4):667. Published 2019 Feb 13. doi:10.3390/molecules24040667

66 - Singh BN, Shankar S, Srivastava RK. Green tea catechin, epigallocatechin-3-gallate (EGCG): Mechanisms, perspectives and clinical applications. *Biochemical Pharmacology.* 2011;82(12):1807-1821. doi:10.1016/j.bcp.2011.07.093

67 - Laschke MW, Schwender C, Scheuer C, Vollmar B, Menger MD. Epigallocatechin-3-gallate inhibits estrogen-induced activation of endometrial cells in vitro and causes regression of endometriotic lesions in vivo. *Human Reproduction.* 2008;23(10):2308-2318. doi:10.1093/humrep/den245

68 - Wang CC, Xu H, Man GCW, et al. Prodrug of green tea epigallocatechin-3-gallate (Pro-EGCG) as a potent anti-angiogenesis agent for endometriosis in mice. *Angiogenesis.* 2012;16(1):59-69. doi:10.1007/s10456-012-9299-4

69 - Matsuzaki S, Darcha C. Antifibrotic properties of epigallocatechin-3-gallate in endometriosis. *Human Reproduction.* 2014;29(8):1677-1687. doi:10.1093/humrep/deu123

70 - Chen X, Man GCW, Hung SW, et al. Therapeutic effects of green

tea on endometriosis. *Critical Reviews in Food Science and Nutrition.* 2021;63(18):3222-3235. doi:10.1080/10408398.2021.1986465

71 - Kamal DAM, Salamt N, Zaid SSM, Mokhtar MH. Beneficial Effects of green tea catechins on female reproductive disorders: a review. *Molecules.* 2021;26(9):2675. doi:10.3390/molecules26092675

72 - Chen Y, Zhu B, Zhang H, Liu X, Guo S. Epigallocatechin-3-Gallate reduces myometrial infiltration, uterine hyperactivity, and stress levels and alleviates generalized hyperalgesia in mice induced with adenomyosis. *Reproductive Sciences.* 2013;20(12):1478-1491. doi:10.1177/193371911134884 55

73 - Park, S., Lim, W., Bazer, F. W., Whang, K. Y., & Song, G. (2019). Quercetin inhibits proliferation of endometriosis regulating cyclin D1 and its target microRNAs in vitro and in vivo. *The Journal of nutritional biochemistry, 63,* 87–100. https://doi.org/10.1016/j.jnutbio.2018.09.024.

74 - Cao Y, Zhuang M, Yang Y, et al. Preliminary study of Quercetin affecting the Hypothalamic-Pituitary-Gonadal axis on rat endometriosis model. *Evidence-based Complementary and Alternative Medicine.* 2014;2014:1-12. doi:10.1155/2014/781684

75 - Ezzati M, Yousefi B, Velaei K, Safa A. A review on anti-cancer properties of Quercetin in breast cancer. *Life Sciences.* 2020;248:117463. doi:10.1016/j.lfs.2020.117463

76 - Vafadar A, Shabaninejad Z, Movahedpour A, et al. Quercetin and cancer: new insights into its therapeutic effects on ovarian cancer cells. *Cell & Bioscience.* 2020;10(1). doi:10.1186/s13578-020-00397-0

77 - Ali A, Kim MJ, Lee HJ, et al. Quercetin induces cell death in cervical cancer by reducing O-GlcNAcylation of adenosine monophosphate-activated protein kinase. *Anatomy & Cell Biology.* 2018;51(4):274. doi:10.51 15/acb.2018.51.4.274

78 - Mlcek J, Jurikova T, Skrovankova S, Sochor J. Quercetin and Its Anti-Allergic Immune Response. *Molecules.* 2016;21(5):623. Published 2016 May 12. doi:10.3390/molecules21050623

The Four Pillars of Health - Movement

1 - Petersen AH, Pedersen BK. The anti-inflammatory effect of exercise. *Journal of Applied Physiology.* 2005;98(4):1154-1162. doi:10.1152/japplphys iol.00164.2004

2 - Dimitrov S, Hulteng E, Hong S. Inflammation and exercise: Inhibition of monocytic intracellular TNF production by acute exercise via β2-adrenergic activation. *Brain, Behavior, and Immunity.* 2017;61:60-68. doi:10.1016/j.bbi.2016.12.017

3 - Thornton LM, Andersen BL. Psychoneuroimmunology examined: The role of subjective stress. *Cellscience.* 2006;2(4):66-91.

4 - Abdurachman, Herawati N. THE ROLE OF PSYCHOLOGICAL WELL-BEING IN BOOSTING IMMUNE RESPONSE: AN OPTIMAL EFFORT FOR TACKLING INFECTION. *Afr J Infect Dis.* 2018;12(1 Suppl):54-61. Published 2018 Mar 7. doi:10.2101/Ajid.12v1S.7

Yoga

1 - Hao M, Liu X, Rong P, Li S, Guo S. Reduced vagal tone in women with endometriosis and auricular vagus nerve stimulation as a potential therapeutic approach. *Scientific Reports.* 2021;11(1). doi:10.1038/s41598-020-79750-9

2 - Santra G. Yoga and the need of its integration in modern medicine. *Journal of Association of Physicians of India.* 2022;70(12):80-84. doi:10.5005/japi-11001-0142

3 - Estevao C. The role of yoga in inflammatory markers. *Brain Behav Immun Health.* 2022;20:100421. Published 2022 Feb 1. doi:10.1016/j.bbih.2 022.100421

4 - Gonçalves AV, Barros NF, Bahamondes L. The Practice of Hatha Yoga for the Treatment of Pain Associated with Endometriosis. *J Altern Complement Med.* 2017;23(1):45-52. doi:10.1089/acm.2015.0343

Lymphatic Movement

1 - Laila F. Jerman, Alison J. Hey-Cunningham, The Role of the Lymphatic System in Endometriosis: A Comprehensive Review of the Literature, *Biology of Reproduction,* Volume 92, Issue 3, 1 March 2015, 64, 1–10,

https://doi.org/10.1095/biolreprod.114.124313.

2 - Morfoisse F, Zamora A, Marchaud E, et al. Sex Hormones in Lymphedema. *Cancers (Basel).* 2021;13(3):530. Published 2021 Jan 30. doi:10.3390/cancers13030530

The Four Pillars of Health – Sleep

1 - Irwin M, Mascovich A, Gillin JC, Willoughby R, Pike J, Smith TL. Partial sleep deprivation reduces natural killer cell activity in humans. *Psychosom Med.* 1994;56(6):493-498. doi:10.1097/00006842-199411000-00004

2 - Imai K, Matsuyama S, Miyaké S, Suga K, Nakachi K. Natural cytotoxic activity of peripheral-blood lymphocytes and cancer incidence: an 11-year follow-up study of a general population. *The Lancet.* 2000;356(9244):1795-1799. doi:10.1016/s0140-6736(00)03231-1

3 - Abramiuk M, Grywalska E, Małkowska P, Sierawska O, Hrynkiewicz R, Niedźwiedzka-Rystwej P. The Role of the Immune System in the Development of Endometriosis. *Cells.* 2022;11(13):2028. Published 2022 Jun 25. doi:10.3390/cells11132028

4 - Garbarino S, Lanteri P, Bragazzi NL, Magnavita N, Scoditti E. Role of sleep deprivation in immune-related disease risk and outcomes. *Communications Biology.* 2021;4(1). doi:10.1038/s42003-021-02825-4

5 - Youseflu S, Sadatmahalleh SJ, Roshanzadeh G, Mottaghi A, Kazemnejad A, Moini A. Effects of endometriosis on sleep quality of women: does life style factor make a difference? *BMC Women's Health.* 2020;20(1). doi:10.1186/s12905-020-01036-z

6 - Ishikura IA, Hachul H, Pires GN, Tufik S, Andersen ML. The relationship between insomnia and endometriosis. *Journal of Clinical Sleep Medicine.* 2020;16(8):1387-1388. doi:10.5664/jcsm.8464

7 - Irwin MR. Sleep disruption induces activation of inflammation and heightens risk for infectious disease: Role of impairments in thermoregulation and elevated ambient temperature. *Temperature (Austin).* 2022;10(2):198-234. Published 2022 Aug 21. doi:10.1080/23328940.2022.2109932

8 - Besedovsky L, Lange T, Born J. Sleep and immune function.

Pflügers Archiv - European Journal of Physiology. 2011;463(1):121-137. doi:10.1007/s00424-011-1044-0

The Four Pillars of Health - Wellbeing

1 - Klussman K, Curtin N, Langer J, Nichols A. The importance of awareness, acceptance, and alignment with the self: A framework for understanding self-connection. *Europe's Journal of Psychology.* 2022;18(1):120-131. doi:10.5964/ejop.3707

2 - Pastore O, Brett BL, Fortier M. Self-Compassion and Happiness: Exploring the influence of the subcomponents of Self-Compassion on happiness and vice versa. *Psychological Reports.* 2022;126(5):2191-2211. doi:10.1177/00332941221084902

3 - Martino J, Pegg J, Frates EP. The Connection Prescription: Using the Power of Social Interactions and the Deep Desire for Connectedness to Empower Health and Wellness. *Am J Lifestyle Med.* 2015;11(6):466-475. Published 2015 Oct 7. doi:10.1177/1559827615608788

4 - Kok BE, Coffey KA, Cohn M, et al. How positive emotions build physical health. *Psychological Science.* 2013;24(7):1123-1132. doi:10.1177/0956797612470827

5 - Mahalingham T, Howell J, Clarke PJF. Attention control moderates the relationship between social media use and psychological distress. *Journal of Affective Disorders.* 2022;297:536-541. doi:10.1016/j.jad.2021.10.071

6 - Reis FM, Coutinho LM, Vannuccini S, Luisi S, Petraglia F. Is stress a cause or a consequence of endometriosis? *Reproductive Sciences.* 2020;27(1):39-45. doi:10.1007/s43032-019-00053-0

Herbal Medicine

1 - Sharifi-Rad J, Rayess YE, Rizk AA, et al. Turmeric and Its Major Compound Curcumin on Health: Bioactive Effects and Safety Profiles for Food, Pharmaceutical, Biotechnological and Medicinal Applications. *Front Pharmacol.* 2020;11:01021. Published 2020 Sep 15. doi:10.3389/fphar.2020.01021

2 - Hewlings SJ, Kalman DS. Curcumin: A Review of Its Effects on Human

Health. *Foods*. 2017;6(10):92. Published 2017 Oct 22. doi:10.3390/foods610 0092

3 - Jafarzadeh E, Shoeibi S, Bahramvand Y, et al. Turmeric for Treatment of Irritable Bowel Syndrome: A Systematic Review of Population-Based Evidence. *Iran J Public Health*. 2022;51(6):1223-1231. doi:10.18502/ijph.v51i 6.9656

4 - Lang A, Salomon N, Wu JCY, et al. Curcumin in combination with mesalamine induces remission in patients with Mild-to-Moderate Ulcerative colitis in a randomized controlled trial. *Clinical Gastroenterology and Hepatology*. 2015;13(8):1444-1449.e1. doi:10.1016/j.cgh.2015.02.019

5 - Coelho MR, Romi MD, Ferreira DMTP, Zaltman C, Soares-Mota M. The use of curcumin as a complementary therapy in ulcerative colitis: A systematic review of randomized controlled clinical trials. *Nutrients*. 2020;12(8):2296. doi:10.3390/nu12082296

6 - Giordano A, Tommonaro G. Curcumin and cancer. *Nutrients*. 2019;11(10):2376. doi:10.3390/nu11102376

7 - Kamal DAM, Salamt N, Yusuf ANM, Kashim MIAM, Mokhtar MH. Potential health benefits of curcumin on female reproductive Disorders: a review. *Nutrients*. 2021;13(9):3126. doi:10.3390/nu13093126

8 - Laschke MW, Elitzsch A, Vollmar B, Vajkoczy P, Menger MD. Combined inhibition of vascular endothelial growth factor (VEGF), fibroblast growth factor and platelet-derived growth factor, but not inhibition of VEGF alone, effectively suppresses angiogenesis and vessel maturation in endometriotic lesions. *Human Reproduction*. 2005;21(1):262-268. doi:10.10 93/humrep/dei308

9 - Mohajeri M, Bianconi V, Ávila-Rodriguez M, et al. Curcumin: a phytochemical modulator of estrogens and androgens in tumors of the reproductive system. *Pharmacological Research*. 2020;156:104765. doi:10.1016/j.phrs.2020.104765

10 - Zhang Y, Cao H, Yu Z, Peng HY, Zhang CJ. Curcumin inhibits endometriosis endometrial cells by reducing estradiol production. *Iran J Reprod Med*. 2013;11(5):415-422.

11 - Boroumand S, Hosseini S, Pashandi Z, Faridi-Majidi R, Salehi

MS. Curcumin-loaded nanofibers for targeting endometriosis in the peritoneum of a mouse model. *Journal of Materials Science: Materials in Medicine*. 2019;31(1). doi:10.1007/s10856-019-6337-4

12 - Kızılay G, Uz YH, Şeren G, et al. In vivo effects of curcumin and deferoxamine in experimental endometriosis. *Advances in Clinical and Experimental Medicine*. 2017;26(2):207-213. doi:10.17219/acem/31186

13 - Reddy PS, Begum N, Mutha S, Bakshi V. Beneficial effect of Curcumin in Letrozole induced polycystic ovary syndrome. *Asian Pacific Journal of Reproduction*. 2016;5(2):116-122. doi:10.1016/j.apjr.2016.01.006

14 - Akazawa N, Choi Y, Miyaki A, et al. Curcumin ingestion and exercise training improve vascular endothelial function in postmenopausal women. *Nutrition Research*. 2012;32(10):795-799. doi:10.1016/j.nutres.2012.09.002

15 - Mahmudi G, Nikpour M, Azadbackt M, et al. The impact of turmeric cream on healing of cesarean scar. *West Indian Medical Journal*. July 2015. doi:10.7727/wimj.2014.196

16 - Sahbaie P, Sun Y, Liang D, Shi X, Clark JD. Curcumin Treatment Attenuates Pain and Enhances Functional Recovery after Incision. *Anesthesia & Analgesia*. 2014;118(6):1336-1344. doi:10.1213/ane.0000000000000189

17 - Ozgoli G, Goli M, Moattar F. Comparison of Effects of Ginger, Mefenamic Acid, and Ibuprofen on Pain in Women with Primary Dysmenorrhea. *Journal of Alternative and Complementary Medicine*. 2009;15(2):129-132. doi:10.1089/acm.2008.0311

18 - Giriraju A, Yunus GY. Assessment of antimicrobial potential of 10% ginger extract againstStreptococcus mutans,Candida albicans, andEnterococcus faecalis: Anin vitrostudy. *Indian Journal of Dental Research*. 2013;24(4):397. doi:10.4103/0970-9290.118356

19 - Ballester P, Cerdá B, Arcusa R, Marhuenda J, Yamedjeu K, Zafrilla P. Effect of ginger on inflammatory diseases. *Molecules*. 2022;27(21):7223. doi:10.3390/molecules27217223

20 - Semwal RB, Semwal DK, Combrinck S, Viljoen A. Gingerols and shogaols: Important nutraceutical principles from ginger. *Phytochemistry*. 2015;117:554-568. doi:10.1016/j.phytochem.2015.07.012

21 - Azgomi RND, Zomorrodi A, Nazemyieh H, et al. Effects ofWithania

somniferaon Reproductive System: A Systematic Review of the Available Evidence. *BioMed Research International*. 2018;2018:1-17. doi:10.1155/2018/4076430

22 - Ni Z, Li Y, Song D, et al. Iron-overloaded follicular fluid increases the risk of endometriosis-related infertility by triggering granulosa cell ferroptosis and oocyte dysmaturity. *Cell Death and Disease*. 2022;13(7). doi:10.1038/s41419-022-05037-8

23 - Tuli HS, Joshi R, Yadav P, Bagwe-Parab S, Buttar HS, Kaur G. Iron Chelation and Antioxidant Properties of Withania somnifera (Ashwagandha) Restore Fertility in Men and Women. *Current Bioactive Compounds*. 2023;19(7). doi:10.2174/1573407219666230210101925

24 - Ajgaonkar A, Jain M, Debnath K. Efficacy and Safety of Ashwagandha (Withania somnifera) Root Extract for Improvement of Sexual Health in Healthy Women: A Prospective, Randomized, Placebo-Controlled Study. *Cureus*. October 2022. doi:10.7759/cureus.30787

25 - Kulkarni SK, Dhir A. Withania somnifera: An Indian ginseng. *Progress in Neuro-Psychopharmacology and Biological Psychiatry*. 2008;32(5):1093-1105. doi:10.1016/j.pnpbp.2007.09.011

26 - Kurapati KRV, Atluri VSR, Samikkannu T, Nair M. Ashwagandha (Withania somnifera) Reverses β-Amyloid1-42 Induced Toxicity in Human Neuronal Cells: Implications in HIV-Associated Neurocognitive Disorders (HAND). *PLOS ONE*. 2013;8(10):e77624. doi:10.1371/journal.pone.0077624

27 - Lopresti AL, Smith SJ, Malvi H, Kodgule R. An investigation into the stress-relieving and pharmacological actions of an ashwagandha (Withania somnifera) extract. *Medicine*. 2019;98(37):e17186. doi:10.1097/md.0000000000017186

28 - Salve J, Pate S, Debnath K, Langade D. Adaptogenic and anxiolytic effects of ashwagandha root extract in healthy adults: a double-blind, randomized, placebo-controlled clinical study. *Cureus*. December 2019. doi:10.7759/cureus.6466

29 - Bhattacharya SK, Bhattacharya A, Krishnamurthy S, Ghosal S. Anxiolytic-antidepressant activity of Withania somnifera glycowithanolides: an experimental study. *Phytomedicine*. 2000;7(6):463-469.

doi:10.1016/s0944-7113(00)80030-6

30 - Ramakanth GSH, Kumar CU, Kishan PV, Pingali U. A random-ized, double blind placebo controlled study of efficacy and tolerability of Withaina somnifera extracts in knee joint pain. *Journal of Ayurveda and Integrative Medicine.* 2016;7(3):151-157. doi:10.1016/j.jaim.2016.05.003

31 - Kort DH, Lobo RA. Preliminary evidence that cinnamon improves menstrual cyclicity in women with polycystic ovary syndrome: a ran-domised controlled trial. *American Journal of Obstetrics and Gynecology.* 2014;211(5):487.e1-487.e6. doi:10.1016/j.ajog.2014.05.009

32 - Jaafarpour M, Hatefi M, Najafi F, Khajavikhan J, Khani A. The effect of cinnamon on menstrual bleeding and systemic symptoms with primary dysmenorrhea. *Iranian Red Crescent Medical Journal.* 2015;17(4). doi:10.581 2/ircmj.17(4)2015.27032

33 - Jaafarpour M, Hatefi M, Khani A, Khajavikhan J. Comparative effect of cinnamon and ibuprofen for treatment of primary dysmenorrhea: a randomized double- blind clinical trial. *Journal of Clinical and Diagnostic Research.* January 2015. doi:10.7860/jcdr/2015/12084.5783

34 - Latif R. Health benefits of cocoa. *Current Opinion in Clinical Nutrition and Metabolic Care.* 2013;16(6):669-674. doi:10.1097/mco.0b013e328365a 235

35 - Lee KW, Kim YJ, Lee HJ, Lee CY. Cocoa Has More Phenolic Phytochem-icals and a Higher Antioxidant Capacity than Teas and Red Wine. *Journal of Agricultural and Food Chemistry.* 2003;51(25):7292-7295. doi:10.1021/jf034 4385

36 - Andújar I, Recio MC, Giner RM, RíOs JL. Cocoa polyphenols and their potential benefits for human health. *Oxidative Medicine and Cellular Longevity.* 2012;2012:1-23. doi:10.1155/2012/906252

Traditional Chinese Medicine (TCM)

1 - Zhou J, Qu F. Treating gynaecological disorders with traditional Chinese medicine: a review. *Afr J Tradit Complement Altern Med.* 2009;6(4):494-517. Published 2009 Jul 3. doi:10.4314/ajtcam.v6i4.57181

2 - Wang, D. Z., Wang, Z. Q., & Zhang, Z. F. (1991). *Zhong xi yi jie he za*

zhi = *Chinese journal of modern developments in traditional medicine*, 11(9), 524–515.

3 - Liu J. X. (1994). *Zhongguo Zhong xi yi jie he za zhi Zhongguo Zhongxiyi jiehe zazhi = Chinese journal of integrated traditional and Western medicine*, 14(6), 337–324.

4 - Yu S. Ninety patients of endometriosis treated with staging method of integrated Chinese and Western medicine. *Chinese Journal of Integrative Medicine*. 1998;4(2):139-141. doi:10.1007/bf02934167

5 - Lian F, Liu H, Wang Y, et al. Expressions of VEGF and Ki-67 in eutopic endometrium of patients with endometriosis and effect of Quyu Jiedu Recipe () on VEGF expression. *Chinese Journal of Integrative Medicine*. 2007;13(2):109-114. doi:10.1007/s11655-007-0109-6

6 - Piriyev E, Gertz MM, Schiermeier S, Römer T. Significance of Ki67 expression in endometriosis for infertility. *European Journal of Obstetrics & Gynecology and Reproductive Biology*. 2022;272:73-76. doi:10.1016/j.ejogrb.2022.03.019

7 - García-Manero M, Alcázar JL, Toledo G. Vascular endothelial growth factor (VEGF) and ovarian endometriosis: correlation between VEGF serum levels, VEGF cellular expression, and pelvic pain. *Fertility and Sterility*. 2007;88(2):513-515. doi:10.1016/j.fertnstert.2006.11.117

8 - Flower A, Liu J, Chen S, Lewith G, Little P. Chinese herbal medicine for endometriosis. *Cochrane Database of Systematic Reviews*. July 2009. doi:10.1002/14651858.cd006568.pub2

9 - Weng Q, Ding ZM, Lv XL, et al. Chinese medicinal plants for advanced endometriosis after conservative surgery: a prospective, multi-center and controlled trial. *Int J Clin Exp Med*. 2015;8(7):11307-11311. Published 2015 Jul 15.

10 - Oku H, Tsuji Y, Kashiwamura SI, et al. Role of IL-18 in pathogenesis of endometriosis. *Human Reproduction*. 2004;19(3):709-714. doi:10.1093/humrep/deh108

11 - Jin Z, Wang L, Zhu Z. Effect of GuiXiong Xiaoyi Wan in treatment of endometriosis on rats. *Evidence-based Complementary and Alternative Medicine*. 2015;2015:1-8. doi:10.1155/2015/208514

Acupuncture

1 - Lu DP, Lu GP. An historical review and perspective on the impact of acupuncture on U.S. medicine and society. *Medical Acupuncture.* 2013;25(5):311-316. doi:10.1089/acu.2012.0921

2 - McDonald J, Cripps AW, Smith P, Smith C, Xue CC, Golianu B. The Anti-Inflammatory Effects of Acupuncture and Their Relevance to Allergic Rhinitis: A Narrative Review and Proposed model. *Evidence-based Complementary and Alternative Medicine.* 2013;2013:1-12. doi:10.1155/2013/591796

3 - Li P, Peng X, Niu XX, et al. Efficacy of acupuncture for endometriosis-associated pain: a multicenter randomized single-blind placebo-controlled trial. *Fertility and Sterility.* 2023;119(5):815-823. doi:10.101 6/j.fertnstert.2023.01.034

4 - Xu Y, Zhao W, Li T, Zhao Y, Bu H, Song S. Effects of acupuncture for the treatment of endometriosis-related pain: A systematic review and meta-analysis. *PLOS ONE.* 2017;12(10):e0186616. doi:10.1371/journal.pone. 0186616

5 - Stener-Victorin E, Waldenström U, Andersson SA, Wikland M. Reduction of blood flow impedance in the uterine arteries of infertile women with electro-acupuncture. *Human Reproduction.* 1996;11(6):1314-1317. doi:10.1093/oxfordjournals.humrep.a019378

6 - Stener-Victorin E, Lundeberg T, Cajander S, et al. Steroid-induced polycystic ovaries in rats: effect of electro-acupuncture on concentrations of endothelin-1 and nerve growth factor (NGF), and expression of NGF mRNA in the ovaries, the adrenal glands, and the central nervous system. *Reproductive Biology and Endocrinology.* 2003;1(1):33. doi:10.1186/1477-7827-1-33

7 - Zhu J, Козовска К. Acupuncture treatment for fertility. *Open Access Macedonian Journal of Medical Sciences.* 2018;6(9):1685-1687. doi:10.3889/oamjms.2018.379

8 - Manheimer E, Zhang G, Udoff LC, et al. Effects of acupuncture on rates of pregnancy and live birth among women undergoing in vitro fertilisation: systematic review and meta-analysis. *The BMJ.* 2008;336(7643):545-549.

doi:10.1136/bmj.39471.430451.be

9 - Kim J, Lee H, Choi T, et al. Acupuncture for Poor Ovarian Response: A Randomized Controlled Trial. *Journal of Clinical Medicine.* 2021;10(10):2182. doi:10.3390/jcm10102182

Homeopathy

1 - Homeopathy and cancer. https://www.cancerresearchuk.org/about-cancer/treatment/complementary-alternative-therapies/individual-therapies/homeopathy.

2 - Wartolowska K, Judge A, Hopewell S, et al. Use of placebo controls in the evaluation of surgery: systematic review. *The BMJ.* 2014;348(may21 2):g3253. doi:10.1136/bmj.g3253

3 - Jonas WB, Crawford C, Colloca L, et al. To what extent are surgery and invasive procedures effective beyond a placebo response? A systematic review with meta-analysis of randomised, sham controlled trials. *BMJ Open.* 2015;5(12):e009655. Published 2015 Dec 11. doi:10.1136/bmjopen-2015-009655

Botox

1 - Abbott JA, Jarvis SK, Lyons SD, Thomson A, Vancaille TG. Botulinum toxin type A for chronic pain and pelvic floor spasm in women: a randomized controlled trial. *Obstet Gynecol.* 2006;108(4):915-923. doi:10.1097/01.AOG.0000237100.29870.cc

2 - Tandon HK, Stratton P, Sinaii N, Shah J, Karp BI. Botulinum toxin for chronic pelvic pain in women with endometriosis: a cohort study of a pain-focused treatment [published online ahead of print, 2019 Jul 8]. *Reg Anesth Pain Med.* 2019;rapm-2019-100529. doi:10.1136/rapm-2019-100529

3 - Witmanowski H, Błochowiak K. The whole truth about botulinum toxin - a review. *Postepy Dermatol Alergol.* 2020;37(6):853-861. doi:10.511 4/ada.2019.82795

Cannabis and CBD

1 - Genovese T, Cordaro M, Siracusa R, et al. Molecular and Biochemical

Mechanism of Cannabidiol in the Management of the Inflammatory and Oxidative Processes Associated with Endometriosis. *International Journal of Molecular Sciences.* 2022;23(10):5427. doi:10.3390/ijms23105427

2 - Ökten SB, Çetin Ç, Tok OE, et al. Cannabidiol as a potential novel treatment for endometriosis by its anti-inflammatory, antioxidative and antiangiogenic effects in an experimental rat model. *Reproductive Biomedicine Online.* 2023;46(5):865-875. doi:10.1016/j.rbmo.2023.01.018

3 - Liang A, Gingher EL, Coleman JS. Medical cannabis for gynecologic pain conditions. *Obstetrics & Gynecology.* 2022;139(2):287-296. doi:10.109 7/aog.0000000000004656

4 - Carrubba AR, Ebbert JO, Spaulding A, DeStephano D, DeStephano CC. Use of Cannabis for Self-Management of Chronic Pelvic Pain. *Journal of Womens Health.* 2021;30(9):1344-1351. doi:10.1089/jwh.2020.8737

5 - Armour M, Sinclair J, Noller G, et al. Illicit Cannabis Usage as a Management Strategy in New Zealand Women with Endometriosis: An Online Survey. *J Womens Health (Larchmt).* 2021;30(10):1485-1492. doi:10.1089/jwh.2020.8668

6 - Mistry M, Simpson P, Morris E, et al. Cannabidiol for the Management of Endometriosis and Chronic Pelvic Pain. *J Minim Invasive Gynecol.* 2022;29(2):169-176. doi:10.1016/j.jmig.2021.11.017

7 - Sinclair J, Collett L, Abbott J, Pate DW, Sarris J, Armour M. Effects of cannabis ingestion on endometriosis-associated pelvic pain and related symptoms. *PLoS One.* 2021;16(10):e0258940. Published 2021 Oct 26. doi:10.1371/journal.pone.0258940

How to Deal With the Day-to-Day

1 - Moseley GL, Butler DS. Fifteen Years of Explaining Pain: The Past, Present, and Future. *J Pain.* 2015;16(9):807-813. doi:10.1016/j.jpain.2015.0 5.005

Toxins to Avoid

1 - Rumph JT, Stephens VR, Archibong AE, Osteen KG, Bruner-Tran KL. Environmental Endocrine Disruptors and Endometriosis. *Adv Anat Embryol*

Cell Biol. 2020;232:57-78. doi:10.1007/978-3-030-51856-1_4

2 - Rubin BS. Bisphenol A: an endocrine disruptor with widespread exposure and multiple effects. *J Steroid Biochem Mol Biol.* 2011;127(1-2):27-34. doi:10.1016/j.jsbmb.2011.05.002

3 - Gao H, Yang BJ, Li N, et al. Bisphenol A and hormone-associated cancers: current progress and perspectives. *Medicine (Baltimore).* 2015;94(1):e211. doi:10.1097/MD.0000000000000211

4 - World Health Organization: WHO. Dioxins and their effects on human health. 2016. https://www.who.int/news-room/fact-sheets/detail/dioxins-and-their-effects-on-human-health.

5 - Institute of Medicine (US) (2003) Committee on the Implications of Dioxin in the Food Supply. Dioxins and Dioxin-like Compounds in the Food Supply: Strategies to Decrease Exposure. Washington (DC): National Academies Press (US); Available from: https://www.ncbi.nlm.nih.gov/books/NBK221714/# Accessed 25 October 2023

6 - DeVito MJ, Schecter A. Exposure assessment to dioxins from the use of tampons and diapers. *Environ Health Perspect.* 2002;110(1):23-28. doi:10.1289/ehp.0211023

7 - Szczęsna D, Wieczorek K, Jurewicz J. An exposure to endocrine active persistent pollutants and endometriosis - a review of current epidemiological studies. *Environ Sci Pollut Res Int.* 2023;30(6):13974-13993. doi:10.1007/s11356-022-24785-w

8 - Terry P, Towers CV, Liu LY, Peverly AA, Chen J, Salamova A. Polybrominated diphenyl ethers (flame retardants) in mother-infant pairs in the Southeastern U.S. *Int J Environ Health Res.* 2017;27(3):205-214. doi:10.1080/09603123.2017.1332344

9 - Costa LG, Giordano G. Polybrominated Diphenyl Ethers. *Elsevier eBooks.* Published online January 1, 2014:1032-1034. doi:https://doi.org/10.1016/b978-0-12-386454-3.00422-x

10 - Halden RU, Lindeman AE, Aiello AE, et al. The Florence Statement on Triclosan and Triclocarban. *Environ Health Perspect.* 2017;125(6):064501. Published 2017 Jun 20. doi:10.1289/EHP1788

11 - Ma K, Cheng Y, Guo H, Wang J, Yu T. Correlation between Triclosan

(TCS) exposure and endometriosis. *Pak J Med Sci.* 2023;39(6):1701-1705. doi:10.12669/pjms.39.6.7170

12 - Zeng W, Xu W, Xu Y, et al. The prevalence and mechanism of triclosan resistance in Escherichia coli isolated from urine samples in Wenzhou, China. *Antimicrob Resist Infect Control.* 2020;9(1):161. Published 2020 Oct 2. doi:10.1186/s13756-020-00823-5

13 - European Commission. (2023). Commission Regulation (EU) .../... of XXX amending Regulation (EC) No 1223/2009 of the European Parliament and of the Council as regards the use of Vitamin A, Alpha-Arbutin and Arbutin and certain substances with potential endocrine disrupting properties in cosmetic products. Available at https://members.wto.org/crnattachments/2023/TBT/EEC/23_10130_00_e.pdf Accessed on 26 October 2023

14 - Engeli RT, Rohrer SR, Vuorinen A, et al. Interference of Paraben Compounds with Estrogen Metabolism by Inhibition of 17β-Hydroxysteroid Dehydrogenases. *Int J Mol Sci.* 2017;18(9):2007. Published 2017 Sep 19. doi:10.3390/ijms18092007

15 - Darbre PD, Harvey PW. Parabens can enable hallmarks and characteristics of cancer in human breast epithelial cells: a review of the literature with reference to new exposure data and regulatory status. *J Appl Toxicol.* 2014;34(9):925-938. doi:10.1002/jat.3027

16 - Jurewicz J, Radwan M, Wielgomas B, et al. Parameters of ovarian reserve in relation to urinary concentrations of parabens. *Environ Health.* 2020;19(1):26. Published 2020 Mar 2. doi:10.1186/s12940-020-00580-3

17 - Peinado FM, Ocón-Hernández O, Iribarne-Durán LM, et al. Cosmetic and personal care product use, urinary levels of parabens and benzophenones, and risk of endometriosis: results from the EndEA study. *Environ Res.* 2021;196:110342. doi:10.1016/j.envres.2020.110342

18 - Meeker JD, Ferguson KK. Urinary phthalate metabolites are associated with decreased serum testosterone in men, women, and children from NHANES 2011-2012. *J Clin Endocrinol Metab.* 2014;99(11):4346-4352. doi:10.1210/jc.2014-2555

19 - Hannon PR, Flaws JA. The effects of phthalates on the ovary. *Front*

Endocrinol (Lausanne). 2015;6:8. Published 2015 Feb 2. doi:10.3389/fendo. 2015.00008

20 - Wieczorek K, Szczęsna D, Jurewicz J. Environmental Exposure to Non-Persistent Endocrine Disrupting Chemicals and Endometriosis: A Systematic Review. *Int J Environ Res Public Health.* 2022;19(9):5608. Published 2022 May 5. doi:10.3390/ijerph19095608

21 - Ribeiro B, Mariana M, Lorigo M, Oliani D, Ramalhinho AC, Cairrao E. Association between the Exposure to Phthalates and the Risk of Endometriosis: An Updated Review. *Biomedicines.* 2024;12(8):1932. Published 2024 Aug 22. doi:10.3390/biomedicines12081932

22 - Kim JH, Kim SH. Exposure to Phthalate Esters and the Risk of Endometriosis. *Dev Reprod.* 2020;24(2):71-78. doi:10.12717/DR.2020.24.2. 71

Medical Research

1 - Tapmeier TT, Rahmioglu N, Lin J, et al. Neuropeptide S receptor 1 is a nonhormonal treatment target in endometriosis. *Sci Transl Med.* 2021;13(608):eabd6469. doi:10.1126/scitranslmed.abd6469

2 - Nishimoto-Kakiuchi A, Sato I, Nakano K, et al. A long-acting anti-IL-8 antibody improves inflammation and fibrosis in endometriosis. *Sci Transl Med.* 2023;15(684):eabq5858. doi:10.1126/scitranslmed.abq5858

3 - Brennan K, Zheng J. Interleukin 8. *xPharm: The Comprehensive Pharmacology Reference.* Published online 2007:1-4. doi:https://doi.or g/10.1016/b978-008055232-3.61916-6

4 - Hirschhaeuser F, Sattler UGA, Mueller-Klieser W. Lactate: A Metabolic Key Player in Cancer. *Cancer Research.* 2011;71(22):6921-6925. doi:https://doi.org/10.1158/0008-5472.can-11-1457

5 - Horne AW, Ahmad SF, Carter R, et al. Repurposing dichloroacetate for the treatment of women with endometriosis. *Proc Natl Acad Sci U S A.* 2019;116(51):25389-25391. doi:10.1073/pnas.1916144116

6 - Bendifallah S, Dabi Y, Suisse S, et al. MicroRNome analysis generates a blood-based signature for endometriosis. *Sci Rep.* 2022;12(1):4051. Published 2022 Mar 8. doi:10.1038/s41598-022-07771-7

7 - Bendifallah S, Suisse S, Puchar A, et al. Salivary MicroRNA Signature for Diagnosis of Endometriosis. *J Clin Med.* 2022;11(3):612. Published 2022 Jan 26. doi:10.3390/jcm11030612

8 - IMAGENDO® – Non Invasive Diagnosis of endometriosis using Artificial Intelligence. Accessed March 1, 2024. https://imagendo.org.au

9 - ClinicalTrials.gov. NIH. https://clinicaltrials.gov/study/NCT0562333 2?cond=NCT05623332&rank=1. Accessed December 27, 2024.